Workbook and Lab Manual for Mosby's® Pharmacy Technician: Principles and Practice

Sixth Edition

Workbook Material Prepared by:

Marcy May, MEd, CPhT, PhTR
Adjunct Professor
Austin Community College
Austin, Texas

ELSEVIER

Elsevier
3251 Riverport Lane
St. Louis, Missouri 63043

Notice

Practitioners and researchers must always rely on their own experience and knowledge in evaluating and
using any information, methods, compounds or experiments described herein. Because of rapid advances
in the medical sciences, in particular, independent verification of diagnoses and drug dosages should be
made. To the fullest extent of the law, no responsibility is assumed by Elsevier, authors, editors or contrib-
utors for any injury and/or damage to persons or property as a matter of products liability, negligence or
otherwise, or from any use or operation of any methods, products, instructions, or ideas contained in the
material herein.

Publishing Director: Kristin Wilhelm
Content Development Specialist: Elizabeth McCormac
Director, Content Development: Laurie Gower
Publishing Services Manager: Shereen Jameel
Senior Project Manager: Kamatchi Madhavan
Design Direction: Gopal Venkatraman

Printed in the United States of America

Last digit is the print number: 9   8   7   6   5   4   3   2   1

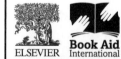

Working together
to grow libraries in
developing countries

www.elsevier.com • www.bookaid.org

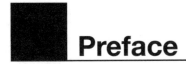

Preface

This student workbook and lab manual is designed to help you master the information and skills presented in your textbook, *Mosby's® Pharmacy Technician: Principles and Practice,* 6th edition. Built to support content mastery of all entry-level and many advanced competencies set forth in the American Society of Health System Pharmacists (ASHP) Pharmacy Technician accreditation standards, the various types of exercises will challenge your knowledge, help further reinforce key content, allow you to gauge your understanding of the subject matter, and demonstrate important concepts in the lab setting. This combination workbook and lab manual is divided into three separate areas for each chapter in the textbook: Reinforce Key Concepts, Reflect Critically, and Relate to Practice. Each of these three sections focuses on activities for students that will maximize their understanding of the content taught in the book. The types of activities available in this workbook and lab manual are listed and described below.

REINFORCE KEY CONCEPTS

Terms and Definitions: Terms and definitions are listed, preceded by a letter. You are to read each statement following the list, and write in the letter that represents the correct response. This exercise helps you recall the many terms that are introduced to you in each chapter. Your textbook conveniently lists this information at the beginning of each chapter. If you find you are not sure of any of your responses, you can easily turn to the appropriate chapter to refresh your memory.

Fill in the Blanks: Complete each statement by filling in the blanks. This exercise gives you the opportunity to specifically apply the vocabulary you have learned within the context of pharmacy.

True or False: Test your knowledge of the validity of the statements. If you think a statement is true, write a "T" in the blank preceding the statement; if you believe it is a false statement, write in an "F." Completing these exercises helps you to recognize immediately content of which you are unsure. You can then review and strengthen your understanding of the material by rereading that section in your textbook.

Multiple Choice: You are to select the one best answer to complete the numbered questions by circling the letter preceding the answer you have selected. This is the type of question in which your first response is usually the correct reply. If you are not sure, then you can easily review the subject in question.

System Identifier: Each chapter devoted to a body system features an illustration of the system with its organs numbered. You are asked to identify the organs contained in the body system. This visual exercise helps further reinforce your knowledge of anatomy. Questions in these chapters test you on the anatomy and physiology of the system, diseases and conditions that may occur within this system, and the medications prescribed to treat such illnesses.

Matching: These exercises provide you with essential practice in matching controlled substance drug schedules with given drug names. Ease of recognition is essential in your chosen profession. If you are not sure of some of your responses, you can then refer to your textbook for further study.

Conversion and Calculation: These questions require you to convert measurements, thereby applying what you have learned.

Research Activities: You are asked to use the Internet as a research tool to assist you in locating essential information. Featured websites address such topics as the scope of practice for pharmacy technicians and where to find information on controlled substances and recalls.

REFLECT CRITICALLY

Critical Thinking: This exercise tests your accumulated knowledge of each chapter by giving you scenarios to solve. You are asked to draw upon your knowledge of pharmacy and direct it to specific situations. This is a good test of your understanding of key concepts. If any of these questions stump you, refer to your textbook for further study or ask your instructor for clarification.

RELATE TO PRACTICE

Lab Activities: Labs for each chapter will help you master such skills as Gram staining, inventory management, compounding, and aseptic technique. These labs offer you many opportunities for hands-on reinforcements of what you have learned in your textbook.

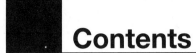

Contents

UNIT ONE   PHARMACY PRACTICE, 1

1 History of Medicine and Pharmacy, **1**
2 Pharmacy, Law, Ethics, and Regulatory Agencies, **6**
3 Competencies, Associations, and Settings for Technicians, **21**
4 Communication and Role of the Technician With the Customer/Patient, **36**
5 Dosage Forms and Routes of Administration, **43**
6 Conversions and Calculations, **61**
7 Drug Information References, **81**
8 Community Pharmacy Practice, **90**
9 Institutional Pharmacy Practice, **121**
10 Additional Pharmacy Practice Settings, **134**
11 Bulk Repackaging and Nonsterile Compounding, **141**
12 Aseptic Technique and Sterile Compounding, **175**
13 Pharmacy Billing and Inventory Management, **203**
14 Medication Safety and Error Prevention, **215**
15 Pharmacy Operations Management, **230**

UNIT TWO   PHARMACOLOGY AND MEDICATIONS, 236

16 Drug Classifications, **236**
17 Therapeutic Agents for the Nervous System, **244**
18 Therapeutic Agents for the Endocrine System, **262**
19 Therapeutic Agents for the Musculoskeletal System, **278**
20 Therapeutic Agents for the Cardiovascular System, **291**
21 Therapeutic Agents for the Respiratory System, **309**
22 Therapeutic Agents for the Gastrointestinal System, **320**
23 Therapeutic Agents for the Renal System, **329**
24 Therapeutic Agents for the Reproductive System, **341**
25 Therapeutic Agents for the Immune System, **351**
26 Therapeutic Agents for the Eyes, Ears, Nose, and Throat, **366**
27 Therapeutic Agents for the Dermatologic System, **380**
28 Therapeutic Agents for the Hematologic System, **393**
29 Over-the-Counter (OTC) Medication, **403**
30 Complementary and Alternative Medicine (CAM), **413**

History of Medicine and Pharmacy

ASHP ACCREDITATION STANDARDS FOR PHARMACY TECHNICIAN EDUCATION AND TRAINING PROGRAMS

Standard 1.3: Demonstrate active and engaged listening skills.
Standard 1.4: Communicate clearly and effectively, both verbally and in writing.
Standard 1.10: Apply critical thinking skills, creativity, and innovation.
Standard 2.3: Describe the pharmacy technician's role, pharmacist's role, and other occupations in the health care environment.
Standard 2.5: Demonstrate basic knowledge of anatomy, physiology and pharmacology, and medical terminology relevant to pharmacy technician's role.
Standard 2.10: Describe further knowledge and skills required for achieving advanced competencies.
Standard 5.10: Describe major trends, issues, goals, and initiatives taking place in the pharmacy profession.

REINFORCEMENT OF CONCEPTS

Terms and Definitions

Select the correct term from the following list and write the corresponding letter in the blank next to the statement.

A. Bloodletting
B. Laudanum
C. Leeches
D. Maggots
E. Medicine
F. Opioid
G. Opium
H. Trephining

_____ 1. Any agent that binds to opioid receptors.

_____ 2. A type of segmented worm with suckers that attaches to the skin of a host and engorges itself on the host's blood.

_____ 3. A practice of making an opening in the head to allow disease to leave the body

_____ 4. A mixture of opium and alcohol used to treat dozens of illnesses through the 1800s

_____ 5. The science and art dealing with the maintenance of health and the prevention, alleviation, or cure of disease.

_____ 6. The practice of draining blood; believed to release illness.

_____ 7. An analgesic that is made from the poppy plant.

_____ 8. Fly larvae that feed on dead tissue; used in medicine to clean wounds not responding to routine antibiotics.

Select the correct term from the following list and write the corresponding letter in the blank next to the statement.

A. Pharmacist
B. Pharmacy clerk
C. Pharmacy technician
D. Shaman

_____ 9. Person who assists the pharmacist at the front counter of the pharmacy; the person who accepts payment for medications.

_____ 10. A person who holds a high place of honor in a tribe as a healer and spiritual mediator.

_____ 11. Person who dispenses drugs and counsels patients on medication use and any interactions it may have with food or other drugs.

_____ 12. Person who assists a pharmacist by filling prescriptions and performing other nondiscretionary tasks.

1

Select the correct term from the following list and write the corresponding letter in the blank next to the statement.

A. Apothecary
B. Caduceus
C. Dogma
D. Hippocratic oath
E. Inpatient pharmacy
F. Pharmacy
G. Pharmacy Technician Certification Board (PTCB)
H. Staff of Asclepius

_____ 13. An oath taken by physicians concerning the ethics and practice of medicine.

_____ 14. Issues a national exam for pharmacy technicians.

_____ 15. Often confused as the symbol of the medical field; it is a staff with two entwined snakes and two wings at the top.

_____ 16. Pharmacies in a hospital or institutional setting.

_____ 17. A principle or set of principles laid down by an authority as incontrovertibly true.

_____ 18. The symbol of the medical profession; it is a wingless staff with one snake wrapped around it.

_____ 19. Latin term for pharmacist; also, a place where drugs are sold.

_____ 20. A place where drugs are sold.

True or False

Write T or F next to each statement.

_____ 1. Military pharmacy technicians have a more limited scope of training than civilian pharmacy technicians.

_____ 2. For licensure, most states require new pharmacists to obtain a Doctor of Pharmacy degree.

_____ 3. All states require pharmacy technicians to complete additional education and on-the-job training.

_____ 4. Over the decades, the pharmacist has become known as a person who can be least trusted to provide truthful information.

_____ 5. It is not important for the patient to be able to trust a technician to provide the best care by filling the correct medication and referring the patient to the pharmacist for appropriate counseling.

_____ 6. National certification for pharmacy technicians is one of the best markers for ensuring a minimum level of competency in pharmacy.

_____ 7. Education, training, and good communication skills, technicians can gain the trust of the patients whom they serve.

_____ 8. Pharmacy technicians do not need be aware of the laws in their state.

_____ 9. Pharmacy technician duties continue to expand and change.

_____ 10. Advanced pharmacy technicians who have additional education may perform tasks that require more responsibility.

Multiple Choice

Complete each question by circling the best answer.

1. Smallpox vaccination was stopped in _____ because the disease had been eradicated worldwide.
   A. 1971
   B. 1932
   C. 1899
   D. 1796

2. _____ is an old remedy that physicians have used successfully in many cases as a means of avoiding amputation.
   A. Bloodletting
   B. Leeches
   C. Honey
   D. Maggots

3. Antibiotics are normally used as the first course of treatment, but physicians have used _____ to do the manual work of restoring the wound to a recoverable stage when antibiotics are ineffective.
   A. phlebotomy
   B. leeches
   C. bees
   D. maggots

4. The division between physicians and pharmacists began after the:
   A. Civil War
   B. Cold War
   C. Vietnam War
   D. Korean War

5. The first 7-Up drink was made with _____ and was sold from soda fountains for conditions such as gout, uremia, and rheumatism.
   A. aspirin
   B. cocaine
   C. opium
   D. lithium

6. The _____ prohibited pharmacists from making cocaine-containing preparations, so they began to sell plain soda drinks.
   A. Omnibus Budget Reconciliation Act of 1990
   B. National Association of Boards of Pharmacy
   C. prohibition in 1919
   D. Harrison Drug Narcotic Act of 1914

7. Some colleges are offering specialized training programs for pharmacy technicians, including the following, *except*:
   A. inventory management
   B. quality improvement
   C. clinical pharmacy
   D. immunization

8. The ASHP created competencies for technicians in organized health care settings and qualifications for entry-level technicians in hospitals in _____ .
   A. 1977
   B. 1982
   C. 1995
   D. 2013

9. The _____ created accreditation standards for training programs in 1982.
   A. American Association of Pharmacy Technicians (AAPT)
   B. American Pharmacists Association (APhA)
   C. Pharmacy Technician Certification Board (PTCB)
   D. American Society of Health-System Pharmacists (ASHP)

10. In _____ the Pharmacy Technician Certification Board (PTCB) was formed, which was responsible for creating a national examination for technicians.
    A. 1976
    B. 1988
    C. 1995
    D. 2013

Fill in the Blanks

Answer each question by completing the statement in the space provided.

1. _____ have been used for centuries for minor ailments such as intestinal problems, arthritis, and gout.

2. Many ancient treatments for illness were based on the _____ or _____ of the believers.

3. In many cultures, the most common form of treatment, _____, has remained as the only way to cure illness.

4. Digestion of the type of _____ that resembled the organ affected by disease also was believed to cure illnesses.

5. As new scientists emerge and new methods are devised to test hypotheses, the results can lead to _____ _____.

6. Remedies used in early American history included cinchona bark (quinine) for the treatment of _____.

7. _____ vaccination was stopped in 1971 because the disease had been eradicated worldwide.

8. Leeches are cared for and stored in the _____ in the pharmacy.

9. Maggots have the ability to eat dead tissue and to kill _____ that are the cause of the infection.

10. _____ was marketed as a tonic and contained extracts of cocaine and caffeine until 1905.

Matching

Match the following pathogen/disease with the vaccine that is administered to prevent the pathogen/disease.

A. Fluzone
B. Varivax
C. Prevnar 13
D. Trumenda
E. Twinrix
F. Gardasil 9
G. Zostavax
H. Enterovirus 71

_____ 1. Hepatitis A and B

_____ 2. Chickenpox

_____ 3. Hand-foot-mouth disease

_____ 4. Meningitis

_____ 5. Influenza

_____ 6. Varicella-zoster virus

_____ 7. Human Papillomavirus

_____ 8. Pneumonia

Short Answer

Write a short response to each question in the space provided.

1. What is the difference between an opioid and opium? What are the side effects of opioids and opiates?

   _____

   _____

   _____

   _____

2. Name four duties of pharmacy technicians in an institutional (inpatient) setting:

   A. _____

   B. _____

   C. _____

   D. _____

3. Name five duties of pharmacy technicians in a community setting:

   A. _____

   B. _____

   C. _____

   D. _____

   E. _____

4. List four skills entry-level pharmacy technicians must possess:

   A. _____

   B. _____

   C. _____

   D. _____

5. Name two areas of pharmacy in which a pharmacist can specialize:

   A. _____

   B. _____

6. Name two areas of pharmacy in which a pharmacy technician can specialize:

   A. _____

   B. _____

7. What must a technician do to gain the trust of the patient?

   _____

   _____

8. What duties do today's pharmacy technician perform that once were included as duties of the traditional pharmacist?

   _____

   _____

Research Activities

Follow the instructions given in each exercise and provide a response.

1. Access the website *http://www.ptcb.org* and investigate the duties outlined for pharmacy technicians.

2. Access the website *http://www.bls.gov/ooh/* and investigate the duties outlined for pharmacy technicians. Do they correspond to the duties the PTCB has outlined for pharmacy technicians? In what type of pharmacy setting are most pharmacy technicians employed?

REFLECT CRITICALLY

Critical Thinking

Reply to each question based on what you have learned in the chapter.

1. One of the most important aspects of a pharmacy technician's job is to gain the trust of the pharmacist. How would you, as a new technician on the job, go about gaining the trust of the pharmacist?

2. Why is it important for all pharmacy technicians to have strong communication and organization skills in any pharmacy setting?

3. What is your experience with the pharmacy? What drug treatments, immunizations, or pharmacy specialty roles are you familiar with or have experience with? How can you use these experiences to help you become a certified pharmacy technician?

RELATE TO PRACTICE

Lab Scenarios
History of Pharmacy

Objective: To allow the pharmacy technician to review the history of pharmacy

Lab Activity #1.1: Answer the following questions as they relate to the history of pharmacy.

Equipment needed:
- Internet access
- Pencil/pen

Time needed to complete this activity: 30 minutes

Access the website *https://pharmacy.wisc.edu/wp-content/uploads/2016/04/timecapsule.pdf* and answer the following questions:

1. What year was the first Hepatitis B vaccine approved?
2. Which pharmaceutical company marketed the first orally active angiotensin-converting enzyme inhibitor Capoten (captopril)?
3. List the conditions that Ritalin (methylphenidate) was first marketed to treat before it was found useful to treat pediatric hyperactivity or ADHD.
4. Which vitamin was successfully isolated from cod liver oil by Paul Karrer in 1931?
5. What novel by Upton Sinclair about the meat-packing industry directly led to the passing of the Pure Food and Drug Act?
6. What year did Louis Pasteur demonstrate the effectiveness of vaccinating sheep against live anthrax?

Pharmacy Technician Future

Objective: To allow the pharmacy technician to gain insight into the current and future pharmacy practice for pharmacy technicians.

Lab Activity #1.2: Answer the following questions about PTCB Credentials as they relate to the current and future pharmacy practice for pharmacy technicians.

Equipment needed:
- Internet access
- Pencil/pen

Time needed to complete this activity: 30 minutes

Access the website https://www.ptcb.org/credentials/ and answer the following questions:

1. What certifications are currently offered? What are the eligibility and educational requirements for each certification offered? What are the continuing education (CE) requirements to maintain each certification?
2. What certificates are currently offered? What are the eligibility and educational requirements for each certificate offered? What are the continuing education (CE) requirements to maintain each certification?
3. Report to your classmates the possible additional certifications and/or certificates you would like to work toward and why.

2 Pharmacy, Law, Ethics, and Regulatory Agencies

Standard 1.1: Demonstrate ethical conduct.

Standard 1.5: Demonstrate a respectful and professional attitude when interacting with diverse populations, colleagues, and professionals.

Standard 1.8: Demonstrate problem solving skills.

Standard 1.10: Apply critical thinking skills, creativity, and innovation.

Standard 2.2: Demonstrate ability to maintain confidentiality of patient information, and understand applicable state and federal laws.

Standard 2.3: Describe the pharmacy technician's role, pharmacist's role, and other occupations in the health care environment.

Standard 5.1: Describe and apply state and federal laws pertaining to processing, handling, and dispensing of medications including controlled substances.

Standard 5.2: Describe state and federal laws and regulations pertaining to pharmacy technicians.

Standard 5.3: Explain that differences exist between states regarding state regulations, pertaining to pharmacy technicians, and the processing, handling, and dispensing of medications.

REINFORCE KEY CONCEPTS

Terms and Definitions

Select the correct term from the following list and write the corresponding letter in the blank next to the statement.

A. Board of Pharmacy
B. Drug Enforcement Agency
C. Food and Drug Administration
D. Health Insurance Portability and Accountability Act of 1996
E. Medicare
F. Medicaid
G. Occupational Safety and Health Administration
H. Omnibus Budget Reconciliation Act of 1990
I. The Joint Commission
J. United States Pharmacopoeia

_____ 1. Federal- and state-operated insurance program that covers health care costs and prescription drugs for low-income children, adults, and elderly and those with disabilities.

_____ 2. An independent, nonprofit organization that establishes documentation on product quality standards, drug quality and information, and health care information on medications, over-the-counter products, dietary supplements, and food ingredients to ensure that they have the appropriate purity, quality, and strength.

_____ 3. Agency within the US Department of Health and Human Services that is responsible for ensuring the safety, efficacy, and security of human and veterinary drugs, biological products, medical devices, the national food supply, cosmetics, and radioactive products.

_____ 4. Federal- and state-managed insurance program that covers health care costs and prescription drugs for individuals older than 65, persons younger than 65 with long-term disabilities, and individuals with end-stage renal disease.

_____ 5. An independent, nonprofit organization that accredits hospitals and other health care organizations in the United States; accreditation is required to be eligible for Medicare and Medicaid payments.

_____ 6. Federal agency within the US Department of Justice that enforces US laws and regulations related to controlled substances.

_____ 7. Congressional act that changed reimbursement limits and mandated drug utilization evaluation, pharmacy patient consultation, and educational outreach programs.

_____ 8. Federal act that protects patients' rights, establishes national standards for electronic health care communication, and ensures the security and privacy of health data.

_____ 9. State board that regulates the practice of pharmacy within the state.

_____ 10. Congressional act that changed reimbursement limits and mandated drug utilization evaluation, pharmacy patient consultation, and educational outreach programs

Select the correct term from the following list and write the corresponding letter in the blank next to the statement.

A. Act
B. Adulteration
C. Amendment
D. Boxed Warning
E. Drug Diversion
F. Ethics
G. Misbranding
H. Morals
I. Negligence
J. Tort

_____ 11. The mishandling of medication that can lead to contamination or impurity, falsification of contents, or loss of drug quality or potency; may cause injury or illness to the consumer.

_____ 12. The intentional misuse of a drug intended for medical purposes; also refers to the channeling of the prescription drug supply away from legal distribution and to the illegal street market.

_____ 13. A legal concept that describes an action taken without the forethought that should have been taken by a reasonable person of similar competency.

_____ 14. An act that causes harm or injury to a person intentionally or because of negligence.

_____ 15. A statutory plan passed by Congress or any legislature that is a "bill" until it is enacted and becomes law.

_____ 16. Labeling of a product that is false or misleading; label information must include directions for use; safe and/or unsafe dosages; manufacturer, packer, or distributor; quantity; and weight.

_____ 17. A change in an original act or law.

_____ 18. Standards concerning or relating to what is right or wrong in human behavior.

_____ 19. The values and morals used within a profession.

_____ 20. Drug warning that is placed in the prescribing information or package insert of the product and indicates a significant risk of potentially dangerous side effects; the strongest warning the FDA can give; often called "Black Box Warnings."

Select the correct term from the following list and write the corresponding letter in the blank next to the statement.

A. Barbiturate
B. Controlled Substances
C. Legend Drug
D. Narcotic
E. Over-the-counter

_____ 21. A drug derived from barbituric acid; acts as a central nervous system depressant and often used in the treatment of seizures and as sedative and hypnotic agents.

_____ 22. Requires a prescription for dispensing; carries the federal legend: "Federal law prohibits the dispensing of this medication without a prescription."

_____ 23. Describes medication that can be purchased without a prescription; non-legend medication.

_____ 24. Any drug or other substance that is scheduled I through V and regulated by the Drug Enforcement Administration.

_____ 25. A nonspecific term used to describe a drug that in moderate doses dulls the senses, relieves pain, and induces profound sleep but in excessive doses causes stupor, coma, or convulsions and may lead to addiction.

Select the correct term from the following list and write the corresponding letter in the blank next to the statement.

A. Drug Utilization Evaluation
B. Monograph
C. National Drug Code
D. Pregnancy categories
E. *Physician's Desk Reference*
F. Protected Health Information
G. Safety Data Sheet
H. *United State Pharmacopeia-National Formulary*

_____ 26. A 10-digit number that indicates specifics the drug manufacturer, the drug product, and the package size of a prescription drug or an insulin product.

_____ 27. Compiles and publishes select manufacturer-provided package inserts and prescribing information useful for health professionals.

_____ 28. A publication of the USP that contains standards for medications, dosage forms, drug substances, excipients, medical devices, and dietary supplements.

_____ 29. A process that ensures that prescribed drugs are used appropriately; main desired outcome is an increase in medication-related efficacy and safety.

_____ 30. A document providing chemical product information.

_____ 31. A system used by the FDA to describe five levels of assessment of fetal effects caused by a drug; a required section of current prescription drug labeling.

_____ 32. Term used to describe a patient's personal health data; protected from being shared or distributed without permission.

_____ 33. Comprehensive information on a medication's actions within that class of drugs; lists generic and trade names, ingredients, dosages, side effects, adverse effects, how the patient should take the medication, and foods or other drugs to avoid while taking the medication.

True or False

Write T or F next to each statement.

_____ 1. The practice of pharmacy is governed by a series of laws, regulations, and rules enforced by federal, state, and local governments.

_____ 2. A good understanding of these laws is not necessary to know the responsibilities of a pharmacy technician.

_____ 3. Manufacturers need to prove the effectiveness of the drugs through methods such as scientific studies.

_____ 4. Hospital pharmacies must send a letter of approval with DEA form 41 two weeks before destruction of controlled substances.

_____ 5. Retail pharmacies disposing of bulk quantities of PSE, phenylephrine, or ephedrine must register with DEA Form 510.

_____ 6. The DEA requires narcotic inventory to be taken every 5 years.

_____ 7. If there are no federal or state laws that require a prescription to dispense schedule V drugs, then dispensing without a prescription is permitted.

_____ 8. A prescriber who has met all conditions to prescribe Suboxone and Subutex will be issued a special number with a Z by the DEA.

_____ 9. VIPPS is a label that indicates to the public that the website from which they are ordering drugs is both legitimate and licensed.

_____ 10. When federal and state law differs, the most lenient law is the one you should follow.

Multiple Choice

Complete each question by circling the best answer.

1. Who has the authority to decide under what schedule a drug should be placed?
   A. RPh
   B. FDA
   C. Attorney general
   D. DEA

2. A C-II drug can be refilled:
   A. 0 times
   B. 2 times
   C. 5 times
   D. 6 times

3. In most states, a prescription for a C-IV drug expires after:
   A. 14 days
   B. 3 months
   C. 6 months or five refills
   D. 12 months

8

4. States that allow schedule V drugs to be sold over-the-counter may dispense
   A. to purchasers at least 17 years of age or older
   B. no more than 120 mL or 24 solid doses of a controlled substance other than opium
   C. no more than a 72-hour supply without a prescription to a purchaser
   D. no more than 480 mL or 96 solid doses of opium to a purchaser

5. Methadone is a C-II controlled substance that is commonly used for opioid addiction but is also prescribed for
   A. Severe depression
   B. Schizophrenia
   C. ADHD
   D. cancer patients to alleviate pain

6. When prescriptions for controlled substances in C-III through C-V will be filed with other non–controlled drug prescriptions, the controlled drug prescriptions are designated in the pharmacy by stamping with a C that must appear:
   A. In red
   B. In black
   C. In green
   D. In blue

7. The following are tamper-proof prescription features *except*:
   A. Thermochromatic ink box shows "SECURE" when rubbed or heated
   B. Each sheet is non-sequentially numbered for internal and state-mandated record keeping
   C. Security feature warning bands are on the front of each script to detail security features
   D. Hidden security "VOID" appears when photocopied on most high-end photocopiers

8. Which medication does not have a dosage limit for filling the prescription without a childproof cap?
   A. Erythromycin tablets
   B. Nitrostat SL tablets
   C. Cholestyramine powder
   D. Prednisone tablets

9. The highest level of a manufacturer recall, which indicates that products could cause serious harm or fatality, is a:
   A. Class 1 recall
   B. Class 2 recall
   C. Class 3 recall
   D. Class 4 recall

10. If a technician is asked a question about the pharmacy's policies and procedures by a representative of the TJC and does not know the answer, the technician should do the following except
    A. make an answer up
    B. pretend they did not hear the question
    C. walk away
    D. give an honest answer

11. To obtain a Schedule II substance from a distributor, which DEA form must be filled out?
    A. 122
    B. 222
    C. 324
    D. 306

12. Which of the following controlled substance schedule drugs can be obtained without a prescription in some states?
    A. C-II
    B. C-III
    C. C-IV
    D. C-V

13. Invoices for C-II drugs must be kept for _____ years.
    A. 2
    B. 4
    C. 5
    D. 7

14. To destroy controlled substances, which DEA form must be used?
    A. 106
    B. 222
    C. 41
    D. 510

15. Record-keeping is regulated by:
    A. Federal law
    B. State law
    C. Company policy
    D. Pharmacists

Fill in the Blanks

Answer each question by completing the statement in the space provided.

1. PPPA specifies that medication should not be able to be opened by at least _____ % of children under the age of 5 and that at least _____ % of adults should be able to open the medication within 5 minutes.

2. The main function of the FDA is to _____ the guidelines for manufacturers to ensure the safety and effectiveness of medications.

9

3. Adverse reactions should be reported to the FDA's

_____ program.

4. The DEA guidelines for controlled C-II substances allow physicians to write up to _____ separate prescriptions at one time for multiple drugs, to be filled sequentially over _____ days.

5. A _____ is distributed by the pharmacy with each prescription and each prescription refill because the information for the patient may change frequently.

6. A _____ mistake can affect a person's ability to continue to work as a technician and also may result in punitive damages.

7. Depending on the state in which the technician works, laws vary as they pertain to the _____ of the technician.

8. More states are enacting laws to make technicians _____ for their actions in the pharmacy.

9. Keeping patients' information _____ and working within the pharmacy's rules and guidelines ensure that patients receive the best service possible.

10. _____ is a key component of professional behavior in the pharmacy.

Matching

Match the controlled substance designations with the correct drugs.

A. C-I
B. C-II
C. C-III
D. C-IV
E. C-V

_____ 1. Tylenol/codeine #3 (acetaminophen/codeine)

_____ 2. LSD

_____ 3. Dormalin (quazepam)

_____ 4. Ritalin (methylphenidate)

_____ 5. Robitussin AC (guaifenesin/codeine)

_____ 6. Heroin

_____ 7. Depo-Testosterone (testosterone)

_____ 8. Lomotil (diphenoxylate/atropine)

_____ 9. Duragesic (fentanyl)

_____ 10. Valium (diazepam)

Match the pharmacy law with the correct description.

A. 1906 Federal Food and Drug Act
B. 1914 Harrison Narcotic Act
C. 1938 Food, Drug, and Cosmetic Act
D. 1951 Durham-Humphrey Amendment
E. 1962 Kefauver-Harris Amendment
F. 1967 Fair Packaging and Labeling Act
G. 1970 Comprehensive Drug Abuse Prevention and Control Act
H. 1970 Poison Prevention Packaging Act

_____ 11. Required practitioner registration, documentation regarding prescriptions and dispensing, and implementation of restrictions regarding the importation, sale, and distribution of opium, coca leaves, and any derivative products.

_____ 12. One of the first laws enacted to stop the sale of inaccurately labeled drugs.

_____ 13. Added more instructions for drug companies, required the labeling "Caution: Federal law prohibits dispensing without a prescription," and made the initial distinction between legend drugs and OTC medications that do not require a physician's order.

_____ 14. Formed the DEA to enforce the laws concerning controlled substances and their distribution and introduced a stair-step schedule of controlled substances.

_____ 15. Label must show net contents; name and place of business of manufacturer, packer, or distributor; and net quantity of contents in terms of weight, measure, or numeric count.

_____ 16. Requires manufacturers and pharmacies to place all medications in containers with childproof caps or packaging, including both over-the-counter and legend drugs.

_____ 17. Ensures the safety and effectiveness of all new drugs on the US market.

_____ 18. Important concepts of this act were adulteration, misbranding, and providing the legal status for the FDA.

Match the pharmacy law with the correct description.

A. 1972 Drug Listing Act
B. 1983 Orphan Drug Act
C. 1987 Prescription Drug Marketing Act
D. 1990 Anabolic Steroids Control Act
E. 1990 The Humanitarian Device Exemption – Safe Medical Devices Act
F. 1990 Nutritional Labeling and Education Act
G. 1990 Omnibus Budget Reconciliation Act
H. 1994 Dietary Supplement Health and Education Act

_____ 19. Helps enforce regulations on the abuse of anabolic steroids.

_____ 20. Provides the FDA with an accurate list of all drugs manufactured, prepared, propagated, compounded, or processed by a drug establishment regulated under the FDA and amends the Federal Food, Drug, and Cosmetic Act and prevents unfair or deceptive packaging and labeling.

_____ 21. Congressional act that changed reimbursement limits and mandated drug utilization evaluation, pharmacy patient consultation, and educational outreach programs.

_____ 22. Better defines the term dietary supplements to include herbs such as ginseng, garlic, fish oil, psyllium, enzymes, glandulars, and mixtures of these.

_____ 23. Encourages discovery and use of devices intended to benefit patients in treatment and diagnosis of diseases or conditions that affect fewer than 4000 individuals in the United States.

_____ 24. Encourages drug companies to develop drugs for rare diseases by providing research assistance, grants, and cost incentives to manufacturers.

_____ 25. Covers food items and their labeling; vitamins, minerals, or other nutrients are on the label and in some cases are highlighted.

_____ 26. Helps to avoid counterfeit drugs and ingredients in the supply chain and also helps limit diversion of pharmaceutical samples and prescription drugs.

Match the pharmacy law with the correct description.

A. 1996 Health Insurance Portability and Accountability Act
B. 1997 Food and Drug Administration Modernization Act
C. 2000 Drug Addiction Treatment Act
D. 2003 Medicare Modernization Act
E. 2005 Combat Methamphetamine Epidemic Act
F. 2010 Patient Protection and Affordable Care Act
G. 2013 Drug Quality and Security Act

_____ 27. Provides a drug discount card to beneficiaries with low incomes who require pharmacy company assistance for obtaining medications.

_____ 28. Makes preventative care more accessible and affordable for many Americans.

_____ 29. Federal act for protecting patients' rights, establishing national standards for electronic health care communication, and ensuring the security and privacy of health data.

_____ 30. Gives greater oversight of bulk pharmaceutical compounding and enhances the agency's ability to track drugs through the distribution process.

_____ 31. Permits physicians to prescribe controlled substances (preapproved by the DEA) in schedules C-III, C-IV, or C-V to persons suffering from opioid addiction, for the purpose of maintenance or detoxification treatments.

_____ 32. Amendment to the Federal Food, Drug, and Cosmetic Act related to the regulation of food, drugs, devices, and biological products by the FDA.

_____ 33. Addresses all areas related to manufacture of, enforcement of laws pertaining to, and sale of pseudoephedrine, which can be used to create methamphetamine.

11

Match the pregnancy category with the correct description.

A. Pregnancy Category A
B. Pregnancy Category B
C. Pregnancy Category C
D. Pregnancy Category D
E. Pregnancy Category X

_____ 34. Animal reproduction studies have shown an adverse effect on the fetus, and there are no adequate and well-controlled studies in humans, but potential benefits may warrant use of the drug in pregnant women despite potential risks.

_____ 35. Studies in animals or humans have demonstrated fetal abnormalities, and/or there is positive evidence of human fetal risk based on adverse reaction data from investigational or marketing experience, and the risks involved in use of the drug in pregnant women clearly outweigh potential benefits.

_____ 36. Adequate and well-controlled studies have failed to demonstrate a risk to the fetus in the first trimester of pregnancy (and there is no evidence of risk in later trimesters).

_____ 37. There is positive evidence of human fetal risk based on adverse reaction data from investigational or marketing experience or studies in humans, but potential benefits may warrant use of the drug in pregnant women despite potential risks.

_____ 38. Animal reproduction studies have failed to demonstrate a risk to the fetus, and there are no adequate and well-controlled studies in pregnant women.

Match the DEA Form with the correct description.

A. Form 224
B. Form 225
C. Form 363
D. Form 222
E. Form 41
F. Form 510
G. Form 106

_____ 39. For loss or theft of a controlled substance

_____ 40. To manufacture or distribute controlled substances

_____ 41. To order or transfer schedule II substances

_____ 42. To manage a controlled substances treatment program or compound controlled substances

_____ 43. For retail pharmacies that want to engage in wholesale distribution of bulk quantities of drugs containing pseudoephedrine, phenylpropanolamine, or ephedrine

_____ 44. To dispense controlled substances

_____ 45. Authorization to destroy damaged, outdated, or unwanted controlled substances

Short Answer

Write a short response to each question in the space provided.

1. Explain what the letters in a DEA number represent. How do you verify that a DEA number is authentic?

_____

_____

_____

_____

_____

_____

2. Under what conditions may a prescription be dispensed in a non–child-resistant container? List five prescription drugs that can be packaged in non–child-resistant bottles.

_____

_____

_____

3. When medication from an original manufacturer's container is repackaged, list the information to be placed on each individual label.

_____

_____

_____

4. List the components of the ACA that involves pharmacy and the components that a pharmacy technician need to be knowledgeable of.

_____

_____

_____

_____

_____

5. Name three characteristics a pharmacy technician should have to demonstrate professional ethics.

_____

_____

6. What does REMS stand for? Which amendment gave the FDA the authority to require REMS from a manufacturer to ensure that the benefits of a drug or biological product outweigh its risks? Name the computer-based risk management program designed to increase awareness of the dangers of isotretinoin to eliminate fetal exposure to the drug.

_____

_____

7. List three dosage forms CBD is available as in the pharmacy and list the treatments CBD is used for.

_____

_____

_____

Research Activities

Follow the instructions given in each exercise and provide a response.

1. Access the website http://www.fda.gov/Safety/MedWatch/. List two drug recalls that have occurred in the last 180 days. What class of recall was it and why was the product recalled?

2. Access the website https://nabp.pharmacy/programs/vipps/. List pharmacies in your area that are VIPPS accredited.

Critical Thinking

Reply to each question based on what you have learned in the chapter.

1. If you could add one more law to the existing laws addressing abuse of prescription medications, what would it be? Why?

2. Marijuana has been the subject of debate lately for possible medicinal use in patients with cancer, AIDS, and multiple sclerosis. Into which controlled substance schedule would you put marijuana if it were approved for such use? Why?

3. Someone presents a C-II prescription in the pharmacy 31 days after it was written. Knowing that the federal law does not put a time limit on when C-II drugs must be filled, how would you tell the patient that this prescription cannot be filled?

4. Everyone is guided and shaped by a code of ethics and morality based on the guidelines (dos/don'ts) you grew up with. As you have developed your own code of ethics, what do you live by? What ethical guideline are a must for you? How important is it to develop a good work ethic and why?

RELATE TO PRACTICE

Lab Scenarios
Pharmacy Law

Objective: To allow the pharmacy technician to develop critical thinking skills when filling prescriptions in keeping with pharmacy laws.

Lab Activity #2.1: Answer the following questions as they relate to pharmacy practice.

Equipment needed:
■ Pencil/pen

Time needed to complete this activity: 60 minutes

1. A physician writes the following prescription:

```
                Dr. Andrew A. Sheen
             1100 Brentwood Blvd, Suite M780
                  St. Louis, MO 63144
                     314-527-0000
                    DEA FS1234563

Brandon Chung                              March 3, 202X


Rx      Tylenol with Codeine #3  #30
        1 tab q-4-6 hr prn pain

Ref x 5                          Dr. Andrew Sheen
```

How many prescription refills are allowed for a Schedule III controlled substance? When must this prescription be filled before it expires?

_____

2. A physician writes the following prescription:

```
                Dr. Andrew A. Sheen
             1100 Brentwood Blvd, Suite M780
                  St. Louis, MO 63144
                     314-527-0000
                    DEA FS1234563

Brandon Chung                           February 17, 202X


Rx      Coumadin 5 mg #30
        1 tab po qd

Ref x 5                          Dr. Andrew Sheen
```

May this prescription be filled with a generic drug? Why or why not?

_____

3. The pharmacy receives the following prescription on a Monday:

```
                Dr. Andrew A. Sheen
             1100 Brentwood Blvd, Suite M780
                  St. Louis, MO 63144
                     314-527-0000
                    DEA FS1234563

Brandon Chung                            April 4, 202X


Rx      Percocet 5 mg #30
        1 tab po q4-6 h prn pain


Ref                              Dr. Andrew Sheen
```

The pharmacy has only 20 tablets of Percocet in stock. What options does the pharmacy have in filling this prescription?

_____

_____

_____

4. A patient has the following prescription filled at a pharmacy:

```
                Dr. Andrew Sheen
             1100 Brentwood Blvd, Suite M780
                  St. Louis, MO 63144
                     314-527-0000
                    DEA FS1234563

Name:  Brandon Chung              Date:  June 15, 202X


Rx      Alprazolam 0.5 mg #30
        i qd prn anxiety


Ref x 5                    Dr. Andrew Sheen
```

The patient now wishes to have the prescription filled at another pharmacy. How many times may the prescription be transferred to another pharmacy? What happens to the prescription at the original pharmacy? What information must be indicated on the original prescription?

_____

_____

_____

_____

5. A patient brings in the following prescription to be filled at your pharmacy:

```
                Dr. Andrew A. Sheen

             1100 Brentwood Blvd, Suite M780

                  St. Louis, MO 63144

                     314-527-0000

                    DEA FS1234563


Brandon Chung                            July 6, 202X



Rx      Hydrochlorothiazide 50 mg #30

        1 tab po qd for fluid retention



Ref  prn                    Dr. Andrew Sheen
```

When will the prescription expire?

_____

6. A patient receives the following prescription:

```
                    Dr. Andrew A. Sheen
                 1100 Brentwood Blvd, Suite M780
                    St. Louis, MO 63144
                       314-527-0000
                      DEA FS1234563

Brandon Chung                          September 14, 202X

Rx    Ambien 10 mg        #30
      1 tab po q hs prn insomnia


Ref x 0                       Dr. Andrew Sheen
```

When will the prescription expire?

_____

7. A female patient brings in a new prescription for amoxicillin 500 mg. As you are entering the prescription into the system, you receive a DUE showing that the patient has filled a prescription for Alesse, an oral contraceptive.

A. What should you do and why?

_____

_____

_____

B. Which pharmacy law would you be enforcing?

_____

C. What auxiliary labels should be applied to this prescription when dispensing?

_____

8. A 16-year-old male comes to the pharmacy counter and asks for a 10-pack of U-30 insulin syringes.

A. How do you handle the situation and why?

_____

_____

B. Why is it important to be familiar with federal and state laws and uphold them?

_____

_____

_____

9. A 21-year-old male approaches the pharmacy counter and asks to buy four boxes of Sudafed tablets that are stocked behind the counter.

A. How would you handle the situation and why?

_____

B. Which pharmacy law would you be enforcing?

_____

10. A 16-year-old female comes to the prescription counter and asks for a 4-ounce bottle of Robitussin AC cough syrup.

A. How would you handle the situation and why?

_____

_____

_____

B. Which pharmacy law would you be enforcing?

_____

11. A. How many times in a year may a retail pharmacy request the destruction of controlled substances? What form would be used to request the destruction in a retail pharmacy?

_____

_____

B. How many times in a year may a hospital pharmacy request the destruction of controlled substances? What form would be used to request the destruction in a hospital pharmacy?

_____

_____

12. Explain the three methods permitted for filing filled prescriptions.

_____

_____

_____

_____

13. How would you handle a patient's request to have a prescription mailed to him or her?

_____

_____

_____

14. What criteria must be evaluated for a medication to be considered a controlled substance?

_____

15. What do the three components of an NDC number represent?

_____

16. What conditions must be met for an individual to purchase an "exempt narcotic"?

_____

_____

_____

17. A. A physician calls in an "emergency" prescription for a Schedule II medication. How much time does the physician have to provide the pharmacy with a handwritten prescription?

_____

B. According to your state laws of pharmacy, how much time does the physician have to provide the pharmacy with a handwritten prescription?

_____

18. Who is permitted to counsel a patient?

_____

19. Which federal agency can issue a drug recall?

_____

20. What organization oversees the practice of pharmacy within a particular state?

_____

Lab Activity #2.2: Using a *Physicians' Desk Reference* book or https://globalrph.com/, identify the pregnancy category for each of the drugs listed.

Equipment needed:
- *Physicians' Desk Reference*
- Computer with Internet
- Pencil/pen

Time needed to complete this activity: 45 minutes

1. Tetracycline

_____

2. Lovastatin

_____

3. Olanzapine

_____

4. Paroxetine HCl

_____

5. Acetaminophen

_____

6. Diphenhydramine

_____

7. Methotrexate

_____

8. Fentanyl

_____

9. Isotretinoin

_____

10. Pantoprazole

_____

11. Ibuprofen

_____

12. Loratadine

_____

13. Liothyronine

_____

14. Nasal Saline

_____

15. Milk of Magnesia

_____

Lab Activity #2.3: Using a *Drug Facts and Comparisons* reference book, identify the control schedule for each of the drugs listed.

Equipment needed:
- *Drug Facts and Comparisons*
- Pencil/pen

Time needed to complete this activity: 45 minutes

1. Clonazepam

_____

2. Diazepam

_____

3. Meperidine

_____

4. Modafinil

_____

5. Morphine

_____

6. Oxycodone/APAP

_____

7. Methyltestosterone

_____

8. Alprazolam

_____

9. Zolpidem

_____

10. Pregabalin

_____

11. Guaifenesin/Codeine

_____

12. Dronabinol

_____

13. Benzphetamine

_____

14. Amphetamine

_____

15. Lorazepam

_____

Lab Activity #2.4: Use the verification process to determine if the listed DEA numbers are valid or invalid. If the DEA number is invalid, explain why it is invalid.

Equipment needed:
- Basic calculator
- Pencil/pen

Time needed to complete this activity: 30 minutes

1. Lucy Garcia, FNP   MG4789270

_____

2. Doug Martinez, MD   MM4921739

_____

3. Tanya Smith, DDS   FS5264813

_____

4. Reyna Reyes, PA   FR3814262

_____

5. Jack Jenson, DO   AJ3875245

_____

6. Daniel de la Rosa, DPM   BR6315750

_____

7. Mary Zepeda, DVM   FZ5783217

_____

8. Shaggy Dog Animal Hospital   BS38752456

_____

9. Kirkland Pharmacy   AP6872313

_____

10. Sarasota Hospital   AS2498637

_____

Chapter **2 Pharmacy, Law, Ethics, and Regulatory Agencies**

Procedural Step	Yes/No
Verified the first letter of the DEA number is either A, B, or F for practitioner's or M for nurse practitioners and physician assistants. Marked DEA set invalid if it did not match.	
Determined if the second letter is the first letter of the practitioner's last name or the first letter of the practitioner's pharmacy/hospital.	
Marked DEA set invalid if it did not match.	
Used the formula to add the first, third, and fifth numbers in the DEA set.	
Continued the formula by adding the second, fourth, and sixth numbers and then multiplied by 2.	
Completed the formula by adding the two sums together.	
Compared the results of the check sum. Marked DEA set valid when the last digit from the check sum matched the last number in the DEA set. Marked DEA set invalid when the last digit from the check sum did not match the last number of the DEA set.	

Role and Responsibilities of the Pharmacy Technician

Objective: To familiarize the pharmacy technician with his or her role and responsibilities as a pharmacy technician in the practice of pharmacy.

The state board of pharmacy oversees the practice of pharmacy within a given state. The state board of pharmacy establishes requirements for an individual to be licensed as a pharmacist. In addition, the board enacts regulations that define the criteria to be met by individuals who seek to be a pharmacy technician, their role in the practice of pharmacy, and the tasks they may perform. These tasks may vary from state to state, and it is the responsibility of the pharmacy technician to become familiar with them.

Lab Activity #2.5: Refer to http://www.nabp.net/boards-of-pharmacy/ for the following information. Identify the tasks permitted by the board of pharmacy in your state.

Equipment needed:
- Computer with Internet access
- Pencil/pen

Time needed to complete this activity: 30 minutes

Task	Yes/No
Accept telephoned prescriptions from physician's office.	
Counsel patients.	
Obtain refill permission from physician's office.	
Order medications.	
Prepare non-sterile (extemporaneous) compounds. If yes, is additional training required?	
Prepare intravenous medications. If yes, is additional training required?	
Prepare radiopharmaceuticals. If yes, is additional training required?	
Prepare total parenteral nutrition products. If yes, is additional training required?	
Prepare hazardous compounds, sterile and non-sterile. If yes, is additional training required?	
Tech-check-tech If yes, is additional training required?	
Administer immunizations If yes, is additional training required?	

Pharmacy Ethics

Objective: To identify those pharmacy situations in which a pharmacy technician will be faced with making ethical decisions.

The practice of pharmacy has established a code of ethics for both pharmacists and pharmacy technicians.

CODE OF ETHICS FOR PHARMACY TECHNICIANS

Preamble

Pharmacy technicians are health care professionals who assist pharmacists in providing the best possible care for patients. The principles of this code, which apply to pharmacy technicians working in any and all settings, are based on application and support of the moral obligations that guide the pharmacy profession in relationships with patients, health care professionals, and society.

Principles

- A pharmacy technician's first consideration is to ensure the health and safety of the patient, and to use knowledge and skills to the best of his or her ability in serving patients.
- A pharmacy technician supports and promotes honesty and integrity in the profession, which includes the duty to observe the law, maintain the highest moral and ethical conduct at all times, and uphold the ethical principles of the profession.
- A pharmacy technician assists and supports pharmacists in the safe and efficacious and cost-effective distribution of health services and health care resources.
- A pharmacy technician respects and values the abilities of pharmacists, colleagues, and other health care professionals.
- A pharmacy technician maintains competency in his or her practice and continually enhances his or her professional knowledge and expertise.
- A pharmacy technician respects and supports the patient's individuality, dignity, and confidentiality.
- A pharmacy technician respects the confidentiality of a patient's records and discloses pertinent information only with proper authorization.
- A pharmacy technician never assists in dispensing, promoting, or distributing medication or medical devices that are not of good quality or that do not meet standards as required by law.
- A pharmacy technician does not engage in any activity that will discredit the profession, and will expose, without fear or favor, illegal or unethical conduct within the profession.
- A pharmacy technician associates with and engages in the support of organizations that promote the profession of pharmacy through the utilization and enhancement of pharmacy technicians.

Lab Activity #2.6: Explain how you would handle the following pharmacy situations and identify the principle of the code of ethics on which you are basing your decision.

Equipment needed:
■ Pencil/pen

Time needed to complete the activity: 45 minutes

1. A friend of your family is diagnosed with a terminal illness and drops off a prescription to be filled. Should you tell your family about this individual's situation? Why or why not?

_____

_____

_____

2. You are not required to be certified as a pharmacy technician to practice in your state. Should you participate in continuing education activities? Why or why not?

_____

_____

_____

3. An individual wishes to purchase insulin syringes, and the pharmacist is not present in the pharmacy at that time. Should you sell the syringes to the customer or wait for the pharmacist to return? Why or why not?

_____

_____

_____

4. You have medication in your inventory that will expire in 8 days. A patient presents a prescription for a 10-day supply of the medication. Should you dispense the medication on your shelf? Why or why not?

_____

_____

_____

5. You have dropped some medication on the floor. What should you do with this medication and why?

_____

_____

_____

6. A woman comes to the pharmacy and asks for a listing of the medications her husband filled last year. What should you do and why?

_____

_____

_____

7. A patient asks you to recommend an OTC medication for respiratory allergies. In the past you have observed the pharmacist recommend Claritin. Should you recommend Claritin to the patient? Why or why not?

_____

_____

_____

8. The FDA has recalled Drug X because of labeling problems, and you have some of the recalled medication on your shelf. An individual requests a refill for this medication on Friday and needs to leave on a plane in the afternoon. Should you dispense the recalled medication that is now on your shelf? Why or why not?

_____

_____

_____

9. You observe the pharmacist preparing an intravenous fluid at a strength that is less than what has been prescribed by the physician. How would you handle this situation?

_____

_____

10. A physician had his license to prescribe medications suspended 5 years ago by both the board of medicine and the pharmacy because of a personal drug problem. His license to practice has been reinstated. A patient brings in a prescription from that physician and casually asks what you know about the physician. How would you handle the situation?

_____

_____

_____

3 Competencies, Associations, and Settings for Technicians

ASHP ACCREDITATION STANDARDS FOR PHARMACY TECHNICIAN EDUCATION AND TRAINING PROGRAMS

Standard 1.2: Present an image appropriate for the profession of pharmacy in appearance and behavior.

Standard 1.3: Demonstrate active and engaged listening skills.

Standard 1.4: Communicate clearly and effectively, both verbally and in writing.

Standard 1.5: Demonstrate a respectful and professional attitude when interacting with diverse populations, colleagues, and professionals.

Standard 2.1: Explain the importance of maintaining competency through continuing education and continuing professional development.

Standard 2.3: Describe the pharmacy technician's role, pharmacist's role, and other occupations in the health care environment.

Standard 5.1: Describe and apply state and federal laws pertaining to processing, handling, and dispensing of medications including controlled substances.

Standard 5.2: Describe state and federal laws and regulations pertaining to pharmacy technicians.

Standard 5.3: Explain that differences exist between states regarding state regulations, pertaining to pharmacy technicians, and the processing, handling, and dispensing of medications.

Standard 5.4: Describe the process and responsibilities required to obtain and maintain registration and/or licensure to work as a pharmacy technician.

Standard 5.10: Describe major trends, issues, goals, and initiatives taking place in the pharmacy profession.

REINFORCE KEY CONCEPTS

Terms and Definitions

Select the correct term from the following list and write the corresponding letter in the blank next to the statement.

A. Accreditation Council for Pharmacy Education (ACPE)
B. Board of pharmacy (BOP)
C. National Association of Boards of Pharmacy (NABP)
D. National Healthcareer Association (NHA)
E. Pharmacy Technician Certification Board (PTCB)

___D___ 1. National board for the certification of pharmacy technicians.

___C___ 2. National agency for the accreditation of professional degree programs in pharmacy and providers of continuing pharmacy education.

___A___ 3. Certification organization for a variety of health care careers, including the Institute for the Certification of Pharmacy Technicians (ICPT).

___E___ 4. A state-managed agency that licenses pharmacists and may either register or license pharmacy technicians to work in pharmacy.

___B___ 5. National organization for members of state boards of pharmacy.

Select the correct term from the following list and write the corresponding letter in the blank next to the statement.

A. American Association of Pharmacy Technicians (AAPT)
B. American Pharmacists Association (APhA)
C. American Society of Health-System Pharmacists (ASHP)
D. American Society of Health-System Pharmacists (ASHP) Model Curriculum for Pharmacy Technician Education and Training
E. The Society for the Education of Pharmacy Technicians (SEPhT)
F. National Pharmacy Technician Association (NPTA)
G. Pharmacy Technician Accreditation Commission (PTAC)

___E___ 6. A national technician organization with free membership that offers tools and useful information used in training and education of students and current practicing pharmacy technicians.

___C___ 7. Oldest pharmacy association; founded in 1852.

___G___ 8. Agency-formed partnership between ASHP and ACPE for review and accreditation of pharmacy technician education and training programs.

___D___ 9. Pharmacy association founded in 1942.

___F___ 10. Pharmacy association primarily for technicians; founded in 1999.

___A___ 11. First pharmacy technician association; founded in 1979.

___B___ 12. A program that provides details on how to meet the ASHP goals for pharmacy technician training curricula.

Select the correct term from the following list and write the corresponding letter in the blank next to the statement.

A. Certified pharmacy technician
B. Competency
C. Continuing education (CE)
D. Registered pharmacy technician
E. Licensed pharmacy technician

___B___ 13. A technician who has passed the national certification examination; the technician can use the abbreviation CPhT after his or her name.

___D___ 14. A pharmacy technician who is licensed by the state board; ensures that an individual has at least the minimum level of competency required by the profession.

___C___ 15. Education beyond the basic technical education, usually required for license or certification renewal.

___E___ 16. The capability or proficiency to perform a function.

___A___ 17. A pharmacy technician who is registered through the state board of pharmacy; helps maintain a list of those working in pharmacies and may require a background check through the legal system.

Select the correct term from the following list and write the corresponding letter in the blank next to the statement.

A. Communication
B. Confidentiality
C. Nondiscretionary duties
D. Professionalism

___C___ 18. The practice of keeping privileged customer information from being disclosed without the customer's consent.

___A___ 19. The ability to express oneself in such a way that one is readily and clearly understood.

___B___ 20. Conforming to the right principles of conduct (work ethics) as accepted by others in the profession.

___D___ 21. Tasks that do not require professional judgment such as repackaging medications, managing inventory, filling automated dispensing machines, and billing.

Select the correct term from the following list and write the corresponding letter in the blank next to the statement.

A. Closed door pharmacy
B. Community pharmacy
C. Inpatient pharmacy
D. Outpatient pharmacy
E. Hyperalimentation
F. Parenteral medications
G. Total parenteral nutrition (TPN)

___G___ 22. A pharmacy that serves patients in community or ambulatory settings.

___D___ 23. A term most used to describe medications administered by injection, such as intravenously, intramuscularly, or subcutaneously.

___B___ 24. Also known as an outpatient or a retail pharmacy; these pharmacies serve patients in their communities; consumers can walk in and purchase a prescription or over-the-counter (OTC) drug.

___F___ 25. Parenteral (intravenous) nutrition for patients who are unable to eat solids or liquids; also known as total parenteral nutrition (TPN).

___C___ 26. A pharmacy in a hospital or institutional setting.

___E___ 27. Large-volume intravenous nutrition administered through the central vein (subclavian vein), which allows for a higher concentration of solutions.

___A___ 28. A pharmacy in which medications are called in from institutions, such as long-term care facilities, and are then delivered; closed-door pharmacies are not open to the public.

True or False

Write T or F next to each statement.

___F___ 1. Pharmacy technician qualifications and job descriptions are same in each state.

___T___ 2. Each state's BOP serves many functions, including registering technicians and licensing pharmacists.

___T___ 3. The number of prescriptions processed per day in a pharmacy is not related to the speed and accuracy of the typist.

___T___ 4. Inventory management is a skill that is normally on the job because it has its own way of handling stock inventory.

___F___ 5. A pharmacy technician is not required to update and improve their computer skills to remain a valuable pharmacy team member.

___F___ 6. Pharmacy technicians do not need to make sure the pharmacist has checked all drugs and/or devices before they leave the pharmacy.

___F___ 7. Certified pharmacy technicians must renew their certification every two years and complete at least 20 hours of pharmacy-related continuing education.

___T___ 8. The ExCPT exam is the only pharmacy technician certification exam accepted in all 50 states.

___T___ 9. How technicians conduct themselves in various situations reveals their professionalism and their personal maturity.

___F___ 10. Pharmacies prefer to hire a pharmacy technician who has graduated from an accredited program and is nationally certified.

Multiple Choice

Complete each question by circling the best answer.

1. If a pharmacy technician violates a pharmacy law, the

   _____ has the authority to revoke their pharmacy license or registration.
   A. Pharmacy Technician Certification Board (PTCB)
   B. American Society of Health-System Pharmacists (ASHP)
   C. National Association of Boards of Pharmacy (NABP)
   D. state board of pharmacy (BOP)

2. The following are nondiscretionary duties pharmacy technicians can perform *except*:
   A. Transcribing prescriptions
   B. Interpret lab results to determine drug therapy effectiveness
   C. Manage inventory
   D. Prepare reports

Chapter **3** **Competencies, Associations, and Settings for Technicians**

3. Which of the following duties would a pharmacy technician in an inpatient setting perform?
   A. Bill prescription insurance companies
   B. Assist patients over the phone
   C. Prepare IV medications
   D. Fill prescriptions for patient pickup

4. Which of the following duties would a pharmacy technician in an outpatient setting perform?
   A. Refill prescriptions
   B. Prepare IV medications
   C. Prepare and deliver a stat dose to the requesting department
   D. Load patient medication drawers

5. Online pharmacies can be verified though:
   A. Pharmacy Checker
   B. VIPPS
   C. FDA
   D. ACPE

6. A candidate may be disqualified for PTCB certification exam upon the disclosure or discovery of:
   A. Receiving a GED instead of a HS diploma
   B. Compliance with all applicable PTCB certification policies
   C. Receiving a passing score on the PTCE
   D. Criminal conduct involving the candidate

7. Pharmacy technicians who meet the requirements of national certification may use initials _____ on their identification tag, indicating they are a certified pharmacy technician.
   A. PT
   B. CPT
   C. CPhT
   D. PhTC

8. Which of the following is *not* a soft skill every employee needs?
   A. Conflict resolution
   B. Inflexibility
   C. Critical observation
   D. Teamwork

9. To be a professional in the workplace, all employees should demonstrate the following quality:
   A. Honesty
   B. Poor work ethics
   C. A sense of entitlement
   D. Rude behavior

10. Which of the following should be avoided to represent a professional appearance in the pharmacy?
    A. Non-visible tattoo
    B. Earrings
    C. Wedding ring
    D. Nose ring

Fill in the Blanks

Answer each question by completing the statement in the space provided.

1. Several states require _____ or _____ certification and have accepted it as their measure of the knowledge base of pharmacy technicians.

2. Technician duties focus on tasks that do not require _____ _____ but instead concentrate on their technical skills and training.

3. Prior knowledge of pharmacy terms, drugs, and procedures are required to perform _____ duties in the pharmacy setting.

4. A knowledge of computers and programs such as Microsoft Word and Excel can make a technician a(n) _____ asset to the pharmacy.

5. Stat doses are to be delivered within _____ minutes or less to the area requesting them.

6. The _____ has been the leader in providing course curriculum and standards and offering students the best foundation for becoming technicians.

7. Association membership is an excellent way for a pharmacy technician to _____ their career and form _____ friendships with pharmacy colleagues.

8. Pharmacy is an important _____, and pharmacy technician is a great _____.

9. A _____ is honest and dependable and displays integrity in all situations.

10. Advanced roles and _____ provide technicians with specialty roles and higher positions.

Matching

Select the correct outpatient pharmacy job opportunity from the following list and write the corresponding letter in the blank next to the description.

A. Insurance billing technician
B. Retail technician
C. Inventory/stock technician
D. Technician recruiter
E. Technician trainer
F. Technician manager

___D___ 1. Recruit other technicians into their company.

___B___ 2. Must know the guidelines of Medicare, Blue Cross, Medicaid, and other insurance companies.

___F___ 3. Supervise the pharmacy technician staff, responsible for interviewing possible new employees, developing and maintaining work schedules, making sure registrations and certifications are current, and working with the pharmacists to continually train and update the skills of the pharmacy technician employees.

___A___ 4. Must know contacts for fast service, be able to obtain products and drugs as soon as possible, and perform proper billing functions for the pharmacy, including processing returns, recalled drugs, and controlled substances.

___C___ 5. Must have excellent communication skills, phone skills, and prescription-filling abilities.

___E___ 6. Train newly hired technicians on computer programs and to master other necessary skills relevant to their specific pharmacy.

Select the correct inpatient pharmacy job opportunity from the following list and write the corresponding letter in the blank next to the description.

A. Inventory technician
B. Robot filler
C. IV technician
D. Chemotherapy technician
E. Anticoagulant technician
F. Technician verifiers
G. Clinical technician
H. Pharmacy informatics analyst
I. Supervisory technician

___F___ 7. Checks the work of other technicians and performs final verification of medication orders and identifies orders on a routine basis that need the pharmacist's intervention to improve the administrative experience.

___B___ 8. Load robots to fill patient medication drawers to keep the pharmacy running smoothly.

___H___ 9. Assists the anticoagulant pharmacist in contacting patients when patient follow-up is necessary, or the patient's anticoagulation medication or dosage needs to be changed.

___G___ 10. Works with the clinical applications specialists to maintain pharmacy software and computers, coordinate hardware and software updates, and work with the pharmacy informatics team.

___E___ 11. Interprets orders and prepares all parenteral medications, in both large and small volumes, and any other special-order intravenous or intramuscular drugs.

___A___ 12. Helps track the patient's medications and compiles important data that the pharmacist needs to monitor and evaluate patient outcomes or the appropriateness of drug therapies or to monitor formulary compliance.

___H___ 13. Schedules other technicians and may even hire prospective technicians by reviewing their skills and backgrounds.

___I___ 14. Orders all stock, handles billing, talks to drug representatives, and may be responsible for ordering lowest cost items.

___C___ 15. Receives orders and prepares all chemotherapeutic agents and their adjunct medications, such as antiemetics.

Short Answer

Write a short response to each question in the space provided.

1. List four responsibilities or competencies a pharmacy technician must have.
   - _Communication Skills_
   - _teamwork_
   - _multi tasking_
   -

2. What are four different types of pharmacy settings in which a pharmacy technician can work?
   Hospital
   Clinic
   store
   pharmacy

3. What are the four different levels of pharmacy technicians?
   CPhT
   PhT
   PhD

4. List four non-traditional positions or roles pharmacy technicians can have.
   Counting pills
   the ngath

5. List four professional associations pharmacy technicians may join.

Research Activities

Follow the instructions given in each exercise and provide a response.

1. Call or visit a local retail or hospital pharmacy. Ask the lead technician or the pharmacist in charge the following questions.

   A. What qualifications do you require for technicians in your pharmacy?

   B. What duties do your technicians perform?

   C. Do you require certification?

2. Call or visit a closed-door pharmacy in your area. Ask the lead technician or the pharmacist in charge the following questions.

   A. What qualifications do you require for technicians in your pharmacy?

   B. What duties do your technicians perform?

   C. Do you require certification?

REFLECT CRITICALLY

Critical Thinking

Reply to each question based on what you have learned in the chapter.

1. You have been asked to advise someone interested in becoming a pharmacy technician. How would you advise this person? What information would be important for this person to know to help them decide?

2. What is your definition of professionalism regarding pharmacy technicians?

3. What is the difference between a profession and a career?

4. How long should new pharmacy technicians receive training when starting a new job? What training do you think would be necessary?

5. What does your state Practice Act require of pharmacy technicians? What do you know about the pharmacy technician's scope of practice in your state? Where could you find this information?

RELATE TO PRACTICE

Lab Scenarios
Working in a Pharmacy

Objective: To make a pharmacy technician student aware of the various career opportunities in their area.

Lab Activity #3.1: Locate different pharmacies in your area that you would be able to begin your career as a pharmacy technician at.

Equipment needed:
- Computer with Internet access
- Paper
- Pencil/pen

Time needed to complete this activity: 45 minutes

For each pharmacy setting, list local pharmacies you could potentially work at as a pharmacy technician. To locate mail order/Internet pharmacies near you, visit *https://nabp.pharmacy/programs/vipps/* or *https://www.safe.pharmacy/buying-safely/*.

Type	Name of Pharmacy	Location(s)
OUTPATIENT		
Community Pharmacy	*Mom & Pop Pharmacy*	*Main Street*
INPATIENT		
CLOSED DOOR		

1. Which type of pharmacy would you prefer to work in? Why?

_____

_____

2. What duties do you expect you will perform at the pharmacy of your choice?

_____

_____

3. Will you need a specialty certification to work for your pharmacy of choice (IV certification, non-sterile compounding certification, etc.)? If a specialty certification is not required, would it be beneficial to obtain a specialty certification?

_____

_____

4. List your skills and attributes that would be beneficial to the pharmacy setting of your choice. Using those skills and attributes, write an elevator speech (a short paragraph with at least three to four sentences) that describes your best attributes and how you would be an asset in the pharmacy. Practice your speech with a partner and help each other refine the speech.

_____

_____

_____

_____

_____

Interviewing for a Pharmacy Technician Position

Objective: To prepare a pharmacy technician student for a pharmacy technician interview.

After completing your pharmacy technician program, you are ready to find your first position as a pharmacy technician. This can be an exciting time in your life. It is extremely important that you are prepared for your interview. Being prepared includes wearing appropriate clothing for the interview, carrying oneself properly, answering questions asked by the interviewer, and asking questions of the interviewer. The interview process is an opportunity for the pharmacy technician and the employer to get to know each other, to determine whether you are the right employee for the position, and for you to discern whether the pharmacy meets your requirements. You will be assessed on what you do, what you say, and what you do not say. You will have only a few moments to impress the employer, so it is important to be prepared. Remember the saying, "Failing to prepare is preparing to fail."

Lab Activity #3.2: Mock interview

Equipment needed:
- Paper
- Pencil/pen

Time needed to complete this activity: 120 minutes

It is extremely important that you are prepared to answer any question that might be asked of you by the interviewer. Your response should be short and concise but should answer the question.

You are a pharmacy technician who has applied for a pharmacy technician position at a local pharmacy. The pharmacy has called and would like you to come in for an interview.

How would you answer the following questions?

1. Tell me about yourself.

_____

_____

2. Why did you decide to become a pharmacy technician?

_____

_____

3. Tell me about the pharmacy technician program that prepared you to become a pharmacy technician. What did you like about it? What did you dislike about it?

_____

_____

_____

_____

4. Did you participate in an externship? Where did you complete your externship? How many hours was it? What types of duties did you perform? Which duty did you find most rewarding? Most challenging? How did you handle the duties that were challenging?

_____

_____

5. Are you certified? If not, when will you be taking the test? Which test will you be taking?

_____

_____

6. Why will you be successful as a pharmacy technician?

_____

_____

7. Why do you want to work for us?

_____

_____

8. What do you know about our company?

_____

_____

9. Why should we hire you?

_____

_____

10. What in your background prepares you for this job?

_____

_____

11. How will your job contribute to the overall goals and mission of this company?

_____

_____

12. What type of job duties do you think you may be performing?

_____

_____

13. What is your vision for yourself in 5 years?

_____

_____

14. How do you feel about what you have accomplished so far?

_____

_____

15. How do you work under pressure? Can you give us some examples?

_____

_____

16. What is your greatest strength?

_____

_____

17. What is your greatest weakness? How have you overcome your weaknesses?

_____

_____

_____

18. What would your references say about you?

_____

_____

19. Who was your best boss or manager? Why?

_____

_____

20. In your last job, what tasks took most of your time?

_____

_____

21. What did you enjoy doing most in your last job? Least?

_____

_____

_____

_____

22. Why did you leave your last job?

_____

_____

23. Have you ever had your work, or your suggestions criticized or attacked? How did you react?

_____

_____

24. What have you done that shows initiative?

_____

_____

25. Tell us about a time when you were completely committed.

_____

_____

26. Explain your role in a team. Tell us about something that you have accomplished working with others.

_____

_____

_____

27. Explain an event that challenged and changed you. Do you think your reaction to the event was different from others?

_____

_____

28. What types of decisions or jobs give you trouble?

_____

_____

29. What skills do you need to improve upon the most? How do you think you could improve those skills?

_____

_____

_____

30. What coursework have you completed that applies to this job?

_____

_____

31. How do you prefer to work: by yourself or with other people?

_____

_____

32. Do you have any questions?

It is customary for the interviewer to ask if the applicant has any questions. This is an opportunity to clarify anything or ask specific question about the job or company. You should have at least two questions prepared for each interview.

_____

_____

During this part of the activity, act as if you are going on an interview. You will be evaluated on your professional attire, body language, and ability to answer questions. The interviewer may ask you questions from the list above, or other questions that might be relevant during an interview and will rate your responses.

Question Being Asked by Interviewer	On a Scale of 1 to 5, with 1 Being the Lowest and 5 Being the Highest, Rate the Potential Employee's Response to the Question:
1.	
2.	
3.	
4.	
5.	
6.	
7.	

Question Being Asked by Interviewer	On a Scale of 1 to 5, with 1 Being the Lowest and 5 Being the Highest, Rate the Potential Employee's Response to the Question:
8.	
9.	
10.	
11.	
12.	
13.	
14.	
15.	

1. Would you hire the individual? Why or why not?

_____

_____

_____

Interview Evaluation	Yes/No
Interviewee arrived on time for interview	
Interviewee introduced themselves to receptionist	
Completed an application legibly and did not leave questions unanswered	
Shook hands with the interviewer(s)	
Provided interviewer with a current resume	
Resume was free of spelling and grammatical errors	
Interviewee had a neat, clean appearance	
Interviewee wore appropriate clothes for an interview	
Jewelry was appropriate for an interview	
Fragrance was subtle, not overwhelming	
Answered interview questions (behavioral and technical) appropriately	
Asked questions of the interviewer	
Thanked interviewer and shook hands as they were leaving	
Sent "Thank-you" note to interviewer within 24 hours	

Pharmacy Technician Certification

Objective: To introduce the pharmacy technician to the process of becoming certified as a pharmacy technician in his/her state.

Certification is the process by which a government agency grants recognition to an individual who has met predetermined qualifications specified by an agency or association. Two pharmacy technician certification organizations are available: (1) Pharmacy Technician Certification Board (PTCB) and (2) National Healthcareer Association (NHA). Not all states require that a pharmacy technician be certified; however, there is a growing trend within the United States for pharmacy technicians to be certified as a prerequisite to working in a pharmacy, regardless of the setting.

Lab Activity #3.3: Visit *www.nabp.net* to obtain the website for your state board of pharmacy. After logging in to your state board of pharmacy, find out the requirements for a pharmacy technician to practice in your state. Complete the following table.

Equipment needed:
- Computer with Internet access
- Pencil/pen
- Paper

Time needed to complete this activity: 30 minutes

Question	Response
Name of state	
Does your state require pharmacy technicians to be certified?	
If yes, what certification tests are approved for your state?	
What is the fee for each test approved by your state?	
Does your state require licensure of pharmacy technicians?	
Is a fee required for licensure? If so, what is the fee? How often does a pharmacy technician need to renew their license?	
Does your state require pharmacy technicians to register with the state board of pharmacy?	
Is a fee associated with the registration? If yes, what is the fee?	
Does your state require formal training (ASHP-accredited coursework, pharmacy technician training program)? If so, what level of training is required?	
Does your state allow compounding of medications, sterile and/or non-sterile? If yes, does your state require additional training or certification? Does your state require continuing education specific to the specialty?	
What continuing education does your state require of pharmacy technicians?	
What fees are required to be paid to the state board of pharmacy for technicians?	
What other requirements does your state necessitate?	

Lab Activity #3.4: Visit *www.ptcb.org* and *www.nhanow.com* to obtain information regarding each of these examinations. Complete the following table for each examination.

Equipment needed:
- Computer with Internet access

Time needed to complete this activity: 30 minutes

PTCB Examination	Response
What is the registration fee for the test?	
How often is the test offered?	
How many questions are included on the test?	
What is the time limit to complete the exam?	
What is the minimum passing score for the examination?	
Where is the test offered in your area?	
If an individual does not pass the exam, when may he or she retake it?	
How long is the certification valid?	
How many continuing education units are required to renew your certification?	
Which states accept this exam?	

ExCPT Examination	Response
What is the registration fee for the test?	
How often is the test offered?	
How many questions are included on the test?	
What is the time limit to complete the exam?	
What is the minimum passing score for the examination?	
If an individual does not pass the exam, when may he or she retake it?	
Where is the test offered in your area?	
How long is the certification valid?	
How many continuing education units are required to renew your certification?	
Which states accept this exam?	

Lab Activity #3.5: Print a copy of the content for the PTCB and ExCPT examinations. Compare and contrast the information included on each examination.

Equipment needed:
- Computer with Internet access
- Computer printer

Time to needed to complete this activity: 30 minutes

1. Which examination will you take? Explain to a partner why you plan to take that exam.

_____

_____

_____

_____

_____

Professionalism as a Pharmacy Technician

Objective: To become familiar with the professional organizations available for membership for pharmacy technicians and the resources that can be used to remain competent as a pharmacy technician.

Two of the principles of the Pharmacy Technician's Code of Ethics state the following:

- A pharmacy technician maintains competency in their practice, and continually enhances their professional knowledge and expertise.
- A pharmacy technician associates with and engages in the support of organizations that promote the profession of pharmacy through the utilization and enhancement of pharmacy technicians.

All certified pharmacy technicians are required to maintain their competency through continuing education. Continuing education may take the form of pharmacy seminars or workshops, webinars, or reading of print materials accredited by the ACPE. A pharmacy technician should become involved with a pharmacy organization that will allow the pharmacy technician to develop professionally as a member of the organization. A pharmacy technician may choose to join many different types of organizations, depending on their interests. These organizations include the following:

- Academy of Managed Care Pharmacy (*www.amcp.org*)
- American Association of Pharmacy Technicians (*www.pharmacytechnician.com*)
- American Pharmacists Association (*www.pharmacist.com*)
- American Society of Health-System Pharmacists (*www.ashp.org*)
- National Community Pharmacy Association (*www.ncpanet.org*)
- National Pharmacy Technician Association (*www.pharmacytechnician.org*)

Lab Activity #3.6: Identify local, state, and national organizations that are available for membership for pharmacy technicians.

Equipment needed:
- Computer with Internet access
- Computer printer
- Paper
- Pencil/pen

Time needed to complete this activity: 45 minutes

Using the Internet, identify state and regional (local) pharmacy associations that you are eligible to join. Complete the following table.

Organization	Open to Pharmacy Technicians	Membership Fee	Continuing Education	Three Benefits of Membership	Career Opportunities
State association					
Regional association					
Academy of Managed Pharmacy (*www.amcp.org*)					
American Association of Pharmacy Technicians (*www.pharmacytechnician.com*)					
American Pharmacist Association (*www.pharmacist.com*)					
American Society of Health-System Pharmacists (*www.ashp.org*)					
National Community Pharmacy Association (*http://www.ncpanet.org/*)					
National Pharmacy Technician Association (*www.pharmacytechnician.org*)					

1. Which association do you plan to join? Why? If you do not plan to join an association, why not?

_____

_____

_____

Lab Activity #3.7: Participate in pharmacy technician continuing education.

Equipment needed:
- Computer with Internet access
- Computer printer
- Paper
- Pencil/pen

Time needed to complete this activity: 90 minutes

Using the Internet, select a pharmacy continuing education article of your choice from one of the following websites.
- *www.freece.com*
- *www.powerpak.com*
- *www.ptcb.org*
- *www.rxschool.com*

Read the article, take the examination, and print out the continuing education certificate. Provide the certificate to your instructor.

1. List 3 key pieces of information you learned from the CE you completed.

_____

_____

2. Explain how you would use the information you learned from the CE in the pharmacy while working as a pharmacy technician.

_____

_____

_____

3. Describe how the CE reinforces or helps you understand trends, issues, goals, and/or initiatives taking place in pharmacy today.

_____

_____

_____

4 Communication and Role of the Technician With the Customer/Patient

REINFORCE KEY CONCEPTS

Terms and Definitions

A. Attitude
B. Channel
C. Communication
D. Compassion
E. Diplomacy
F. Etiquette
G. Perception
H. Nonverbal communication
I. Tact
J. Verbal communication

__F__ 1. The skill of dealing with others without causing bad feelings

__G__ 2. The ability to do or say things without offending or upsetting other people

__B__ 3. The ability to express oneself in such a way that one is understood readily and clearly

__E__ 4. The way a person thinks about or understands someone or something

__C__ 5. The sharing of information by individuals through the use of speech

__H__ 6. The act of giving or exchanging information without using spoken words

__A__ 7. A means of communication that can be a written message, spoken words, or body language

__H__ 8. An unwritten guideline or rule of behavior

__I__ 9. A mental disposition or feeling a technician adopts toward customers, co-workers, or duties at work

__D__ 10. A feeling of wanting to help someone who is sick or in trouble

True or False

Write T or F next to each statement.

__T__ 1. Effective communication skills are critical to achieve optimal patient satisfaction and trust.

__T__ 2. All employers require basic communication abilities as a prerequisite to hiring.

__F__ 3. Good communication is not important for patient safety.

__T__ 4. Sometimes just listening to a person is all that is required.

__F__ 5. It is not important for pharmacy technicians to always behave professionally.

__F__ 6. Arguing with a customer can de-escalate a misunderstanding.

__T__ 7. The way in which you emphasize a word in a sentence does not make a big difference in how it is perceived.

__T__ 8. Always treat customers as you would want to be treated.

36

_____ T 9. Technicians who speak multiple languages are in high demand and can play an important role on the pharmacy team.

_____ T 10. The pharmacy technician can influence the development of a positive atmosphere in the pharmacy setting by maintaining an inappropriate attitude.

Multiple Choice

Complete each question by circling the best answer:

1. Pharmacy technicians are expected to use the following skills when communicating *except*:
   A. tact
   B. sensitivity
   C. compassion
   D. indifference

2. If a customer is angry about a medication, regardless of the problem, a pharmacy technician can ease the person's frustration by doing the following:
   A. respond with frustration
   B. show impatience while listening
   C. just listen
   D. roll their eyes

3. Most people make an instant judgment of others within the first _____ of meeting.
   A. 30 seconds
   B. minute
   C. minute and a half
   D. 5 minutes

4. Which of the following could improve your vocal communication skills?
   A. Use a monotone voice all the time.
   B. Do not talk too rapidly.
   C. Talk with an extremely soft voice.
   D. Use slang.

5. The following may alienate the patient and result in a loss of business *except* for:
   A. Giving the patient warm and friendly customer service
   B. Making patient feel embarrassed
   C. Causing the patient to become angry
   D. Belittling the patient's opinion

6. When all things are equal, what is the deciding factor for customers to have their prescriptions filled at a pharmacy?
   A. Location of the pharmacy
   B. Cost of medications
   C. Generic drug availability
   D. Pharmacy staff

7. All of the following can help optimize your communication *except*:
   A. Use open-ended questions
   B. Provide empathetic responses
   C. Mumble and mispronounce words
   D. Minimize distractions

8. If the call must be placed on hold, the technician should check back with the caller in _____ intervals to reassure the patient that she or he has not been forgotten.
   A. 30-second
   B. 1- to 2-minute
   C. 3-minute
   D. 5-minute

9. Which of the following is *not* a stage that terminally ill patients experience?
   A. Regret
   B. Denial
   C. Anger
   D. Bargaining

10. To be an effective team player, a pharmacy technician should do the following *except*:
    A. Take the time to discuss the pharmacy's goals with the team.
    B. Stay informed.
    C. Become a negative part of the decision-making process.
    D. Understand the job duties and responsibilities of a pharmacy technician.

Fill in the Blanks

Answer each question by completing the statement in the space provided.

1. Pharmacy technicians communicate _____ with co-workers, health care professionals, and customers.

2. A competent technician will possess _____ written and verbal communication skills.

3. The communication cycle involves two or more individuals _____ information.

4. Active listening is a communication technique in which the listener confirms understanding by _____ what was heard in his or her own words.

5. Rolling your eyes or sighing loudly shows _____ and a lack of _____ for the customer.

6. The primary goal of pharmacy personnel is to _____, which can be accomplished by being friendly and remaining calm.

7. _____ can choose where they want to fill their medication.

8. The way the pharmacy technician answers the phone can set the _____ for the remainder of the conversation.

9. Technicians must be careful not to talk or text on their cell phone while _____.

10. Trust and communication are key components of a _____ team.

Matching

Select the correct form of communication and write the corresponding letter in the blank next to the correct example.

A. Nonverbal communication
B. Vocal communication
C. Verbal communication

__A__ 1. Frowning at a customer

__A__ 2. Smiling as a customer walks up to counter

__B__ 3. Tone of voice

__C__ 4. Use positive words when talking with a patient

__A__ 5. Rolling your eyes

__C__ 6. Talking very fast to customers

__B__ 7. Inflection of your voice

__B__ 8. Using belittling words to a customer

__A__ 9. Folding your arms while speaking with a customer

__B__ 10. Talking loudly to all customers

__C__ 11. Using comforting words while talking with a patient

__C__ 12. Telling a patient they are wrong

Short Answer

Write a short response to each question in the space provided.

1. List six skills pharmacy technicians are expected to use while communicating.

_____

_____

_____

2. Explain the communication cycle and the importance of having a clear understanding of the cycle.

_____

_____

_____

3. If a customer is angry about a situation, name two things you can do to ease the person's frustration.

_____

_____

_____

4. Name four nonverbal ways stress can manifest itself.

_____

_____

_____

5. List four aspects of your voice (how you sound) that can affect the customer or person to whom you are talking.

_____

_____

_____

_____

6. List four things you can do to help improve your verbal skills.

_____

_____

_____

_____

7. List four guidelines for interacting with patients and medical personnel over the phone.

_____

_____

_____

_____

8. Identify two ways to help eliminate barriers to effective communication and the best defense against any communication barrier.

_____

_____

_____

9. List five guidelines for cell phone use in the pharmacy workplace.

_____

_____

_____

_____

Research Activities

Follow the instructions given in each exercise and provide a response.

1. Access the USP Pictogram Library at http://www.usp.org/usp-healthcare-professionals/related-topics-resources/usp-pictograms. Review the pictograms available.

   A. Do you think the pictograms would be useful for those who speak English as a second language? Why or why not?

   B. What other pictograms should be available? Draw an example of what it should look like.

2. Access the website https://www.uspnf.com/notices/gc-17-rx-container-labeling-prospectus. How can a standardized prescription label help with communication and reduce medication errors?

REFLECT CRITICALLY

Critical Thinking

Reply to each question based on what you have learned in the chapter.

1. What is a benefit of empathizing with a patient to show them that you can see the situation from their point of view?

2. When talking with a customer, why would using open-ended questions help prevent potential errors?

3. The slogan "The customer is always right" has been used to convey to consumers that a company is willing to give good customer service and that employees of the company should offer good customer service. Is this true for customer service in the pharmacy? Is the customer always right when they are a customer in the pharmacy? Can you think of an instance when a customer would be wrong, but they insist they are right? How would you handle a situation in which a customer is upset about something they are "not right" about?

4. Our society is culturally diverse. As a pharmacy technician, you will often encounter patients who do not speak English as their first language. What other language may be beneficial for you to know or become familiar with to serve your patients better in your area when working in the pharmacy?

RELATE TO PRACTICE

Lab Scenarios
Recognizing and Responding to Verbal and Nonverbal Communications

Objective: To be able to recognize and respond to verbal and nonverbal communications in a professional manner

To be an effective communicator in the pharmacy, a pharmacy technician must be able to read nonverbal cues and control his or her own nonverbal communication cues. Additionally, pharmacy technicians must be able to communicate clearly so that the patient's message is heard and the pharmacy technician's response is understood by the patient. This will not only help improve the communications process between health care professionals, other staff members, and patients, but will also help earn their trust.

Lab Activity #4.1: Read each scenario and answer each question. With a partner, take turns role-playing each scenario. Use learned verbal and nonverbal techniques to respond to each scenario appropriately, to make sure your message is understood properly.

Equipment needed:
- Paper
- Pencil/pen

Time needed to complete this activity: 45 minutes

1. Select a classmate as a partner or your instructor who will play the role of a patient or health care provider for this procedure. Take turns role-playing each scenario provided and act out an appropriate response. Ask your instructor questions or ask for guidance when needed.
2. Use appropriate body language and other nonverbal skills in communicating with patients, family, and staff.
3. Demonstrate sensitivity appropriate to the message being delivered.
4. Demonstrate empathy.
5. Apply active listening skills.
6. Restate the receiver's response.
7. Analyze communications in providing appropriate responses and feedback.
   - Try not to escalate a situation.
   - Involve the pharmacist when needed.
   - Do not be afraid to ask for help if needed.
   A. Scenario #1: A customer walks up to the pharmacy counter to pick up a prescription. After looking up the prescription, the pharmacy technician notices it is not ready. The pharmacy technician informs the customer they will have to wait to pick it up. The customer states, "Why did I even bother to call it in ahead of time?"
   B. Scenario #2: Nurse Johnson calls the pharmacist to ask if the two drugs Nurse Johnson is about to administer are compatible and is in a hurry. The pharmacy technician scribbles down the question but does not get the nurse's name or telephone extension. By the time the nurse calls back to contact the pharmacist, the dose is late, and the patient has been in pain while waiting for a response. The nurse asks, "Why didn't you ask the pharmacist?"
   C. Scenario #3: A patient calls the pharmacy to ask about their medication during a busy time at the pharmacy. The patient states they are calling because their medication looks different from before, and they need to know if it is the same drug or not. The pharmacy technician asks the patient if they could be placed on hold, but the patient states they are in a hurry and cannot hold.
   D. Scenario #4: A patient walks up to the counter to have their prescription filled and asks whether it can be done within 5 minutes because the bus will be leaving. The pharmacy technician informs the patient that this may not be possible because of other prescriptions needing to be filled first. The patient rolls their eyes and shakes her head.
   E. Scenario #5: You are working at a hospital and it is your job to refill the automated dispensing system (ADS) at the end of your shift. You will need a nurse's help because some of the medications are controlled substances. You are running behind schedule with your other duties and this is your last ADS to fill. You ask the nurse to help you load the ADS, but the nurse tells you to come back later because they cannot help you right now.

F. Scenario #6: A patient has called your pharmacy to refill their prescription during a morning rush. You quickly write down the patient's name, date of birth, and the prescription they are requesting for refill. After the rush is over, you begin to process the refill but notice the prescription does not have any refills remaining.

G. Scenario #7: Act out a scenario that you have been a part of during a pharmacy visit. Be sure to use nonverbal and verbal cues for your partner to pick up on and to respond to.

Procedural Step	Yes/No
Selected a classmate as a partner to play the role of a patient for this procedure.	
Took turns with partner role-playing each nonverbal cue provided.	
Used appropriate body language and other nonverbal skills in communicating with patients, family, and staff.	
Demonstrated sensitivity appropriate to the message being delivered.	
Demonstrated empathy.	
Applied active listening skills.	
Restated the patient's response.	
Determined whether the receiver understood the message correctly.	
Analyzed communications in providing appropriate responses and feedback.	
Did not escalate a negative situation.	
Involved the pharmacist when needed.	
Asked for help when communication tactics did not work.	

Communicating in Spanish

Objective: To be able translate prescription medication directions into Spanish

Lab Activity #4.2: Using the *Drug Topics Red Book or the website* http://www.spanishdict.com/translation translate common prescription directions and phrases into Spanish.

Equipment needed:
- Computer with Internet connection
- *Drug Topics Red Book*
- Pencil/pen

Time needed to complete this activity: 30 minutes

1. Take one tablet by mouth daily.

   _____

2. Take one capsule by mouth two times a day.

   _____

3. Instill three drops in the left eye four times a day.

   _____

4. Put four drops in each ear three times a day.

   _____

5. Take one tablespoon two times a day.

   _____

6. Take one-half teaspoon three times a day.

   _____

7. Do not refrigerate.

   _____

8. Shake gently and keep in refrigerator.

   _____

9. Use as needed.

   _____

10. Apply to affected area.

    _____

11. Inject 40 units subcutaneously.

_____

12. Do not take at same time as other medicine.

_____

13. Do not drink alcoholic beverages while taking this medicine.

_____

14. Do not drive while taking this medicine.

_____

15. Take with food or milk.

_____

16. Take on an empty stomach.

_____

17. Avoid sunlight.

_____

18. Do not use after this date.

_____

19. Hi, how are you?

_____

20. How may I help you today?

_____

21. What is your name?

_____

22. What is your date of birth?

_____

23. What is your address?

_____

24. What is your telephone number?

_____

25. Are you allergic to any medications?

_____

26. Are you allergic to any foods?

_____

27. Do you have prescription insurance?

_____

28. Your prescription will cost:

_____

29. Do you have any questions for the pharmacist about your medications?

_____

30. Thank you. Have a nice day.

_____

31. Are you fluent in another language? Share these same translations with a partner in the language you are fluent in and/or familiar with.

Communicating Using Sign Language

Objective: To be able translate common pharmacy terms using sign language

Lab Activity #4.3: Access the website http://www.signingsavvy.com/ to look up common pharmacy terms in sign language. Practice using sign language for each term with a partner.

Equipment needed:
- Computer with Internet connection

Time needed to complete this activity: 30 minutes

1. Pharmacy
2. Teaspoon
3. Tablespoon
4. Tablet
5. Capsule
6. Ointment
7. Medicine
8. Take pill
9. AM
10. PM
11. Twice or two times
12. Three times
13. Four times
14. Daily
15. Bedtime
16. Morning
17. With
18. At
19. At once
20. Food
21. Avoid sunlight
22. Inject or injection
23. Apply
24. Help or help you
25. Thank you

What other signs can you find? Act out these signs with a partner. Can you put them together to communicate a sentence?

5 Dosage Forms and Routes of Administration

ASHP ACCREDITATION STANDARDS FOR PHARMACY TECHNICIAN EDUCATION AND TRAINING PROGRAMS

Standard 1.4: Communicate clearly and effectively, both verbally and in writing.
Standard 1.10: Apply critical thinking skills, creativity, and innovation.
Standard 2.5: Demonstrate basic knowledge of anatomy, physiology and pharmacology, and medical terminology relevant to pharmacy technician's role.

REINFORCE KEY CONCEPTS

Terms and Definitions

Select the correct term from the following list and write the corresponding letter in the blank next to the statement.

A. Absorption
B. Bioavailability
C. Bioequivalence
D. Distribution
E. Elimination
F. First-pass effect
G. Half-life
H. Metabolism
I. Pharmacokinetics

_____ 1. The relationship between two drugs that have the same dosage and dosage form and that have similar bioavailability

_____ 2. A process in which a portion of the drug dose is metabolized before the drug has a chance to be distributed systemically

_____ 3. The processes by which the body breaks down or converts medications to active or inactive substances

_____ 4. The time required for a chemical to be decreased by one half, or for half the amount of a substance, such as a drug in a living system, to be eliminated or disintegrated by natural processes, or for the concentration of a substance in a body fluid (blood plasma) to decrease by half

_____ 5. The movement of a medication throughout the blood, organs, and tissues after administration

_____ 6. The study of the absorption, metabolism, distribution, and elimination of drugs

_____ 7. The degree to which a drug or other substance becomes available to the target tissue after administration

_____ 8. The final evacuation of a drug or other substance from the body via normal body processes, such as kidney elimination (urine), biliary excretion (bile to stool), sweat, respiration, or saliva

_____ 9. The taking in of nutrients and drugs into the body from food and liquids

Select the correct term from the following list and write the corresponding letter in the blank next to the statement.

A. Behind-the-counter (BTC)
B. Enteral
C. Instill
D. Legend drugs
E. Over-the-counter (OTC)
F. Parenteral
G. Pro-drug

_____ 10. Drugs that require a prescription; these drugs carry the federal legend: "Federal law prohibits the dispensing of this medication without a prescription"

_____ 11. A route of administration by way of the intestine, such as orally, rectally, or sublingually

_____ 12. Nonprescription drugs that are kept behind the pharmacy counter; limited amounts may be sold, or the customer may require the permission of a pharmacist to purchase them

_____ 13. Medications that can be purchased without a prescription

_____ 14. An inactive substance that is converted to a drug in the body by the action of enzymes or other chemicals

_____ 15. To place into; commonly used for ophthalmic or otic drugs

_____ 16. A term used to describe a medication that is usually given by injection into a vein, the skin, or muscle that bypasses the gastrointestinal system

True or False

Write T or F next to each statement.

_____ 1. To become proficient in the medical profession, a technician must be able to interpret orders correctly.

_____ 2. Much of the terminology used in pharmacy comes from the Latin and Greek languages.

_____ 3. It is not necessary for the pharmacy technician to learn all dosage forms and abbreviations to decipher a physician's orders.

_____ 4. The number of errors resulting from physicians' poor handwriting or from transcription of orders is of little concern.

_____ 5. A dosage form refers to how a drug is available for use or the vehicle by which the drug is delivered.

_____ 6. Enteric coated tablets dissolve in the stomach.

_____ 7. Dosage forms that are especially made to release over time can be crushed or broken into pieces.

_____ 8. Troches are oral tablets that should be swallowed immediately.

_____ 9. An emulsifier binds oil and water together in a mixture.

_____ 10. The most common parenteral medications are given IV, IM, or SUBCUT.

_____ 11. Physicians often use eye solutions to treat ear conditions.

_____ 12. Otic drugs (ear preparations) are always sterile.

_____ 13. If inhalers are not used properly, the medication is swallowed rather than inhaled into the lungs.

_____ 14. When the outside of a box is labeled "refrigerate or keep frozen," the contents can be left at room temperature.

_____ 15. New dosage forms are always being invented both for convenience and to achieve the best results.

Multiple Choice

Complete each question by circling the best answer.

1. The directions for use of a medication are "ii gtts os bid." The route of administration is:
   A. Right eye
   B. Left eye
   C. Right ear
   D. Left ear

2. Which of the following is the abbreviation for "before meals"?
   A. ac
   B. pc
   C. hs
   D. au

3. The directions for use of a medication are "Tylenol 80 mg pr q6h prn." What dosage form should be dispensed?
   A. Chew tab
   B. Syrup
   C. Suppository
   D. Capsule

4. The directions for use are "Nitrostat 1/200 gr sl prn." How should this be administered?
   A. In the left ear
   B. Very slowly
   C. Under the tongue
   D. Under the skin

5. When a drug is processed by the liver, this is referred to as:
   A. Absorption
   B. Distribution
   C. Metabolism
   D. Excretion

6. Which of the following dosage forms should generally be stored in the refrigerator?
   A. Suppositories
   B. Patches
   C. Enemas
   D. Tablets

7. Which route of administration has the quickest onset of action?
   A. IM
   B. PR
   C. IV
   D. PO

8. The directions for use are "i gtt ad qd." The medication may be:
   A. Ear drops
   B. Eye drops
   C. Suppositories
   D. Vaginal tablets

9. The abbreviation NGT refers to:
   A. Nitroglycerin
   B. Nothing by gastrostomy tube
   C. Nasogastric
   D. Nasogastric tube

10. The pharmaceutical abbreviation CD refers to:
    A. Controlled drug
    B. Compact disk
    C. Controlled diffusion
    D. Continuous drip

11. A positive aspect of taking tablets, capsules, or any agent by mouth is:
    A. Convenience to the patient
    B. Physicians mainly write for those forms
    C. Injectable forms are expensive
    D. Medication can be taken with water

12. Respiratory solutions are often:
    A. Refrigerated
    B. Packaged in unit dose ampules
    C. For adult use only
    D. Purchased over-the-counter

13. Patients with diabetes may be instructed to buy drug products that are:
    A. Sterile only
    B. Additive free
    C. Sugar-free
    D. Preservative free

14. This unique vial keeps the medication separate from the diluent until it is time to reconstitute, which can save waste when an expensive drug is used that has a short shelf life after preparation:
    A. Ampule
    B. ADD-Vantage container
    C. MDI
    D. Glass vial

15. The following dose forms can be used vaginally *except*:
    A. Suppositories
    B. Creams
    C. Gels
    D. Patches

Matching

Matching I

Match the following abbreviations with their meanings.

A. Intravenous	_____ 1. INH
B. Rectal	_____ 2. PV
C. Sublingual	_____ 3. SUBCUT
D. By mouth	_____ 4. IV
E. Inhalant	_____ 5. Top
F. Subcutaneous	_____ 6. NAS
G. Intramuscular	_____ 7. BUC
H. Vaginal	_____ 8. PR
I. Topical	_____ 9. IM
J. Buccal	_____ 10. PO
K. Nasal	_____ 11. IT
L. Intrathecal	_____ 12. SL

Match the following abbreviations with their meanings.

A. Elixir
B. Tincture
C. Suppositories
D. Enteric-coated tablet
E. Suspension
F. Diluent
G. Powder
H. Lotion
I. Syrup
J. Spirit
K. Solution
L. Injection
M. Metered dose inhaler
N. Ointment

_____ 1. Pdr

_____ 2. elix

_____ 3. Ung

_____ 4. lot

_____ 5. dil

_____ 6. Inj

_____ 7. Sp

_____ 8. tinc

_____ 9. MDI

_____ 10. syr

_____ 11. EC tab

_____ 12. Soln

_____ 13. susp

_____ 14. sup

Fill in the Blanks

Answer each question by completing the statement in the space provided.

1. Many of the top-selling drugs are available in several

   different _____ _____

2. To substitute a different dosage form for the one ordered,

   the prescriber must give _____

3. When administered enterally, _____ agents can be given orally, rectally, or sublingually.

4. _____ tablets are convenient for persons who have difficulty swallowing tablets and for children who are unable to swallow large tablets.

5. _____ are sterile, solid dosage forms that consist of drugs and rate-controlling excipients and are usually intended for insertion into a body cavity or under the skin.

6. The best approach to discarding a transdermal patch is to fold it, so the adhesive side sticks to itself, wrap it,

   and discard the patch in such a way that a _____

   or _____ would not be able to grasp it.

7. _____ are sugar-based solutions, and _____ are sweetened solutions in a water and alcohol base.

8. _____ may be used for rectal, vaginal, and urethral conditions.

9. Oral administration is one of the _____ ways to give medication, because if too much is given there may be time to react before the drug begins to work.

10. _____ is the most used sublingual tablet that treats anginal attacks.

11. Technicians need to pay close attention the _____ requirements for injectable drugs.

12. Most of the final _____ of a drug takes place in the liver.

13. A reference source that can be used to determine whether the _____ drug is rated as bio-equivalent to the brand name drug is the Orange Book.

14. All manufactured types of _____ must be approved by the Food and Drug Administration

15. Medications are _____ according to manufacturers' specifications to ensure the effectiveness and shelf life of the drug.

Short Answer

Write a short response to each question in the space provided.

1. List three classifications of drugs that describe their availability to consumers.

   _____

   _____

2. List five general classifications of medications and a related body system for the classification.

   _____

   _____

   _____

3. List five examples of solid dose forms.

_____

_____

4. List five examples of liquid dose forms.

_____

_____

5. List five examples of semisolid dose forms.

_____

_____

6. List five abbreviations and its meaning for agents that release medication over different periods of time and in different quantities and should therefore not be crushed.

_____

_____

7. List the common uses for transdermal patches.

_____

_____

8. Explain the difference between pharmacokinetics and pharmacodynamics.

_____

_____

_____

_____

9. Describe the "first-pass" effect of drugs in the liver and its importance in drug delivery.

_____

_____

_____

10. List four different influences than can alter drug metabolism.

_____

_____

11. List five routes of drug elimination.

_____

_____

12. List five examples of additives and the reason they are used in the production of medications.

_____

_____

_____

_____

_____

Research Activities

Follow the instructions given in each exercise and provide a response.

1. Visit a local pharmacy. Locate the cough and cold section. Select one brand of medication with the following dosage forms: tablet, capsule, and liquid. What are the active ingredients in all three dosage forms?

2. Visit a local pharmacy. Locate the pain management section. Select one brand of medication with the following dosage forms: tablet, capsule, and liquid. What are the active ingredients in all three dosage forms?

REFLECT CRITICALLY

Critical Thinking

Reply to each question based on what you have learned in the chapter.

1. List as many dosage forms as you can. Write two advantages and two disadvantages of each.
   Example: Tablet—advantage, easy to carry; disadvantage, tastes bad

2. Interpreting prescriptions can be challenging because of the various handwriting styles of physicians. Think of three rules that can make this task easier.

3. Compounding medications unavailable commercially is much like creating a good recipe in the kitchen. Compare and contrast the two tasks. How are they similar, and how do they differ?

4. How could you encourage prescribers to not use abbreviations on the **ISMP's** *List of Error-Prone Abbreviations, Symbols, and Dose Designations*?

Lab Scenarios

Medical Abbreviations

Objective: To introduce the pharmacy technician to the many abbreviations that may be encountered in the practice of pharmacy, regardless of the pharmacy setting.

Lab Activity #5.1: Write the meanings of the following medical abbreviations.

Equipment needed:
- Pencil/pen
- Medical dictionary

Time needed to complete this activity: 45 minutes

Abbreviation	Meaning	Abbreviation	Meaning
ADHD		ADR	
AIDS		BBB	
BM		BP	
BPH		BS	
BUN		CABG	
CAD		CBC	
CCU		CHD	
CHF		COPD	
CP		CVD	
DOA		DOB	
DJD		DNR	
DVT		Dx	
EEG		EENT	
EKG		ER	
FX		GERD	
GI		HA	
HBP		HIV	
HPV		hr	
HTN		ICU	
IDDM		KVO	
LBP		LLL	

Abbreviation	Meaning	Abbreviation	Meaning
MI		N&V	
NICU		NIDDM	
NPO		OA	
OBGYN		OR	
PPN		PT	
PVCs		RA	
RBC		RLS	
SARS		SBO	
SLE		SOB	
Sx		TB	
TED		TIA	
TKO		TPN	
TX		UC	
UNG		URI	
UTI		WBC	

Medical Terminology

Objective: To become familiar with the meanings of prefixes, suffixes, and root words used in medical terminology.

Lab Activity #5.2: Interpreting the meanings of prefixes, suffixes, and root words that are found in medical literature associated with the practice of pharmacy.

Equipment needed:
- Medical terminology book
- Pencil/pen

Time needed to complete this activity: 60 minutes

Complete the following table of prefixes used in medical terminology.

Prefix	Meaning	Prefix	Meaning
a-; an-; ana-		micro-	
ab-		multi-	
ante-		neo-	
anti-		non-	
auto-		oligo-	
bi-		pan-	
brady-		para-	
carcin-		per-	
contra-		peri-	

Continued

Prefix	Meaning	Prefix	Meaning
dys-		poly-	
ect-		post-	
en-		pre-	
endo-		primi-	
epi-		retro-	
ex-		semi-	
hemi-		sub-	
hyper-		super-	
hypo-		supra-	
infra-		sym-	
inter-		syn-	
intra-		tachy-	
iso-		tri-	
macro-		uni-	
mal-		xero-	

Complete the following table of suffixes found in medical terminology.

Suffix	Meaning	Suffix	Meaning
-ac; -al; -ar; -ary		-paresis	
-algia		-pathy	
-cele		-penia	
-centesis		-pepsia	
-crine		-phagia	
-crit		-phobia	
-cyte		-phonia	
-cytosis		-phoresis	
-desis		-phoria	
-ectomy		-plasty	
-emesis		-plegia	
-emia		-pnea	
-genesis		-poiesis	
-globin; -globulin		-r/rhage; -r/rhagia	

Suffix	Meaning	Suffix	Meaning
-gram		-rrhea	
-graph		-rhexis	
-graphy		-scler/o	
-ia; -iac; -ic		-scope	
-ism		-scopy	
-itis		-somnia	
-lysis; -lytic		-spasm	
-malacia		-stasis	
-megaly		-sten/o	
-oid		-therapy	
-logist		-thorax	
-logy		-tocia	
-oma		-tripsy	
-osis		-trophy	
-stomy		-tropin	

Complete the following table of root words found in medical terminology.

Root Word—Combining Forms	Meaning	Root Word—Combining Forms	Meaning
Abdomen/o		mast/o	
aden/o		melan/o	
adipo/o		men/o	
amino		metacarp/o	
andr/o		metatars/o	
angi/o		morph/o	
aque/o		muc/o	
arteri/o		my/o	
arteriol/o		myc/o	
arthr/o		myel/o	
ather/o		myring/o	
audi/o		narc/o	
aur/o		nat/o	
bil/i		nephr/o	

Continued

Root Word—Combining Forms	Meaning	Root Word—Combining Forms	Meaning
blephar/o		neur/o	
bronch/o		noct/o	
bronchiol/o		nyctal/o	
bucc/o		ocul/o	
calc/i		onch/o	
capn/o		oophor/o	
carcin/o		ophthalm/o	
cardi/o		opt/o	
carp/o		or/o	
cephal/o		orch/o	
cerebr/o		orchi/o	
chol/e		orchid/o	
cholangi/o		orth/o	
cholecyst/o		oste/o	
chondr/o		ot/o	
coagul/o		ovari/o	
cochle/o		ox/o	
col/o		pachy/o	
conjunctiv/o		pancreat/o	
cor/o		par/o	
corne/o		part/o	
coron/o		patell/o	
cost/o		pector/o	
crani/o		ped/o	
cry/o		pelv/i	
cut/o		perine/o	
cutane/o		peritone/o	
cyan/o		phag/o	
cyst/o		phalang/o	
cyt/o		pharyng/o	
dacry/o		phleb/o	
dent/i		phot/o	

Root Word—Combining Forms	Meaning	Root Word—Combining Forms	Meaning
derm/o		phren/o	
dermat/o		pil/o	
dipl/o		pneum/o	
dips/o		pod/o	
duoden/o		proct/o	
dur/a		psych/o	
electr/o		pub/o	
embry/o		pulmon/o	
encephal/o		py/o	
enter/o		pyel/o	
eosin/o		quadr/i	
epis/i		radi/o	
erythr/o		rect/o	
esophag/o		ren/o	
fasci/o		retin/o	
femor/o		rhabdomy/o	
fet/o		rheumat/o	
fibul/o		rhin/o	
fund/o		salping/o	
gastr/o		sarc/o	
gingiv/o		semin/o	
glauc/o		septi	
gli/o		sial/o	
glomerul/o		sinus/o	
gloss/o		somat/o	
gluc/o		spermat/o	
glyc/o		spher/o	
gonad/o		sphygm/o	
gravid/a		spir/o	
gyn/o		splen/o	
gynec/o		spondyl/o	
hem/o		steth/o	

Continued

Root Word—Combining Forms	Meaning	Root Word—Combining Forms	Meaning
hemangi/o		stomat/o	
hemat/o		synovi/o	
hepat/o		tars/o	
hidr/o		ten/o	
humer/o		tendon/o	
hydr/o		test/o	
hyster/o		testicul/o	
ile/o		thorac/o	
ili/o		thromb/o	
immune/o		thyr/o	
is/o		trache/o	
jejun/o		tympan/o	
kal/i		ur/o	
kinesi/o		urethr/o	
lacrim/o		vas/o	
lact/o		ven/o	
lapar/o		xanth/o	
laryng/o		lip/o	
ligament/o		lumb/o	
lingu/o		mamm/o	

Dosage Forms, Routes of Administration, and Storage

Objective: To become familiar with dosage forms, routes of administration, and storage requirements for drugs commonly prescribed.

Lab Activity #5.3: Using a pharmacy reference book, find the dosage form availability, route of administration, and storage requirements for each drug listed.

Equipment needed:
- *Drug Facts and Comparisons* or *USP DI* reference book
- Pencil/pen

Time needed to complete this activity: 60 minutes

Complete the following table for drugs commonly prescribed.

Drug	Dosage Forms Available	Routes of Administration	Storage
acetaminophen			
albuterol			
amoxicillin			

Drug	Dosage Forms Available	Routes of Administration	Storage
budesonide			
ciprofloxacin			
clindamycin			
clonidine			
diphenhydramine			
erythromycin			
fluticasone			
furosemide			
insulin detemir			
ipratropium bromide			
isosorbide mononitrate			
lantanoprost			
levalbuterol			
lidocaine			
lorazepam			
marinol			
MMR Vaccine			
MMRV Vaccine			
montelukast			
nitroglycerin			
penicillin			
promethazine			
succinylcholine			
tiotropium bromide			
triamcinolone			

Lab Activity #5.4: Using the drug labels provided, identify the dose form, route of administration for drug, and storage information when available.

Equipment needed:
- Pencil/pen

Time needed to complete this activity: 30 minutes

1. **Dosage Form** _____

   Route of Administration _____

   Storage Information _____

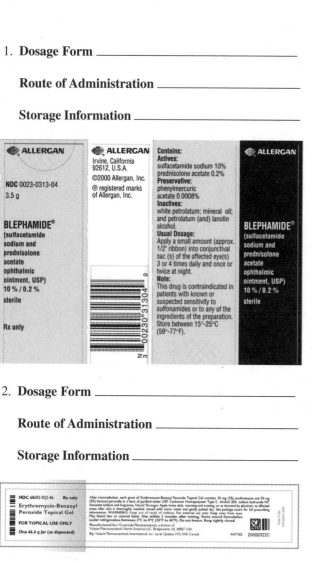

2. **Dosage Form** _____

   Route of Administration _____

   Storage Information _____

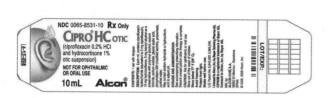

3. **Dosage Form** _____

   Route of Administration _____

   Storage Information _____

4. **Dosage Form** _____

   Route of Administration _____

   Storage Information _____

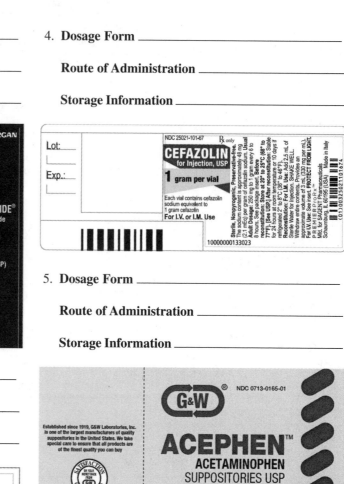

5. **Dosage Form** _____

   Route of Administration _____

   Storage Information _____

6. Dosage Form _____

   Route of Administration _____

   Storage Information _____

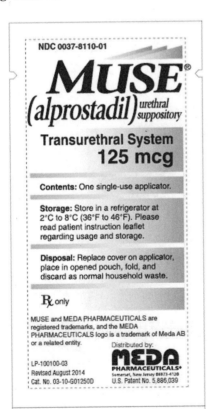

NDC 43598-409-25

Levalbuterol Inhalation Solution, USP

1.25 mg/ 3 mL

Each 3 mL unit-dose vial contains 1.25 mg (0.042%) of levalbuterol as the hydrochloride salt in an aqueous solution containing edetate disodium, sodium chloride and sulfuric acid to adjust the pH of the solution to 4.0.

Contains no preservatives.

Attention Pharmacist: Detach "Patient's Instructions for Use" from package insert and dispense it with product.

Use only as directed by your physician. Do not exceed recommended dosage.

Protect from light. Avoid excessive heat.

Store at 20° to 25°C (68° to 77°F) [See USP Controlled Room Temperature].

Keep out of reach of children.

Unit-dose vials should remain stored in the protective foil pouch at all times. Once the foil pouch is opened, the vials should be used within two weeks. Once removed from the foil pouch, the individual vials should be used within one week. Discard if the solution is not colorless.

℞ONLY

NDC 43598-409-25

Levalbuterol Inhalation Solution, USP

1.25 mg/ 3 mL

For Oral Inhalation Only.

Sterile Unit – Dose Vial

Carton contains:
25 x 3 mL Sterile Unit – Dose Vials (5 pouches of 5 x 3 mL vials each)

M.L. 25/2/2010

Manufactured by: Cipla Ltd.
Plot 9 & 10, Indore SEZ
Pithampur, M.P. - 454 775, INDIA

Manufactured for:
Dr. Reddy's Laboratories, Inc.
Princeton, NJ 08540

Rev. 06/14   ℞ONLY

7. Dosage Form _____

   Route of Administration _____

   Storage Information _____

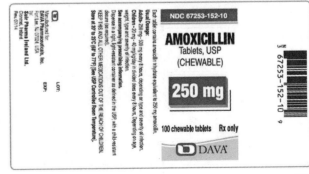

NDC 0037-8110-01

MUSE®

(alprostadil) urethral suppository

Transurethral System

125 mcg

Contents: One single-use applicator.

Storage: Store in a refrigerator at 2°C to 8°C (36°F to 46°F). Please read patient instruction leaflet regarding usage and storage.

Disposal: Replace cover on applicator, place in opened pouch, fold, and discard as normal household waste.

℞ only

MUSE and MEDA PHARMACEUTICALS are registered trademarks, and the MEDA PHARMACEUTICALS logo is a trademark of Meda AB or a related entity.

Distributed by:

MEDA
PHARMACEUTICALS®
Somerset, New Jersey 08873-4120

LP-100100-03
Revised August 2014
Cat. No. 03-10-G01250D
U.S. Patent No. 5,886,039

8. Dosage Form _____

   Route of Administration _____

   Storage Information _____

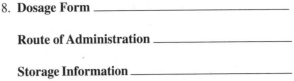

Each buccal tablet contains 50 mg of miconazole.

Usual Dosage: Read enclosed Patient Package Insert.

Do not chew, crush or swallow tablets. KEEP THIS AND ALL DRUGS OUT OF REACH OF CHILDREN.

Storage:
Store at 20° to 25°C (68° to 77°F).

Distributed by:
Midatech Pharma US Inc.
8601 Six Forks Rd., Suite 160
Raleigh, NC 27615

Made in Germany
04/2016

NDC 89141-250-14

once-daily
ORAVIG®
(miconazole) buccal tablets 50 mg

3 89141 25014 8

9. Dosage Form _____

   Route of Administration _____

   Storage Information _____

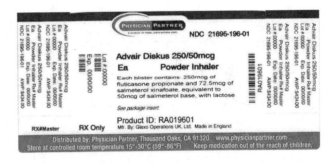

PHYSICIAN PARTNER   NDC 21695-196-01

Advair Diskus 250/50mcg
Ea   Powder Inhaler

Each blister contains: 250mcg of fluticasone propionate and 72.5mcg of salmeterol xinafoate, equivalent to 50mcg of salmeterol base, with lactose

See package insert.

Product ID: RA019601

RX#Master   RX Only   Mfr. By: Glaxo Operations UK, Ltd. Made in England

Distributed by: Physician Partner, Thousand Oaks, CA 91320   www.physicianpartner.com
Store at controlled room temperature 15°-30°C (59°-86°F)   Keep medication out of the reach of children.

10. Dosage Form _____

   Route of Administration _____

   Storage Information _____

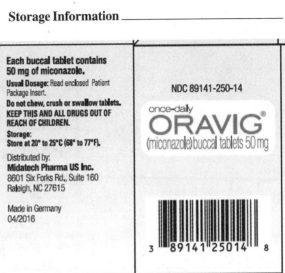

NDC 67253-152-10

AMOXICILLIN
Tablets, USP
(CHEWABLE)

250 mg

100 chewable tablets   Rx only

DAVA®

3 67253 152-10 9

57

11. **Dosage Form** _____

   Route of Administration _____

   Storage Information _____

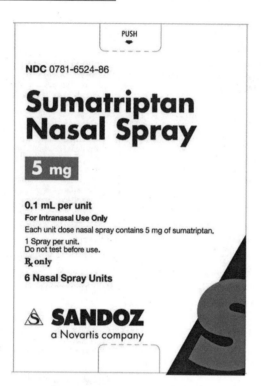

12. **Dosage Form** _____

   Route of Administration _____

   Storage Information _____

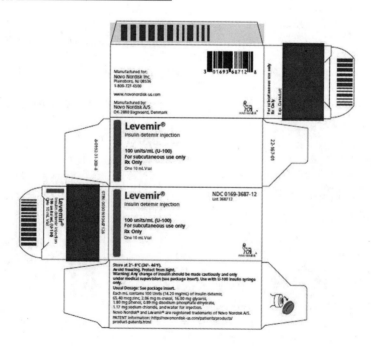

13. Dosage Form _____

    Route of Administration _____

    Storage Information _____

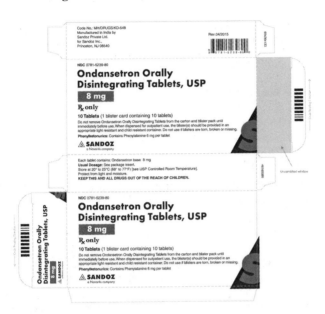

14. Dosage Form _____

    Route of Administration _____

    Storage Information _____

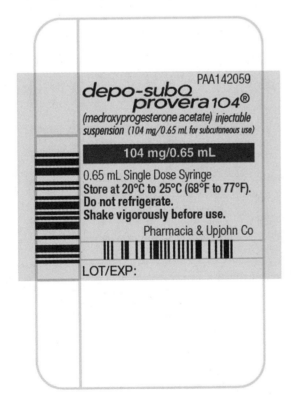

15. Dosage Form _____

    Route of Administration _____

    Storage Information _____

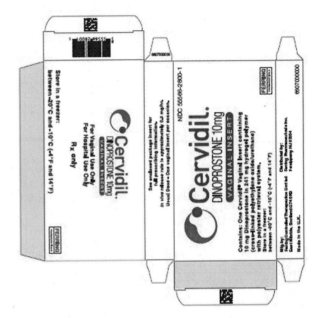

FDA Drug Ratings

Objective: To introduce the pharmacy technician to FDA drug ratings to determine whether a generic drug is rated as bioequivalent to the brand name drug.

Lab Activity #5.5: Using a pharmacy reference book or the FDA Orange Book website located at *https://www.accessdata.fda.gov/scripts/cder/ob/default.cfm*, find the drug rating for each drug listed.

Equipment needed:
- *Red Book* reference book or Internet access
- Pencil/pen

Time needed to complete this activity: 45 minutes

1. Alprazolam 0.25-mg tablets, Mylan Pharmaceuticals

    _____

2. Amoxicillin 250-mg capsules, Teva Pharmaceuticals

    _____

3. Budesonide; Formoterol Fumarate Dihydrate 0.08 mg/0.0045 mg/INH, Astra Zenica LPC _____

    _____

4. Acyclovir 200-mg capsules, Teva Pharmaceuticals

    _____

5. Warfarin 1-mg tablets, Barr Laboratories Inc _____

6. Levothyroxine Sodium Powder, 100 mcg/vial, Dr. Reddy's Laboratories LTD _____

7. Carvedilol 6.25-mg tablet, Smith Kline Beecham LTD _____

8. Bimatoprost 0.03% Ophthalmic Solution, Sandoz LTD _____

9. Diflorasone Diacetate 0.05% Cream, Taro Pharmaceuticals _____

10. Indomethacin Sodium 1-mg/vial Injection, Hospira Inc _____

11. Carisoprodol 350-mg Tablet, Watson Laboratories Inc _____

12. Fluoxetine HCl 20-mg Capsule, Teva Pharmaceuticals _____

13. Clindamycin Phosphate 1% Gel, Bausch Health US LLC _____

14. Citalopram HBr 10 mg/5 mL Oral Solution, Hikma Pharmaceuticals USA Inc. _____

15. Rimegepant Sulfate 75 mg ODT, Biohaven Pharmaceutical _____

Cleaning Nebulizer Equipment

Objective: To learn the steps to properly clean a nebulizer and its tubing in order to avoid infection.

Lab Activity #5.6: Properly explain and demonstrate, to your partner, how to clean a nebulizer kit.

Equipment needed:
- Nebulizer kit (tubing and nebulizer chamber)
- Warm water
- Soap
- Vinegar
- Paper towels
- Plastic resealable bag

Time needed to complete this activity: 30 minutes

Procedural Steps

1. After each treatment, rinse nebulizer cup with warm water.
2. Empty nebulizer cup of excess water and let air dry.
3. At the end of the day, wash nebulizer cup, mask, or mouthpiece in warm soapy water; rinse and allow to air dry.
4. Every third day disinfect the equipment using a vinegar/water solution (½ cup white vinegar with 1½ cups water).
5. Soak for 20 minutes and rinse well under a steady stream of water.
6. Remove excess water and allow to air dry on a paper towel.
7. Make sure all equipment is completely dry before storing in a plastic resealable bag.

Procedural Step	Yes/No
Gathered all necessary supplies for demonstration.	
Explained and demonstrated how to rinse nebulizer cup with warm water after each treatment.	
Explained and demonstrated how to empty nebulizer cup of excess water and let air dry.	
Explained and demonstrated how to wash nebulizer cup, mask or mouthpiece in warm soapy water, rinse and allow to air dry at the end of each day.	
Explained and demonstrated how to disinfect the equipment using a vinegar/water solution (½ cup white vinegar with 1 ½ cups water) every third day.	
Explained and demonstrated how to soak for 20 minutes and rinse well under a steady stream of water.	
Explained and demonstrated how to remove excess water and allow to air dry on a paper towel.	
Explained and demonstrated how to make sure all equipment is completely dry before storing in a plastic resealable bag.	

6 Conversions and Calculations

ASHP ACCREDITATION STANDARDS FOR PHARMACY TECHNICIAN EDUCATION AND TRAINING PROGRAMS

Standard 2.6: Perform mathematical calculations essential to the duties of pharmacy technicians in a variety of settings.

REINFORCE KEY CONCEPTS

Terms and Definitions
Select the correct term from the following list and write the corresponding letter in the blank next to the statement.

A. Diluent/solvent
B. Dilution
C. Drip rate (DR) or drop rate
D. Drop factor
E. Flow rate
F. International time
G. Milliequivalent (mEq)
H. Units
I. Volume

_____ 1. A 24-hour method of keeping time; hours are not distinguished as AM or PM, but rather are counted continuously throughout the day

_____ 2. The amount of liquid enclosed within a container

_____ 3. The number of drops (gtt) administered over a specific time via an intravenous infusion

_____ 4. A unit of measurement assigned to medications called "biologicals," which have been tested for potency in biological systems; specific to each medication

_____ 5. The amount of intravenous (IV) solution administered over a specific period; eg, mL/min, mL/hr, gtt/min

_____ 6. The process of adding a diluent or solvent to a compound, resulting in a product of increased volume or weight and lower concentration

_____ 7. A type of unit used in the United States to express the concentration of electrolytes such as sodium, potassium, magnesium, and calcium

_____ 8. The size of drops (gtts/mL) coming through the tubing

_____ 9. An inert product, either liquid or solid, that is added to a preparation to reduce the strength of the original product

Select the correct term from the following list and write the corresponding letter in the blank next to the statement.

A. Alligation alternate
B. Apothecary system
C. Avoirdupois system
D. Conversion factor
E. Dimensional analysis (DA)
F. Household system
G. International System of Units (SI)
H. Markup
I. Metric system
J. Retail price
K. Wholesale cost

_____ 10. A method used to solve complicated pharmaceutical calculations that would require numerous sets of ratio and proportion problems

_____ 11. A mathematical method of solving problems that involves the mixing of two solutions or two solids with different percentage weights to achieve a desired third strength

_____ 12. The approved system of measurement for pharmacy in the United States based on multiples of 10

_____ 13. A system of measurement commonly used in the United States; it measures volumes using household utensils

_____ 14. A system of measurement once used in the practice of pharmacy to measure both volume and weight; this system has been mostly replaced by the metric system

_____ 15. The wholesale price plus markup

16. A system of measurement based on seven base units with prefixes that change units by multiples of 10; the prefixes for the modern metric system are taken from the French Système International d'Unités and were adopted to provide a single worldwide system of weights and measures

_____ 17. A system of measurement previously used in pharmacy for the determination of weight in ounces and pounds

_____ 18. The purchase price of a product (in this case, medicine), which is then marked up for resale

_____ 19. The amount added to a wholesale price (usually a percentage) to make a profit

_____ 20. A fraction with the numerical value of 1, which is used to convert 1 unit to another without changing the value of the number

True or False

Write T or F next to each statement.

_____ 1. The ability to manipulate conversions is a required competency of pharmacy technicians.

_____ 2. Not all transcriptions and calculations need to be checked by a pharmacist.

_____ 3. A pharmacy technician can assume that a person understands the meaning of a measurement.

_____ 4. It is important to place the proper units (mL, L, mg, or g) next to the number amount.

_____ 5. One of the least common errors made in pharmacy is the improper use of the decimal point.

_____ 6. A pharmacy technician should convert measurements to the metric system because it is the approved system of measurement for pharmacy in the United States.

_____ 7. Calculations should be checked at least three times before asking a pharmacist to check them.

_____ 8. The pharmacy technician should show the parent of a pediatric patient how to measure the correct dosage.

_____ 9. If you round off at each step of a calculation, your answer will be very accurate.

_____ 10. If an IM dose is calculated to be greater than 5 mL, an error has occurred in either the prescribed amount or the calculation.

Multiple Choice

Complete each question by circling the best answer.

1. The cost of 100 g of hydrocortisone powder is $36.00. What would be the cost of 12 g?
   A. $5.42
   B. $4.32
   C. $10.60
   D. $8.94

2. A 125-pound patient weighs how many kilograms?
   A. 0.125 kg
   B. 125,000 kg
   C. 56.82 kg
   D. 275 kg

3. Convert 1200 mg to grams.
   A. 12,000 g
   B. 12 g
   C. 120 g
   D. 1.2 g

4. Of the following, volume best refers to the measurement of:
   A. Liquids
   B. Dry ingredients
   C. Distance
   D. Temperature

5. The weight of 1 grain is:
   A. 60 mg
   B. 64.8 mg
   C. 65 mg
   D. All of the above; different measurement systems define grains in different weights

6. Phenobarbital 200 mg/3 mL is prescribed with a sig gr iss IV. What volume is needed for this dose? (Use 65 mg/1 gr)
   A. 0.98 mL
   B. 1.5 mL
   C. 4.3 mL
   D. 3 mL

7. Amoxicillin 250 mg/5 mL is prescribed with a sig 200 mg po bid for 10 days. How many milliliters will need to be dispensed for this treatment regimen?
   A. 100 mL
   B. 80 mL
   C. 40 mL
   D. 200 mL

8. Humulin N U-100 insulin is prescribed with a sig 25 units qd. What volume is needed for this dose?
   A. 0.025 mL
   B. 25 mL
   C. 2.5 mL
   D. 0.25 mL

9. A pharmacy wants to increase the price of a product by 35%. How much would an item cost with this markup if its original cost was $6.75?
   A. $6.95
   B. $8.21
   C. $12.50
   D. $9.11

10. The approximate size of a container used to dispense 120 mL of a liquid medication would be:
    A. 6 fl oz
    B. 4 fl oz
    C. 8 fl oz
    D. 2 fl oz

11. A physician orders cefuroxime 0.5 g PO q12h. The medication available is cefuroxime 250 mg/5 mL. What is the quantity of medication to be administered per dose?
    A. 10 mL
    B. 1 mL
    C. 0.1 mL
    D. 0.01 mL

12. The physician orders atropine 1/150 gr PO bid. The atropine available is 0.4 mg per tablet. The nurse will administer how many tablets per dose? (Use 60 mg/1 gr.)
    A. ½ tablet
    B. 1 tablet
    C. 1.5 tablet
    D. 2 tablets

13. A prescription is written for Pen VK 500 mg tabs PO qid for 10 days. The patient, who has throat cancer and cannot swallow, requests a liquid form. What volume of a 250 mg/5 mL suspension should be dispensed to fulfill the prescription?
    A. 4 mL
    B. 40 mL
    C. 400 mL
    D. 4000 mL

14. A pharmacist dispenses 150 mL of amoxicillin 250 mg/5 mL suspension. The sig is 250 mg PO tid. How many days will the prescription last?
    A. 7 days
    B. 10 days
    C. 12 days
    D. 14 days

15. The physician's order is for Timoptic ii gtts ou bid. How many drops will the patient get in 12 days?
    A. 4 gtt
    B. 48 gtt
    C. 69 gtt
    D. 96 gtt

16. You receive an order for Kaopectate 15 mL bid prn. One dose equals how many tablespoonfuls?
    A. 2 Tbsp
    B. 3 Tbsp
    C. 1 Tbsp
    D. 1.5 Tbsp

17. Mylanta and Donnatal are to be combined in a 2:1 ratio. How many milliliters of each is required to make 120 mL of the suspension?
    A. 70 mL/50 mL
    B. 50 mL/70 mL
    C. 80 mL/40 mL
    D. 40 mL/80 mL

18. An IV solution is ordered to run at 3.5 gtts/min. It contains 875 mg in a total of 250 mL. How many milligrams will the patient receive per hour if the set is calibrated to deliver 12 gtts/mL?
    A. 0.16 mg/hr
    B. 16 mg/hr
    C. 61 mg/hr
    D. 610 mg/hr

19. The Roman numeral XLVIII is equivalent to:
    A. 43
    B. 48
    C. 53
    D. 68

20. Convert 12:14 AM to military (international) time.
    A. 1214
    B. 0214
    C. 0014
    D. 0140

21. The Roman numeral LVIII is equivalent to:
    A. 58
    B. 48
    C. 43
    D. 68

22. How many days will the following prescription last if taken as prescribed?
Rx: Zoloft 100 mg #90
Sig: 1 PO bid
A. 55 days
B. 30 days
C. 45 days
Ď. 90 days

23. A dose is written for 10 mg/kg every 12 hours for 1 day. The adult taking this medication weighs 165 pounds. How much drug will be needed for this order?
A. 425 mg
B. 950 mg
C. 750 mg
D. 1500 mg

24. How many tablets would be needed for the following prescription?
Rx: Prednisone tablets 10 mg
Sig: One qid for 6 days; one tid for 3 days; one bid for 1 day; then stop
A. 35 tabs
B. 15 tabs
C. 25 tabs
D. 45 tabs

25. The doctor has ordered Regular Insulin 30 units subcut qam. What volume is needed for this dose?
A. .3 mL
B. 0.3 mL
C. 3 mL
D. 3.0 mL

26. A dosage of 0.75 g is prescribed. You have in stock 250 mg/mL. How many milliliters would be given using the dosage strength on hand?
A. 1 mL
B. 15 mL
C. 3 mL
D. 500 mL

27. How many milligrams of epinephrine is needed to prepare 3 L of a 1:30,000 solution?
A. 0.1 mg
B. 1 mg
C. 10 mg
D. 100 mg

28. How many liters of a 0.9% normal saline solution can be made from 90 g of NaCl?
A. 10 L
B. 100 L
C. 1,000 L
D. 10,000 L

29. If 5 mL of diluent is added to a vial containing 2 g of a drug for injection, resulting in a final volume of 5.8 mL, what is the concentration in milligrams per milliliters of the drug in the reconstituted solution?
A. 0.3 mg/mL
B. 345 mg/mL
C. 444 mg/mL
D. 2035 mg/mL

30. Which prescription instructions would require 21 tablets to be dispensed?
A. One tab PO bid for 8 d
B. One tab ac and hs for 4 d
C. One tab tid for 3 d; one tab bid for 3 d; one qd for 3 d
D. Three tabs bid for 2 d; two tabs qd for 3 d; one tab qd for 3 d

31. How many grams of potassium permanganate is required to prepare 2 quarts of a 1:750 solution of potassium permanganate?
A. 1.28 g
B. 3 g
C. 2.56 g
D. 5 g

32. If the dosage of a drug is 35 mg/kg/day in six divided doses, how much would be given in each dose to a 38-pound child?
A. 17.3 mg
B. 60.4 mg
C. 101 mg
D. 604 mg

33. To make 300 mL of a 5% dextrose solution, using 10% dextrose solution and water, how much of each do you need?
A. 150 mL dextrose 10% solution and 150 mL water
B. 175 mL dextrose 10% solution and 125 mL water
C. 180 mL dextrose 10% solution and 120 mL water
D. 200 mL dextrose 10% solution and 100 mL water

34. How many capsules, each containing 1.5 gr of a drug, can be filled completely from a 28 g bottle of the drug? (Use 60 mg/gr.)
A. 24 caps
B. 32 caps
C. 311 caps
D. 431 caps

35. An IV solution containing 20,000 units of heparin in 500 mL of 0.45% NaCl solution is to be infused to provide 1000 units of heparin per hour. Roughly how many drops per minute should be infused to deliver the desired dose if the IV set calibrates at 15 gtt/mL?
    A. 0.42 gtt/min
    B. 6.3 gtt/min
    C. 0.16 gtt/min
    D. 44.4 gtt/min

36. How many days will the following prescription last if taken as prescribed?
    Rx: KCl 20 mEq tablets #60
    Sig: 1 PO bid
    A. 120 days
    B. 60 days
    C. 30 days
    D. 20 days

37. You ordered 2 cases of diphenhydramine liquid. Each case contains 12 bottles of 120 mL each. The supplier will give the pharmacy a 10% discount if the invoice is paid in full in 5 days. If each case is $24 and the invoice is paid within 5 days, how much will be paid to the supplier for this invoice?
    A. $52.80
    B. $43.20
    C. $45.60
    D. $50.40

38. How many grams of cream base must be added to 60 g of 2% (w/w) hydrocortisone to prepare 1.5% hydrocortisone cream?
    A. 20 g
    B. 80 g
    C. 45 g
    D. 5 g

39. A compounding pharmacy receives an order for a 1% ointment. The technician weighs out 2 g of the active ingredient. What is the final weight of the correctly compounded prescription?
    A. 0.02 g
    B. 0.2 g
    C. 200 g
    D. 20 g

40. A technician is filling a medication for a 4-year-old child weighing 45 pounds. The average adult dose is 250 mg. How much medication should the child receive?
    A. 62.5 mg
    B. 27 mg
    C. 83 mg
    D. 75 mg

Fill in the Blanks
Conversions
Convert the following measurements.

1. 6 fl oz = _____ mL

2. 120 mL = _____ oz

3. 4 kg = _____ g

4. 4 pints = _____ cups

5. 1.5 = _____ %

6. 0.25 = _____ %

7. 1.5 gr = _____ mg

8. 55 lb = _____ kg

9. 125 kg = _____ lb

10. 5500 mL = _____ L

11. 0.15 mg = _____ mcg

12. 3600 mL = _____ pts

13. 78 mg = _____ gr

14. 33% = _____ decimal

15. 40% = _____ decimal

Roman Numerals and Arabic Numbers
Interpret the following.

1. XVI _____

2. XCIX _____

3. 250 _____

4. 44 _____

5. MDX _____

6. XXIII _____

7. 125 _____

8. 60 _____

9. IX _____

10 CC _____

Chapter **6** **Conversions and Calculations**

International Time

Convert each time to either international or standard time.

1. 0330 = _____

2. 4:45 PM = _____

3. 1430 = _____

4. 1715 = _____

5. 8:20 PM = _____

6. 9:40 AM = _____

7. 2300 = _____

8. 9:10 PM = _____

9. 1925 = _____

10. 11:30 AM = _____

Temperature

Convert to Fahrenheit or Celsius as appropriate.

1. 212° F = _____ ° C

2. 32° C = _____ ° F

3. 66° C = _____ ° F

4. 104° F = _____ ° C

5. 32° F = _____ ° C

6. 2° C = _____ ° F

7. 8° C = _____ ° F

8. 48° F = _____ ° C

9. 25° C = _____ ° F

10. 85° F = _____ ° C

Matching

Match the conversion factors with their correct equivalents.

A. 5 mL
B. 15 mL
C. 30 mL
D. 480 mL
E. 3840 mL
F. 454 g
G. 1 oz
H. 8 fl oz
I. 2.2 lb

_____ 1. 1 gallon

_____ 2. 30 grams

_____ 3. 1 tablespoon

_____ 4. 1 pint

_____ 5. 1 cup

_____ 6. 1 kg

_____ 7. 1 teaspoon

_____ 8. 1 fluid ounce

_____ 9. 1 pound

Match the pharmacy abbreviation with their correct dosing schedule.

A. bid
B. q12h
C. tid
D. q8h
E. qid
F. q6h

_____ 10. 3 times daily

_____ 11. every 6 hours

_____ 12. every 8 hours

_____ 13. 2 times daily

_____ 14. 4 times daily

_____ 15. every 12 hours

Short Answer

Write a short response to each question in the space provided.

1. Give the units used in the metric system for the following:

   A. Volume

   _____

   B. Weight

   _____

2. Give the units used in the household system for the following:

   A. Volume

   _____

   B. Weight

   _____

3. Give the units used in the apothecary system for the following:

A. Liquids

_____

B. Dry weights

_____

4. Give the units used in the avoirdupois system for the following:

A. Liquids

_____

B. Weights

_____

Research Activities

Follow the instructions given in each exercise and provide a response.

1. Access the website *http://www.medcalc.com/body.html*. Use the BSA calculator to determine the BSA of the following:

A. Patient: length 62 inches; weight 59 kg

BSA = _____

B. Patient: length 65 inches; weight 145 lb

BSA = _____

C. Patient: length 21 inches; weight 7 lb

BSA = _____

D. Patient: length 48 inches; weight 20 kg

BSA = _____

E. Patient: length 68 inches; weight 170 lb

BSA = _____

2. Access the website *http://www.pharmacopeia.cn/v29240/usp29nf24s0_c1079.html*. Fill in the table with the recommended storage temperatures outlined by the USP.

Storage Condition	Temperature
Freezer	
Cold	
Controlled cold temperature	
Room temperature	
Controlled room temperature	
Warm	
Excessive heat	

REFLECT CRITICALLY

Critical Thinking

Reply to each question based on what you have learned in the chapter.

1. Bobbi is a second-semester pharmacy technician student and is having difficulty with the calculations course. Although the instructor assures Bobbi it is necessary to have a solid working knowledge of pharmacy math, Bobbi is not sure the calculations will really ever have to be used on the job. How would you convince Bobbi of the importance of a strong calculations foundation?

2. Proper decimal notation is crucial in pharmacy calculations. Therefore, technicians cannot afford to misread a prescription. What would be the outcome if a pharmacy technician mistook 5 mcg for 5 mg and the pharmacist did not catch the error?

RELATE TO PRACTICE

Lab Scenarios
Pharmacy Conversions

Objective: To introduce and review various pharmacy math conversions with the pharmacy technician

Prescribers write prescriptions and medication orders using a variety of measurement systems, which include metric, household, apothecary, and avoirdupois systems. Two advantages of the metric system are (1) that its tables are simple to understand because they are based on the decimal system, and (2) that the greater of two consecutive denominations is always ten times the lesser amount.

The basic units of measurements of the metric system are as follows:

- The meter (m) for length
- The liter (L) for volume
- The gram (g) for weight

The metric system is the official system of the United States Pharmacopeia (USP). However, the pharmacy technician must be familiar with the other systems of measurement when interpreting prescription and medication orders.

Lab Activity #6.1: Identify the meaning of the following metric prefixes.

Equipment needed:
- Pencil/pen

Time needed to complete this activity: 5 minutes

1. nano- _____

2. micro- _____

3. milli- _____

4. centi- _____

5. deci- _____

6. deca- _____

7. hecto- _____

8. kilo- _____

Lab Activity #6.2: Convert the following measurements. Make sure to use decimals with the metric system! It is common practice to use fractions with household measurements.

Equipment needed:
- Pencil/pen
- Calculator

Time needed to complete this activity: 30 minutes

1. 250 mcg = _____ mg

2. 100 mg = _____ g

3. 10 g = _____ mg

4. 12 fl oz = _____ pt

5. 3 pt = _____ gal

6. 2500 g = _____ kg

7. 10 Tbsp = _____ fl oz

8. 480 mL = _____ qt

9. 5 kg = _____ g

10. 12 tsp = _____ Tbsp

11. 3 gr = _____ mg

12. 96 tsp = _____ gal

13. 6 Tbsp = _____ mL

14. 1500 mcg = _____ g

15. 30 mL = _____ tsp

16. 6 fl oz = _____ tsp

17. 16 fl oz = _____ cup

18. 0.4 kg = _____ mg

19. 360 mL = _____ cup

20. 0.5 g = _____ mcg

21. 480 mL = _____ gal

22. 8 tsp = _____ mL

23. 0.1 mg = _____ mcg

24. 1 pt = _____ tsp

25. 12 tsp = _____ cup

26. 720 mL = _____ pt

27. 32 fl oz = _____ qt

28. 325 mg = _____ gr

29. 48 tsp = _____ pt

30. 1 cup = _____ pt

31. 12 Tbsp = _____ tsp

32. 180 mL = _____ fl oz

33. 4 cup = _____ gal

34. 24 tsp = _____ fl oz

35. 4 pt = _____ qt

36. 24 Tbsp = _____ cup

37. 4 fl oz = _____ mL

38. 90 mL = _____ Tbsp

39. 8 fl oz = _____ Tbsp

40. 0.5 kg = _____ mcg

41. 64 fl oz = _____ gal

42. 2 cup = _____ mL

43. 1/2 gal = _____ pt

44. 1/2 cup = _____ Tbsp

45. 1 qt = _____ fl oz

46. 1 cup = _____ fl oz

47. 96 Tbsp = _____ qt

48. 1/4 gal = _____ fl oz

49. 2 cup = _____ qt

50. 96 tsp = _____ qt

51. 2 pt = _____ mL

52. 1 pt = _____ fl oz

53. 1 cup = _____ tsp

54. 2 pt = _____ cup

55. 2 gal = _____ cup

56. 2 qt = _____ mL

57. 1½ qt = _____ tsp

58. 1 qt = _____ Tbsp

59. 2 qt = _____ pt

60. 6 qt = _____ gal

61. 2 gal = _____ mL

62. 1/4 gal = _____ tsp

63. 1 gal = _____ Tbsp

64. 8 pt = _____ Tbsp

65. 48 Tbsp = _____ pt

66. 1 gal = _____ qt

69

Reducing and Enlarging a Formula

Objective: To introduce and review with the pharmacy technician the steps needed to enlarge or reduce a prescription

A pharmacy technician may receive a prescription or medication order that requires enlargement or reduction of the formula for a compound. The technician may be required to calculate the quantity of each ingredient in the compound. A ratio and proportion may be expressed in specific quantities for each ingredient or in parts. To enlarge or reduce a formula using specific quantities, the following formula may be used:

$$\frac{Quantity\ of\ ingredient\ in\ original\ formula}{Total\ quantity\ of\ original\ formula} = \frac{Quantity\ of\ ingredient\ desired}{Total\ Quantity\ desired}$$

Normally this will be solved with X as the unknown *quantity of ingredient desired* to make a reduced or increased amount of medication.

If the order is written using parts, the following formula can be used:

$$\frac{Number\ of\ parts\ of\ ingredient\ in\ original\ formula}{Total\ number\ of\ parts\ in\ original\ formula} = \frac{Number\ of\ parts\ of\ ingredient\ desired}{Total\ number\ of\ parts\ desired}$$

Normally this will be solved with X as the unknown *number of parts of ingredients desired*.

Lab Activity #6.3: Reducing and enlarging a prescription. Calculate the correct quantities of each ingredient needed to prepare the following compounds.

Equipment needed:
- Pencil/pen
- Calculator

Time needed to complete this activity: 30 min

1. Following is the formula to compound 1000 g of yellow ointment, USP:

Yellow wax	50 g
Petrolatum	950 g

How much of each ingredient should be used to prepare 2 ounces of yellow ointment, USP?

Yellow wax _____

Petrolatum _____

2. Following is the formula for calamine lotion:

Calamine	80 g
Zinc oxide	80 g
Glycerin	20 g
Bentonite magma	250 mL
Calcium hydroxide qs	1000 mL

How much of each ingredient should be used to prepare 8 fluid ounces of calamine lotion?

Calamine _____

Zinc oxide _____

Glycerin _____

Bentonite magma _____

Calcium hydroxide qs _____

3. Following is the formula for benzoin tincture compound:

Benzoin	100 g
Aloe	20 g
Storax	80 g
Tolu balsam	40 g
Alcohol qs	1000 mL

How much of each ingredient should be used in this preparation to make one quart of benzoin tincture compound?

Benzoin _____

Aloe _____

Storax _____

Tolu balsam _____

Alcohol qs _____

4. Following is the formula for coal tar ointment:

Coal tar	5 parts
Zinc oxide	10 parts
Hydrophilic ointment	50 parts

How much of each ingredient should be used to make one pound of coal tar ointment?

Coal tar _____

Zinc oxide _____

Hydrophilic ointment _____

5. Following is the formula to prepare 1000 g of hydrophilic petrolatum, USP:

Cholesterol	30 g
Stearyl alcohol	30 g
White wax	80 g
White petrolatum	860 g

How much of each ingredient should be used to prepare ½ pound of hydrophilic petrolatum, USP?

Cholesterol _____

Stearyl alcohol _____

White wax _____

White petrolatum _____

6. Following is the formula to prepare about 1000 g of hydrophilic ointment, USP:

Methylparaben	0.25 g
Propylparaben	0.15 g
Sodium lauryl sulfate	10 g
Propylene glycol	120 g
Stearyl alcohol	250 g
White petrolatum	250 g
Purified water	370 g

How much of each ingredient should be used to prepare 4 oz of hydrophilic ointment, USP?

Methylparaben _____

Propylparaben _____

Sodium lauryl sulfate _____

Propylene glycol _____

Stearyl alcohol _____

White petrolatum _____

Purified water _____

7. Following is the formula to prepare 1000 mL of benzyl benzoate lotion:

Benzyl benzoate	250 mL
Triethanolamine	5 mL
Oleic acid	20 mL
Purified water qs	1000 mL

How much of each ingredient should be used to prepare one pint of benzyl benzoate lotion?

Benzyl benzoate _____

Triethanolamine _____

Oleic acid _____

Purified water qs _____

8. Following is the formula to prepare 1000 mL of phenobarbital elixir:

Phenobarbital	4 g
Orange oil	0.25 mL
Certified red color	qs
Alcohol	200 mL
Propylene glycol	100 mL
Sorbitol solution	600 mL
Water qs	1000 mL

How much of each ingredient should be used to prepare 2 gallons of phenobarbital elixir?

Phenobarbital _____

Orange oil _____

Certified red color _____

Alcohol _____

Propylene glycol _____

Sorbitol solution _____

Water qs _____

71

Chapter **6** **Conversions and Calculations**

9. Following is the formula to prepare 1 liter of white lotion, USP:

Zinc sulfate	40 g
Sulfurated potash	40 g
Purified water qsad	1000 mL

How much of each ingredient should be used to prepare 1 cup of white lotion, USP?

Zinc sulfate _____

Sulfurated potash _____

Purified water qsad _____

10. Following is the formula to prepare 1 liter of iodine topical solution, USP:

Iodine	20 g
Sodium iodide	24 g
Purified water qsad	1000 mL

How much of each ingredient should be used to prepare sixty 15-mL bottles of iodine topical solution, USP?

Iodine _____

Sodium iodide _____

Purified water qsad _____

Medication Concentrations (Strengths)

Objective: To become familiar with the concepts of percent weight-weight, weight-volume, and volume-volume

A medication's concentration (strength) can be expressed mathematically in several different manners, which include a fraction, a ratio, or a percent. The term *percent* or its corresponding sign (%) means "by the hundred," and percentage means "rate per 100." A percent may also be expressed as a ratio represented as a common or decimal fraction. Percents are usually changed to equivalent decimal fractions.

A medication expressed as a percent can be a solid dissolved in another solid, a solid dissolved in a liquid, or a liquid dissolved in another liquid.

- w/w% is defined as the number of grams of solute dissolved in 100 grams of vehicle base.
- w/v% is defined as the number of grams of solute dissolved in 100 milliliters of vehicle base.
- v/v% is defined as the number of milliliters of solute dissolved in 100 milliliters of vehicle base.

The following formula can be used in calculating the amount of solute, the total amount of vehicle base, or its percent.

$$\frac{amount\ of\ solute}{amount\ of\ vehicle\ base} = \frac{x}{100}$$

$$x = \%\ strength$$

The concentration of a weak solution or liquid preparation is frequently expressed in terms of ratio strength. Because all percentages represent a ratio of parts per hundred, ratio strength is another way of expressing the percentage strength of solutions or liquid preparations. For example, 10% means 10 parts per 100 or 10:100. Although 10 parts per 100 designates a ratio strength, it is customary to translate the designation; therefore, 10:100 : 1:10.

When a ratio strength is used to designate a concentration, it is *always* expressed in the form of 1:*x*.

For example, the ratio strength 1:1000 is to be interpreted as the following:

- For solids in liquids, 1 g of solute in 1000 mL of solution or liquid preparation
- For liquids in liquids, 1 mL of solute in 1000 mL of solution or liquid preparation
- For solids in solids, 1 g of solute in 1000 g of mixture

The following formula can be used to calculate the number of parts, the total number of parts, or the percent of a ratio strength problem:

$$\frac{\#\ parts}{total\ parts} = \frac{x}{100}$$

$$x = \%\ strength$$

Lab Activity #6.4: In the following table, convert the percent strength to ratio strength and ratio strength to percent strength.

Equipment needed:
- Calculator
- Pencil/pen

Time needed to complete this activity: 15 minutes

Percent Strength	Ratio Strength
25%	
	1:200
15%	
	1:400
50%	
	1:1000
4%	
	1:500
2%	
	1:175

Lab Activity #6.5: Solve the following problems involving percent strength and ratio strength.

Equipment needed:
- Calculator
- Pencil/pen
- Paper

Time needed to complete this activity: 45 minutes

1. How many grams of antipyrine should be used in preparing the prescription?

_____

Rx:
Antipyrine	5%
Glycerin, USP	qsad 90 mL
Sig: gtt v in right ear tid	

2. How many grams of resin of podophyllum should be used in preparing the prescription?

_____

Rx:
Resin of Podophyllum	25%
Compound Benzoin Tincture	qsad 60 mL
Sig: Apply to papillomas tid	

3. How many grams of potassium iodide and ephedrine sulfate should be used in preparing the prescription?

_____

_____

Rx:
Potassium Iodide Solution	10%	
Ephedrine Sulfate Solution	3%	aa 45 mL
Sig: Place five drops in water as directed		

4. What is the percentage strength (w/w) each of iodochlorhydroxyquin and hydrocortisone in the prescription?

_____

_____

Rx:
Iodochlorhydroxyquin	1.8 g
Hydrocortisone	0.3 g
Cream base	qsad 60 g
Sig: Apply to the affected areas of skin once a day.	

5. How many milligrams of methylparaben are needed to prepare 16 fluid ounces of a solution containing 0.12% (w/v) of methylparaben?

_____

6. A formula for a mouth rinse contains 1/10% (w/v) of zinc chloride. How many grams of zinc chloride should be used in preparing 20 liters of the mouth rinse?

_____

7. If 425 g of sucrose is dissolved in enough water to make 500 mL, what is the percentage strength (w/v) of the solution?

_____

8. How many milliliters of 0.9% (w/v) sodium chloride solution can be made from 1 lb of sodium chloride?

_____

9. One gallon of a certain lotion contains 946 mL of benzyl benzoate. Calculate the percentage (v/v) of benzyl benzoate in the lotion.

_____

10. A liniment contains 15% of methyl salicylate. How many milliliters of the liniment can be made from 1 quart of methyl salicylate?

_____

11. How many grams each of resorcinol and hexachlorophene should be used in preparing 2 pounds of an acne ointment that is to contain 2% resorcinol and 0.25% of hexachlorophene?

_____

_____

12. How many milligrams of procaine hydrochloride should be used in preparing 60 suppositories, each weighing 2 grams and containing 1/4% of procaine hydrochloride?

_____

13. If a topical cream contains 1.8% (w/w) of hydrocortisone, how many milligrams of hydrocortisone should be used in preparing 1 ounce of the cream?

_____

14. A pharmacist incorporates 6 grams of coal tar into 120 grams of a 6% coal tar ointment. Calculate the percentage (w/w) of coal tar in the finished product.

_____

73

15. Express each of the following concentrations as a ratio strength:

   A. 2 mg of active ingredient in 1 mL of solution

   _____

   B. 0.125 mg of active ingredient in 5 mL of solution

   _____

   C. 2 g of active ingredient in 500 mL of solution

   _____

   D. 100 mg of active ingredient in 100 mL of solution

   _____

16. A vaginal cream contains 0.01% (w/v) of dienestrol. Express this concentration as a ratio strength.

   _____

   _____

17. How many milligrams each of menthol and hexachlorophene should be used in compounding the prescription?

   _____

   _____

Rx:

Menthol	1:500
Hexachlorophene	1:800
Hydrophilic ointment base	qsad 60 g

Sig: Apply to hands bid

18. Hepatitis B virus vaccine inactivated is inactivated with 1:4000 (w/v) of formalin. Express this ratio strength as a percentage strength.

   _____

19. Versed injection contains 5 mg of midazolam per milliliter of injection. Calculate the ratio strength of midazolam in the injection.

   _____

20. A sample of white petrolatum contains 10 mg of tocopherol per kilogram as a preservative. Express the amount of tocopherol as a ratio strength.

   _____

Dilution Calculations

Objective: To become familiar with calculations used in the dilution of a product

A pharmacy may receive a prescription for a medication in which the prescribed concentration is less than what is currently stocked in the pharmacy. The concentration may be written in the form of a percent, fraction, or ratio. In a dilution problem, the initial strength (the stock strength) is greater than the final strength (the desired strength). A diluent (an inert substance that does not have strength—such as water or petrolatum) is added to the initial volume or weight to make the final volume or weight. In other words, the amount of diluent can be calculated by using the following formula:

Final volume (weight) − Initial volume (weight) = Amount of diluent to be added

A dilution problem may be solved using the following formula:

(Initial volume) (Initial strength) = (Final volume) (Final strength)

or

(Initial weight) (Initial strength) = (Final weight) (Final strength)

It is important to remember that both initial and final strengths must be expressed in the same unit of concentration and that initial and final volumes (weight) must be expressed in the same unit of measurement. It is easiest to change all strengths to percent before solving dilution problems, so you may see the equations written as:

(Stock volume/weight) (Stock percent) = (Desired volume/weight) (Desired percent) or

$SV \cdot SP = DV \cdot DP$ where amount of diluent needed = DV − SV

$SW \cdot SP = DW \cdot DP$ where amount of diluent needed = DW − SW

Lab Activity #6.6: Calculate the quantity of the ingredient needed to prepare the following prescriptions.

Equipment needed:
- Calculator
- Pencil/pen
- Paper

Time to complete this activity: 45 minutes

1. Rx 1:

```
                    Dr. Andrew A. Sheen
                 1100 Brentwood Blvd, Suite M780
                      St. Louis, MO 63144
                         314-527-0000
                        DEA FS1234563

Dr. Andrew A. Sheen                        January 12, 202X
1100 Brentwood Blvd Suite M780             St. Louis, MO 63144

                       FOR OFFICE USE

Rx    Isopropyl Alcohol 30%      1 gallon
      To be used in office for soaking sponges

Refills: 0                          Dr. Andrew Sheen
```

The pharmacy has in stock 70% isopropyl alcohol. How much of the 70% concentration and diluent is needed to prepare this prescription?

Isopropyl alcohol 70%: _____

Diluent: _____

2. Rx 2:

```
                    Dr. Andrew A. Sheen
                 1100 Brentwood Blvd, Suite M780
                      St. Louis, MO 63144
                         314-527-0000
                        DEA FS1234563

Dr. Andrew A. Sheen                        January 12, 202X
1100 Brentwood Blvd Suite M780             St. Louis, MO 63144

                       FOR OFFICE USE

Rx    Zephiran 7.5%        1 gallon
      For office use

Refills: 0                          Dr. Andrew Sheen
```

The pharmacy has in stock Zephiran chloride 20%. How much of the 20% Zephiran chloride and diluent is needed to prepare this prescription?

Zephiran chloride 20%: _____

Diluent: _____

3. Rx 3:

```
                    Dr. Andrew A. Sheen
                 1100 Brentwood Blvd, Suite M780
                      St. Louis, MO 63144
                         314-527-0000
                        DEA FS1234563

Dr. Andrew A. Sheen                        January 12, 202X
1100 Brentwood Blvd Suite M780             St. Louis, MO 63144

                       FOR OFFICE USE

Rx    Hypochlorous acid 1:10      4 liters
      For office use

Refills: 0                          Dr. Andrew Sheen
```

The pharmacy has in stock 25% hypochlorous acid. How much of the 25% hypochlorous acid and diluent is needed to prepare this order?

Hypochlorous acid 25%: _____

Diluent: _____

4. How many milliliters of a ½% solution of gentian violet should be used in preparing the prescription?

_____

Rx Gentian violet solution   1:100,000   500 mL
Sig: Use as a mouthwash

5. How many milliliters of a 17% solution of benzalkonium chloride should be used in preparing the prescription?

_____

Rx Benzalkonium chloride solution   240 mL
Make a solution such that 10 mL diluted to a liter equals a 1:5000 solution.
Sig: 10 mL diluted to a liter for external use

6. How many milliliters of a 1:50 (w/v) boric acid solution can be prepared from 500 mL of a 5% (w/v) boric acid solution?

_____

7. How many milliliters of water must be added to 250 mL of a 25% (w/v) stock solution of sodium chloride to prepare a 0.9% (w/v) sodium chloride solution?

_____

8. How many milliliters of a 1% (w/v) solution of phenyl mercuric nitrate may be used in preparing a 100-mL prescription requiring 1:50,000 (w/v) of phenyl mercuric nitrate as a preservative?

_____

75

9. How many milliliters of water should be added to 1 gallon of 70% isopropyl alcohol to prepare a 30% solution for soaking sponges?

_____

10. How many milliliters of water should be added to a liter of 1:3000 (w/v) solution to make a 1:8000 (w/v) solution?

_____

11. How many milliliters of water for injection must be added to 10 liters of a 50% (w/v) dextrose injection to reduce the concentration to 30% (w/v)?

_____

12. A physician orders 1 pint of 10% ethyl alcohol. The stock solution is 200 mL of 95% ethyl alcohol. How many milliliters of the 95% stock solution would be necessary to prepare the 10% solution?

_____

13. The pharmacy has 300 mL of a 50% solution. 200 mL is added to this solution to reduce the concentration. How many grams of active ingredient would be included in 4 fluid ounces of the diluted solution?

_____

14. How many grams of salicylic acid should be added to 75 g of a polyethylene glycol ointment to prepare an ointment containing 6% (w/w) of salicylic acid?

_____

15. How many grams of petrolatum (diluent) should be added to 250 g of ichthammol ointment to make a 5% ointment?

_____

Lab Activity #6.7: Calculate the final strength of the compound to appear on the prescription label from the following prescription.

Equipment needed:
- Calculator
- Pencil/pen
- Paper

Time needed to complete this activity: 30 minutes

1. If 250 mL of a 1/800 (v/v) solution is diluted to 1 liter, what will be the ratio strength (v/v)?

_____

2. Aluminum acetate topical solution contains 5% (w/v) of aluminum acetate. When 100 mL is diluted to a 0.5 liter, what will be the resulting ratio strength?

_____

3. If 500 mL of a 10% (w/v) solution is diluted to 2 liters, what will be the ratio strength (w/v)?

_____

4. If 2 tablespoonfuls of povidone-iodine solution (10% w/v) is diluted to 1 quart with purified water, what is the ratio strength of the dilution?

_____

5. If 400 mL of a 20% (w/v) solution is diluted to 2 liters, what will be the ratio strength?

_____

6. If a 0.067% (w/v) methylbenzethonium chloride lotion is diluted with an equal volume of water, what will be the ratio strength (w/v) of the dilution?

_____

7. In preparing a solution for a wet dressing, two 0.3-g tablets of potassium permanganate are dissolved in 1 gallon of purified water. What will be the percentage strength (w/v) of the solution?

_____

8. If 150 mL of a 17% (w/v) concentrate of benzalkonium chloride is diluted to 5 gallons, what will be the ratio strength?

_____

9. If a pharmacy technician adds 3 g of hydrocortisone to 60 g of a 5% (w/w) hydrocortisone cream, what is the final percentage strength of hydrocortisone in the product?

_____

10. If 20 mL of a 2% (w/v) solution is diluted with water to 8 pints, what is the ratio strength (w/v) of the solution?

_____

Alligation Calculations

Objective: Perform pharmacy calculations using both alligation medial and alligation alternate in compounding prescriptions with multiple strengths of a medication.

Alligation medial is a method by which the "weighted average" percentage strength of a mixture of *two or more* substances of known quantity and concentration may be easily calculated. By this method, the percentage strength of each component expressed as a decimal fraction is multiplied by its corresponding quantity (volume or weight); then the sum of the products is placed over the total quantity and a ratio and proportion is solved to find the amount per 100 or the percent strength. Alligation medial can be used with both solids and liquids.

For example, consider the following problem. What is the percentage strength in a mixture of 300 mL of a 40% (v/v) alcohol, 100 mL of a 60% (v/v) alcohol, and 100 mL of a 70% alcohol?

$$0.4 \times 300 \text{ mL} = 120 \text{ mL}$$

$$0.6 \times 100 \text{ mL} = 60 \text{ mL}$$

$$0.7 \times 100 \text{ mL} = 70 \text{ mL}$$

500 mL total quantity and 250 mL alcohol

$$250 \text{ mL}/500 \text{ mL} = x/100$$

x = 50 so the resultant solution is 50% strength

Alligation alternate, which uses a tic-tac-toe style, is a method by which we calculate the number of parts of two components of a given strength needed to prepare a mixture of a different desired strength. The desired strength of the compound must be between the strengths of the two medications on hand. This method is demonstrated in detail in the textbook.

Lab Activity #6.8: Practice pharmacy calculations using alligation medial and alligation alternate.

Equipment needed:
- Calculator
- Pencil/pen
- Paper

Time needed to complete this activity: 45 minutes

1. Four equal amounts of belladonna extract, containing 1.15%, 1.3%, 1.35%, and 1.2% of alkaloids, respectively, were mixed. What was the percentage strength of the mixture?

_____

2. What is the percentage of alcohol in a mixture containing 150 mL of witch hazel (14% alcohol), 200 mL of glycerin, and 500 mL of 50% alcohol?

_____

3. A pharmacy technician mixes 20 g of 10% ichthammol ointment, 45 g of 5% ichthammol ointment, and 100 g of petrolatum (diluent). What is the percentage of ichthammol in the finished compound?

_____

4. Calculate the percentage of alcohol in the lotion.

_____

Rx Coal tar solution (85% alcohol)	80 mL
Glycerin	160 mL
Alcohol (95% alcohol)	500 mL
Boric acid qs	1000 mL

Sig: Use as a medicated lotion once a day.

5. A manufacturing pharmacy has four lots of ichthammol ointment, containing 50%, 25%, 10%, and 5% ichthammol. How many grams of each should be used in preparing 1 pound of 20% ichthammol ointment? (Hint: There are 4 possible combinations using alligation alternate.)

_____

_____

_____

_____

6. How much 95% and 30% alcohol should be mixed to make 1 pint of 70% alcohol?

_____

_____

7. How many grams of 5% and 1% hydrocortisone should be mixed to make 1 pound of 2½% hydrocortisone ointment?

_____

_____

8. Prepare 1 liter of 0.75% sodium chloride solution from normal saline (0.9%) and half-normal saline (0.45%). How much of each strength would be required to fill this order?

_____

_____

9. Prepare 1 liter of $D_{10}W$ using both D_5W and $D_{20}W$. How much of each is required to fill this order?

_____

_____

10. Prepare 1 pound of 20% ointment using both 10% and 30% of the ointment. How much of each should be used?

_____

_____

IV Drip Rate Calculations

Objective: Calculate the flow rates or the amount of drug found in intravenous fluid administered to a patient.

Small-volume parenterals are generally considered to be 100 mL or less in volume. Some are injected into the body site slowly using a handheld syringe and needle. The medication is drawn into a syringe from a single-dose ampule or a multidose vial. Some syringes are packaged prefilled by the manufacturer or hospital pharmacist or pharmacy technician. Other small-volume doses are piggybacked through a large-volume IV.

Large-volume parenterals for continuous administration are hung at the patient's bed and are allowed to drip slowly into a vein by gravity flow or through the use of electrical or battery-operated volumetric infusion pumps. Some of these pumps can be calibrated to deliver "micro infusion" volumes such as 0.1 mL per hour or up to 2000 mL per hour, depending on the drug and the requirements. Solutions of additive drugs can be placed directly into large-volume parenterals, or small-volume parenterals (minibags) containing the additive drug, may be hung piggyback and allowed to enter the tubing of the primary intravenous fluid and then enter the patient at a controlled rate. In either situation, the physician specifies the rate of flow of intravenous fluids as milliliters per minute, drops per minute, or total volume to be delivered over a number of hours.

In a hospital, the pharmacy is responsible for preparing fluids to be injected intravenously into a patient. The pharmacy technician may be required to calculate the flow or drip rate of an intravenous solution. The rate that a volume is infused per hour can be calculated by setting the following information equal to x mL/hr and solving for x:

$$\frac{\text{Volume (mililiters)}}{\text{Time (hours)}}$$

At times, a pharmacy technician may be required to calculate the number of drops per minute that a patient is to receive. In this situation, the technician will need to know the flow rate and drop factor (number of drops per milliliter of the substance that the tubing delivers) and must use a conversion factor to convert hours to minutes. This can be done using the following formula:

Drops/min = (Drop factor) (Flow rate) (Conversion factor)

or

gtt/min = (gtt/mL) (mL/hr) (1 hr/60 min)

At other times, the pharmacy technician may need to calculate the amount of drug delivered over a specified period of time. This can be done using the following formula:

(amount of drug in IV/total volume) (rate of administration)

A conversion factor for time may be needed depending on whether the rate is given per hour or per minute and a conversion factor may be needed for weight depending on how it is given (example: mg or g).

Lab Activity #6.9: Complete the following questions.

Equipment needed:
- Calculator
- Pencil/pen
- Paper

Time needed to complete this activity: 30 minutes

1. 500 mL of a 2% sterile solution is to be administered by intravenous infusion over a period of 4 hours; how many milliliters will be administered over 1 hour?

_____

2. A physician orders 1 liter of normal saline infused over 24 hours; how many milliliters of the intravenous solution will the patient receive after 8 hours?

_____

3. How many mL are delivered per hour in question #2?

_____

4. A physician prescribes 1 liter of $D_{20}W$ to be administered over 8 hours using an infusion kit with a drop factor of 10 gtt/mL. What will be the number of drops per minute?

_____

5. A physician writes a medication order for $D_{10}W$. The drop factor is set at 60 gtt/mL and the flow rate is 50 mL/hr. How many liters of fluid would be required to fill this order for 1 day?

_____

6. A physician prescribes 1-liter of 1/2 NS to be infused at 6 mL/min, and the drop factor is 20 gtt/mL. How many drops per minute will the patient receive?

_____

7. A physician prescribes 1000 mL of lactated Ringer's solution to be infused over 8 hours using a drop factor of 20 gtt/mL. How many gtt/min will the patient receive?

_____

8. A physician orders a 2-g vial of a drug to be added to 500 mL of D_5W (5% dextrose in water for injection). If the administration rate is set at 125 mL per hour, how many milligrams of the drug will a patient receive per minute?

_____

9. A certain hyperalimentation fluid measures 1 liter. If the solution is to be administered over 8 hours and if the administration set is calibrated at 25 drops/mL, at what rate should the set be calibrated to administer the solution during the designated time interval?

_____

10. Five hundred (500) milliliters of an intravenous solution contains 0.2% of succinylcholine chloride in sodium chloride injection. At what rate should the infusion be administered to provide 2.5 mg of succinylcholine chloride per minute?

_____

Special Dosing Calculations

Objective: Calculate doses using Clark's Rule, Young's Rule, BSA, and body weight.

Lab Activity #6.10: Complete the following questions about individualized doses.

Equipment needed:
- Calculator
- Pencil/pen
- Paper

Time needed to complete this activity: 30 minutes

1. Drug Y has a recommended dose of 5 mg/kg of body weight given as a single daily dose. How many milligrams should this patient take daily if the patient weighs 120 lb?

_____

2. The dose of a drug is 500 mcg per kg of body weight. How many milligrams should be given to a child weighing 40 lb?

_____

3. The dose of gentamicin sulfate is 1.7 mg per kg of body weight every 8 hours. How many milliliters of an injectable solution containing 40 mg of gentamicin per mL should be administered per dose to a person weighing 176 lb?

_____

4. If the adult dose of a drug is 5 gr, what is the dose in mg for a child who weighs 50 lb and is 8 years old?

A. Use Young's Rule to calculate the dose.

B. Use Clark's Rule to calculate the dose.

5. The adult dose of a medication is 500 mg. What is the dose for a 3-year-old who weighs 32 lb?

A. Use Young's Rule to calculate the dose.

B. Use Clark's Rule to calculate the dose.

6. The adult dose of a medication is 200 mg, three times a day. What would be the daily dose for a 5-year-old child who weighs 55 lb?

A. Use Young's Rule to calculate the dose.

B. Use Clark's Rule to calculate the dose.

7. The pediatric dose is 25 mg/m^2. What would be the dose if the child is 18 kg, 36 inches, and has a BSA of 0.65 m^2?

_____

8. The adult dose is 150 mg/m^2. What would be the dose if the adult is 100 kg, 73 inches, and has a BSA of 2.24 m^2?

_____

9. The adult dose of a drug is 250 mg/m^2. If the drug is available as 150 mg/mL, what would be the dose in mL if the adult is 67 inches, 175 lb, and has a BSA of 1.91 m^2?

_____

79

10. The adult dose of a drug is 100 mg/m^2. If the drug is available as 50 mg/mL, what would be the dose in mL if the adult has a BSA of 1.8 m^2?

_____

Business Calculations

Objective: Calculate retail prices.

Lab Activity #6.11: Complete the following questions about retail pricing.

Equipment needed:
- Calculator
- Pencil/pen
- Paper

Time needed to complete this activity: 15 minutes

1. You order 6 cases of anti-itch cream. Each case has 12 tubes of cream and costs $14.50 per case. Your drug wholesaler will give you a discount of 25% if the invoice is paid within 2 weeks. What would be the total paid for this order if the invoice is paid within 2 weeks?

_____

2. Your pharmacy is having a 20% off sale for all antihistamines. Calculate the cost of each of the following items:

A. Benadryl Allergy, $6.50 _____

B. Children's Allegra, $9.99 _____

C. Claritin, $18.99 _____

D. Zyrtec, $21.99 _____

E. Alavert, $8.49 _____

3. Your pharmacy has Ben-Gay cream on sale at 10% off the price of $6.79 per tube. How much will the customer save?

_____

4. All new customers are being given 30% off new prescriptions. What is the dollar amount lost by the pharmacy if all the new prescriptions for the day added up to $1,327.27?

_____

5. Your pharmacy received an order of 10 cases of cough medicine. Each case contains 15 bottles and costs $25 per case. If each bottle is sold for $5.50, what is the percent markup?

_____

7 Drug Information References

ASHP ACCREDITATION STANDARDS FOR PHARMACY TECHNICIAN EDUCATION AND TRAINING PROGRAMS

Standard 2.5: Demonstrate basic knowledge of anatomy, physiology, and pharmacology, and medical terminology relevant to pharmacy technician's role.

REINFORCE KEY CONCEPTS

Terms and Definitions

Select the correct term from the following list and write the corresponding letter in the blank next to the statement.

A. Brand name
B. Chemical structure
C. Drug classification
D. *Drug Facts and Comparisons*
E. Formulary
F. Generic name
G. Monograph
H. Nonformulary
I. Package insert
J. Trade name

_____ 1. Reference book found in pharmacies that contains detailed information on more than 22,000 prescription and 6000 over-the-counter medications; drugs are divided into therapeutic groups for easy comparison

_____ 2. A list of drugs that are not included in the list of preferred medications that a committee of pharmacists and physicians deems to be the safest, most effective, and most economical; they are drugs not included in the drug list approved for reimbursement by the health care plans

_____ 3. The makeup of a chemical, including the elements, the shape, the bonding types, the molecular configurations, charges, and so on; the nature of the chemical's structure has much to do with the chemical's stability, reactivity, and physical and chemical properties

_____ 4. The official prescribing information for a prescription drug; the medication information sheet provided by the manufacturer that includes side effects, dosage forms, indications, and other important information

_____ 5. Name assigned to a medication or nonproprietary name of a drug

_____ 6. Categorization based on various characteristics, including the chemical structure of a drug, the action of a drug, and/or the therapeutic or anatomic use of a drug

_____ 7. Comprehensive information on a medication's actions within that class of drugs

_____ 8. Trademark of a drug or device held by the originating manufacturing company

_____ 9. The proprietary or brand name given to a drug by the company that developed it; the trade name may be related to the function or main use of the drug

_____ 10. A list of approved drugs to be stocked by the pharmacy; also a list of drugs covered by an insurance company

True or False

Write T or F next to each statement.

_____ 1. Pharmacists rely on credible, accurate, and up-to-date reference resources to help give the correct information to others.

_____ 2. Knowing which book to choose for referencing and how to access the information is not an important skill for pharmacists and technicians.

_____ 3. Pharmacy technicians should not provide patients with information about side effects, dosing, or compatibility.

_____ 4. The last date of update for a drug monograph is listed directly on the official product labeling.

_____ 5. Most generic drug names typically begin with J or W.

_____ 6. Most pharmacies carry the unbound *Drug Facts and Comparisons* to allow for monthly updates.

_____ 7. It is important for technicians to carry a good pocket guide.

_____ 8. All pharmacy reference books have an app for electronic devices.

_____ 9. Finding websites at universities and through publishing companies is not a good way to look for information.

_____ 10. Accessing personal websites will give you a person's perspective and will always provide medically sound information.

Multiple Choice

Complete each question by circling the best answer.

1. A reference text familiar to most pharmacists and available in hardback, loose-leaf hardback, pocket-sized, or by electronic subscription is:
   A. *Drug Facts and Comparisons*
   B. *Physicians' Desk Reference*
   C. *Drug Topics Red Book*
   D. *United States Pharmacopeia*

2. Although pharmacies have this reference book, physicians are the primary users:
   A. *Pharmacists' Drug Reference*
   B. *Physicians' Desk Reference*
   C. *Pharmacists' Desk Reference*
   D. *Pharmacy Dosage Regulations*

3. The PDR does not contain which of the following:
   A. Manufacturers' addresses and phone numbers
   B. Manufacturer-provided package inserts for select FDA-approved drugs
   C. Products listed by classification or method of action
   D. Average and wholesale drug costs

4. The diagnostic product information section of the PDR contains:
   A. A key to controlled substances
   B. A key to FDA pregnancy ratings
   C. An FDA telephone directory
   D. Information on drug products used as diagnostic agents

5. Of the sources listed here, which would be best for determining if a drug can be crushed?
   A. *Physicians' Desk Reference*
   B. *Drug Topics Red Book*
   C. *Drug Facts and Comparisons*
   D. *Ident-A-Drug*

6. If a technician must know the upper limit price and rules or the billing units for each type of drug under state AIDS drug assistance programs, he or she would use:
   A. *Drug Facts and Comparisons*
   B. *Physicians' Desk Reference*
   C. *Drug Topics Red Book*
   D. *Orange Book*

7. A patient has taken a drug in tablet form but does not know what it is; the technician might use which reference to find out what the drug is?
   A. *American Hospital Formulary Service Drug Information*
   B. *United States Pharmacopeia Drug Information*
   C. *Ident-A-Drug*
   D. *The Injectable Drug Handbook*

8. The book used to reference the compatibility of various parenteral agents is:
   A. *American Hospital Formulary Service Drug Information*
   B. *United States Pharmacopeia Drug Information*
   C. *Ident-A-Drug*
   D. *Trissel's Handbook on Injectable Drugs*

9. This book can be used to find pharmaceutical excipients:
   A. *Physicians' Desk Reference*
   B. *Ident-A-Drug*
   C. *United States Pharmacopeia Drug Information*
   D. *Martindale's the Complete Drug Reference*

10. This book can be used to reference the laws pertaining to compounding:
    A. *Geriatric Dosing Handbook*
    B. *Clinical Pharmacology*
    C. *Handbook of Nonprescription Drugs*
    D. *United States Pharmacists' Pharmacopeia*

11. Of the sources listed here, which would be best for finding the spectrum resistance for antibiotics?
    A. *American Hospital Formulary Service Drug Information*
    B. *The Injectable Drug Handbook*
    C. *The Purple Book*
    D. *American Drug Index*

12. Of the sources listed here, which would be best for finding a recommendation for a sugar-free and alcohol-free cough syrup?
    A. *Physicians' Desk Reference*
    B. *Drug Topic Red Book*
    C. *Drug Facts and Comparisons*
    D. *Ident-A-Drug*

13. Which of the following references is only available electronically?
    A. *Physicians' Desk Reference*
    B. *Pediatric Dosage Handbook*
    C. *Remington's Pharmaceutical Sciences: The Science and Practice of Pharmacy*
    D. *Orange Book*

14. Which of the following references is *not* available electronically?
    A. *Clinical Xpert*
    B. *Clinical Pharmacology*
    C. *United States Pharmacopoeia–National Formulary (USP-NF)*
    D. *American Hospital Formulary*

15. _____ offers basic free drug information that can be downloaded onto a personal computer or handheld device.
    A. *Epocrates*
    B. *Remington's Pharmaceutical Sciences*
    C. *American Drug Index*
    D. *Drug Topics Red Book*

Fill in the Blanks

Answer each question by completing the statement in the space provided.

1. It is important for technicians to be proficient in _____ accurate drug references and materials.

2. When a new drug is in the experimentation phase, the creators or the company give the drug a _____ or investigational drug name based on its chemical attributes.

3. Many times, drugs in the same class have the same _____.

4. Knowing how to use the _____ properly allows the technician to find the correct information in a timely manner.

5. One of the best books to keep is one in which a drug can be looked up by trade or brand name without having to check the _____.

6. The _____ has a lot of information, but it is up to the reader to determine whether the information is reliable and accurate.

7. Pharmacy organizations have websites on the Internet, and many have _____ news boards that reference important information concerning pharmacy.

8. Journals allow the technician to stay _____ on the most recent drugs being developed.

9. Seminars and continuing education dinners, provided by pharmacy associations, are a good source of information on drug topics, new drugs, and fulfilling _____ requirements.

10. Knowing the proper book to reference is important, not only for finding the correct information, but also for saving _____ and frustration.

Matching

Match the following drug reference books with their correct description.

A. *Drug Facts and Comparisons*
B. *Physicians' Desk Reference*
C. *Drug Topics Red Book*
D. *Orange Book*
E. *American Hospital Formulary Service Drug Information*
F. *USP–NF*
G. *United States Pharmacists' Pharmacopeia*
H. *Clinical Pharmacology*
I. *Ident-A-Drug*
J. *The Purple Book*

_____ 1. Provides access to official standards of the FDA

_____ 2. A good source of information pertaining to average and wholesale drug costs and prices

_____ 3. A comprehensive listing used to determinate whether a generic drug is the same as a brand drug

_____ 4. A comprehensive compilation of information on compounding products and ingredients and their safety as well as products used to treat specific medical conditions

_____ 5. Includes more than 38,000 listings of tablet and capsule identifications

_____ 6. Contains quick and accurate reference and drug comparison and is the most frequently used book by pharmacists

_____ 7. A compilation of package inserts with a complete description of each drug listed, including its chemical structure and study results

_____ 8. Provides drug monographs that list drug information; used mainly by hospitals

_____ 9. An electronic drug compendium commonly encountered in retail and health system pharmacy settings and an officially recognized compendium by the Centers for Medicare and Medicaid Services

_____ 10. A comprehensive list of approved biological products with biosimilar and interchangeable products

Match the following drug reference books with their correct description.

A. *Micromedex Healthcare Evidence*
B. *Trissel's Handbook on Injectable Drugs*
C. *American Drug Index*
D. *Goodman & Gilman's The Pharmacological Basis of Therapeutics*
E. *Handbook of Nonprescription Drugs*
F. *Martindale's The Complete Drug Reference*
G. *Remington's Pharmaceutical Sciences: The Science and Practice of Pharmacy*
H. *Pediatric and Neonatal Dosage Handbook*
I. *Geriatric Dosage Handbook*

_____ 11. A well-known reference used for information on parenteral agents; used mostly in the hospital setting

_____ 12. Provides information on suggested current dosages for geriatric patients

_____ 13. Contains information for both prescription and OTC products; covers pronunciation of drugs, active ingredients, dosage forms, and packaging, to name a few

_____ 14. Provides self-care options for nonprescription medications, nutritional supplements, medical foods, and complementary and alternative therapies to name a few

_____ 15. Covers the entire scope of pharmacy, from the history of pharmacy and ethics to the specifics of industrial pharmacy and pharmacy practice

_____ 16. Lists pharmacokinetics and pharmacodynamics, drug transport/drug transporters, drug metabolism

_____ 17. Provides information on suggested current dosages for pediatric patients

_____ 18. Provides information on drugs in clinical use worldwide

_____ 19. Provides an online and mobile application that can be used by physicians, pharmacists, and nurses within a health care facility through several different software programs that can be purchased

Short Answer

Write a short response to each question in the space provided.

1. List three key points to consider when you beginning to look for information in a drug reference book.

   _____

   _____

   _____

2. Explain how you would locate a drug in the *Drug Facts and Comparisons* and the information you could find about that drug.

   _____

   _____

   _____

   _____

3. List the sections of the *American Hospital Formulary Service Drug Information*.

   _____

   _____

   _____

   _____

4. List five components of drug information included in the *American Drug Index*.

   _____

   _____

   _____

   _____

   _____

5. List five self-care options in the *Handbook of Nonprescription Drugs*.

   _____

   _____

   _____

   _____

   _____

Research Activities

Follow the instructions given in each exercise and provide a response.

1. Access the websites listed in Table 7.2 of the textbook. Describe the type of information provided on each website.

2. Access the websites listed in Table 7.3 of the textbook. Describe the type of information provided on each website.

REFLECT CRITICALLY

Critical Thinking

Reply to each question based on what you have learned in the chapter.

1. Of all the reference books discussed in this chapter, which one seems to be the easiest to use and understand?

2. Download the *Epocrates* app to your electronic device. Describe the type of information provided in the app. How do you think this app would be useful while working in the pharmacy?

3. Do you plan to carry a pocket-sized reference book? Why or why not? If you plan to use an app as reference, when would having a book reference be beneficial over an app?

Lab Scenarios

Reference Materials

Objective: To familiarize the pharmacy technician with various forms of reference materials and the terminology associated with each.

Each pharmacy, regardless of the setting, is required by state boards of pharmacy to maintain a library relevant to its practice. State boards of pharmacy require that a pharmacy maintain a current edition of the *USP-NF* (the official compendium in the United States) and a copy of the United States Controlled Substance Act.

A pharmacy technician must be familiar with proper usage of these reference materials, which may consist of books, journals, and pharmacy magazines. In many situations, these materials may be found in an electronic format.

Lab Activity #7.1: Use the *Physicians' Desk Reference (PDR)* or *Drug Facts and Comparisons* to define the terms found in these reference materials.

Equipment needed:
- *Physicians' Desk Reference (PDR)* or *Drug Facts and Comparisons*
- Pencil/pen

Time needed to complete this activity: 15 minutes

Define the following terms used in pharmacy reference materials.

1. Adverse reactions

_____

2. Clinical pharmacology

_____

3. Contraindication

_____

4. Description

_____

5. Dosage and administration

_____

6. How supplied

_____

7. Indication

_____

8. Mechanism of action

_____

9. Monograph

_____

10. Pharmacokinetics

_____

11. Precautions

_____

12. Teratogenic effects

_____

13. Warnings

_____

14. Black Boxed Warning

_____

Lab Activity #7.2: Use *Approved Drug Products with Therapeutic Equivalence Evaluations (Orange Book)* to define the following terms found in drug monographs.

Equipment needed:
- Computer with Internet connection (*http://www.fda.gov*)
- Pencil/pen

Time needed to complete this activity: 10 minutes

Define the following terms.

1. Pharmaceutical equivalents

_____

2. Pharmaceutical alternatives

_____

3. Therapeutic equivalent

_____

4. Bioavailability

_____

5. Bioequivalent drug products

_____

86

Chapter **7 Drug Information References**

Lab Activity #7.3: Use *Approved Drug Products with Therapeutic Equivalence Evaluations (Orange Book)* to define the following therapeutic equivalent evaluation codes.

Equipment needed:
- Computer with Internet connection (*www.fda.gov*) to access *Approved Drug Products with Therapeutic Evaluations (Orange Book)*
- Pencil/pen

Time needed to complete this activity: 30 minutes

Define the following therapeutic equivalent evaluation codes.

1. A

_____

2. AA

_____

3. AB

_____

4. AN

_____

5. AO

_____

6. AP

_____

7. AT

_____

8. B

_____

9. BC

_____

10. BD

_____

11. BE

_____

12. BN

_____

13. BP

_____

14. BR

_____

15. BS

_____

16. BT

_____

17. BX

_____

Lab Activity #7.4: Use *Approved Drug Products with Therapeutic Equivalence Evaluations (Orange Book)* to determine the following therapeutic equivalent evaluation codes.

Equipment needed:
- Computer with Internet connection (*http://www.fda.gov*) to access *Approved Drug Products with Therapeutic Evaluations (Orange Book)*
- Pencil/pen

Time needed to complete this activity: 30 minutes

1. Atorvastatin calcium 10-mg tablet

_____

2. Mirtazapine 45 mg ODT

_____

3. Levofloxacin 250 mg/10 mL oral solution

_____

4. Montelukast sodium 5-mg chewable tablet

_____

5. Zolpidem tartrate extended release 6.25-mg tablet

_____

6. Levetiracetam 100-mg/mL injection

_____

7. Lorazepam 2-mg/mL oral solution

_____

8. Clotrimazole 1% topical solution

_____

9. Lopinavir/Ritonavir 100 mg/25 mg oral tablet

_____

10. Rosiglitazone maleate 4-mg oral tablet

_____

11. Clindamycin phosphate/tretinoin 1.2%/0.025% topical gel

_____

12. Nebivolol HCl 20-mg tablet

_____

13. Indomethacin sodium 1-mg base/vial injection

_____

14. Diclofenac sodium 0.1% ophthalmic solution

_____

15. Desvenlafaxine 50-mg extended release oral tablet

_____

Lab Activity #7.5: Use the electronic reference *Epocrates* to determine the following drugs from their description.

Equipment needed:
■ Computer with Internet connection to access *http://www.Epocrates.com* or download the *Epocrates* App to use the *Pill Identification Tool*.
■ Pencil/pen

Time needed to complete this activity: 30 minutes

1. This drug is a peach, oblong, scored tablet imprinted with "A CS"

_____

2. This drug is a pink tablet imprinted with "J" and "49"

_____

3. This drug is a dark grayish tablet imprinted with "DXL" and "NVR"

_____

4. This drug is a white, oblong, film-coated tablet imprinted with "XR 150"

_____

5. This drug is a white, round, scored, film-coated tablet imprinted with "A ms"

_____

6. This drug is a tan, triangle tablet imprinted with "5" and "FL"

_____

7. This drug is a yellow, hexagonal, film-coated tablet imprinted with "logo and 5" and "5121."

_____

8. This drug is a orange, double-scored tablet imprinted with "M 2540"

_____

9. This drug is a brown, diamond-shaped tablet imprinted with "L190"

_____

10. This drug is a dark orange, oblong capsule imprinted with "R50."

_____

Lab Activity #7.6: Use the electronic reference *Epocrates* or *Drug Facts and Comparisons* to access drug monograph information.

Equipment needed:
■ Computer with Internet connection to access *http://www.Epocrates.com* or *Drug Facts and Comparisons*
■ Pencil/pen

Time needed to complete this activity: 30 minutes

Answer the following questions based on the drug your instructor assigned to you by reading the drug monograph:

Generic Name: _____

1. What is the chemical name?

_____

2. Do you see a correlation (or common word) between the chemical name of the drug and the generic name of the drug? If so, what is it?

_____

3. What are the inactive ingredients?

_____

_____

4. What are the indications?

_____

_____

5. What is the dosage and administration?

_____

_____

6. How is the drug supplied?

_____

_____

7. How should the drug be stored?

_____

8. What are the side effects?

_____

_____

9. What are the drug interactions?

_____

_____

10. What is the pregnancy category?

_____

11. What is the mechanism of action?

_____

_____

12. List the patient information:

_____

_____

_____

8 Community Pharmacy Practice

Standard 1.2: Present an image appropriate for the profession of pharmacy in appearance and behavior.

Standard 1.4: Communicate clearly and effectively, both verbally and in writing.

Standard 1.5: Demonstrate a respectful and professional attitude when interacting with diverse patient populations, colleagues, and professionals.

Standard 1.7: Apply interpersonal skills, including negotiation skills, conflict resolution, customer service, and teamwork.

Standard 1.10: Apply critical thinking skills, creativity, and innovation.

Standard 1.12: Demonstrate the ability to effectively and professionally communicate with other health care professionals, payors and other individuals necessary to serve the needs of patients and practice.

Standard 2.2: Demonstrate the ability to maintain confidentiality of patient information, and understand applicable state and federal laws.

Standard 2.3: Describe the pharmacy technician's role, pharmacist's role, and other occupations in the health care environment.

Standard 2.6: Perform mathematical calculations essential to the duties of pharmacy technicians in a variety of settings.

Standard 2.7: Explain the pharmacy technician's role in the medication-use process.

Standard 3.1: Assist pharmacists in collecting, organizing, and recording demographic and clinical information for the *Pharmacists' Patient Care Process.*

Standard 3.2: Receive, process, and prepare prescriptions/medication orders for completeness, accuracy, and authenticity to ensure safety.

Standard 3.3: Assist pharmacist in the identification of patients who desire/require counseling to optimize the use of medication, equipment, and devices.

Standard 3.4: Prepare patient-specific medications for distribution.

Standard 3.6: Assist pharmacist in preparing, storing, and distributing medication products including those requiring special handling and documentation.

Standard 3.7: Assist the pharmacist in the monitoring of medication therapy.

Standard 3.11: Apply quality assurance practices to pharmaceuticals, durable and non-durable medical equipment, devices, and supplies.

Standard 3.13: Use current technology to ensure the safety and accuracy of medication dispensing.

Standard 3.31: Manage drug product inventory stored in equipment or devices used to ensure the safety and accuracy of medication dispensing.

Standard 4.1: Explain the Pharmacists' Patient Care Process and describe the role of the pharmacy technician in the patient care process.

Standard 4.2: Apply patient- and medication-safety practices in aspects of the pharmacy technician's roles.

Standard 4.7: Explain pharmacist and pharmacy technician roles in medication management services.

Standard 4.8: Describe best practices regarding quality assurance measures according to leading quality organizations.

Standard 5.1: Describe and apply state and federal laws pertaining to processing, handling, and dispensing of medications including controlled substances.

Standard 5.2: Describe state and federal laws and regulations pertaining to pharmacy technicians.

Standard 5.3: Explain that differences exist between states regarding state regulations, pertaining to pharmacy technicians, and the processing, handling, and dispensing of medications.

Standard 5.9: Participate in pharmacy compliance with professional standards and relevant legal, regulatory, formulary, contractual, and safety requirements.

REINFORCE KEY CONCEPTS

Terms and Definitions

Select the correct term from the following list and write the corresponding letter in the blank next to the statement.

A. Aphasia
B. Behind-the-counter (BTC) medications
C. Chain pharmacy
D. Dysarthria
E. Franchise
F. Nonproprietary (generic) name
G. Over-the-counter (OTC) medication
H. Proprietary (brand or trade) name
I. Sole proprietorship
J. Therapeutic alliance

_____ 1. A form of business organization in which a firm that already has a successful product or service (the franchisor) enters into a continuing contractual relationship with other businesses (franchisees) operating under the franchisor's trade name and usually with the franchisor's guidance, in exchange for a fee

_____ 2. A communication disorder that results from damage or injury to the language parts of the brain; it is more common in older adults, particularly those who have had a stroke

_____ 3. A brand name or trademark under which a drug product is marketed

_____ 4. A speech deficiency that interferes with the normal control of the speech mechanism

_____ 5. A trust relationship between a health care professional and a patient, incorporating patient perceptions of the acceptability of interventions and mutually agreed upon goals for treatment

_____ 6. Medications kept behind the pharmacy counter that require a pharmacist's intervention before dispensing to a patient; BTC medications are not considered prescription medications

_____ 7. A medication that does not require a physician's order or prescription for the patient to purchase

_____ 8. An unincorporated business owned by one person

_____ 9. A corporate-owned group of pharmacies that share a brand name and central management and usually have standardized business methods and practices

_____ 10. A short name coined for a drug or chemical that is not subject to proprietary (trademark) rights and is recommended or recognized by an official body

Select the correct term from the following list and write the corresponding letter in the blank next to the statement.

A. Auxiliary label
B. Dispense as Written (DAW) codes
C. Drug utilization evaluation (DUE)
D. e-Prescribing
E. Federal Legend
F. Inscription
G. Prescription
H. Refills
I. Repackage
J. Signatura *(signa* or *sig)*
K. Subscription
L. Superscription

_____ 11. A statement required on the labeling of all prescription medications: "Federal law prohibits dispensing without a prescription"

_____ 12. An authorized, structured, ongoing review of health care provider prescribing, pharmacist dispensing, and patient use of medication

_____ 13. The part of the prescription that provides specific instructions to the pharmacist on how to compound the prescription

_____ 14. The computer-to-computer transfer of prescription data between pharmacies, prescribers, and payers

_____ 15. To reduce the amount of medication taken from a bulk bottle

_____ 16. A numeric set of codes, created by the National Council for Prescription Drug Programs (NCPDP), that is used when filling prescriptions; they can affect reimbursement amounts from insurance companies

_____ 17. An order for medication issued by a physician, dentist, or other properly licensed practitioner, such as a physician assistant or nurse practitioner

_____ 18. The heading of a prescription, represented by the Latin symbol *Rx*, meaning "take thou" or "you take"; the symbol has come to represent prescription or pharmacy

_____ 19. The name, dosage form, strength, and quantity of the medication prescribed

_____ 20. A label that provides supplementary information about proper and safe administration, use, or storage of a medication

_____ 21. Permission by a prescriber to replenish a prescription

_____ 22. The directions on a prescription that explain how the patient is to take the prescribed medication; a Latin expression meaning to "write on label"

Select the correct term from the following list and write the corresponding letter in the blank next to the statement.

A. Adjudication
B. Bank identification number (BIN)
C. Drug Enforcement Administration (DEA) number
D. Help Desk
E. National Drug Code (NDC) number
F. National Provider Identifier (NPI)

_____ 23. A unique 10-digit identification number for covered health care providers that is issued by the Centers for Medicare and Medicaid Services

_____ 24. A six-digit number on a prescription drug card that is used for routing and identification to process a prescription claim

_____ 25. A unique 10- or 11-digit number, composed of three segments, that is assigned to a medication

_____ 26. The process by which a prescription is submitted electronically to a third-party payer for the pharmacy to be reimbursed for the medication dispensed

_____ 27. A toll-free hotline to an insurance company, available 24 hours a day, 7 days a week, so that pharmacists can call in specific questions about insurance claims and coverage and pharmacy-specific inquiries

_____ 28. An alphanumeric number consisting of two letters and seven numbers that is assigned to prescribers authorized by the DEA to prescribe controlled substances

True or False

Write T or F next to each statement.

_____ 1. The success of a community pharmacy is very dependent on the knowledge and training of its pharmacy technicians.

_____ 2. The pharmacy technician typically has the initial contact with the patient when the person drops off a new prescription or requests a refill of a prescription.

_____ 3. The Pure Food and Drug Act requires that every ambulatory pharmacy maintain patient profiles.

_____ 4. The apothecary system is the official system of measurement for weights and volumes in the United States.

_____ 5. Only the pharmacist is responsible for inputting the patient's information into the pharmacy's computer information system.

_____ 6. Submitting a prescription claim using the incorrect DAW code will not affect the pharmacy being reimbursed properly for the medication that was dispensed.

_____ 7. State laws require that patient product information (PPI) be provided to the patient when specific medications are dispensed.

_____ 8. The technician does not need to check the medication against the script and the label when selecting medication from the shelf.

_____ 9. A controlled substance inventory should be done twice yearly and when there is a change of the pharmacist-in-charge.

_____ 10. When the prescription is being picked up, the pharmacy technician will ask the patient if he or she has any questions for the pharmacist.

Multiple Choice

Complete each question by circling the best answer.

1. When taking in a prescription, neither the technician nor the pharmacist can decipher the physician's writing; therefore:
   A. The technician should guess what to fill
   B. The technician should ask the patient
   C. The pharmacist should call the physician
   D. The technician should tell the patient to go back to the doctor and get a prescription that can be read

2. Which of the following is *not* the duty of a technician upon taking in a prescription?
   A. Translating the prescription
   B. Entering information into the database
   C. Filling the prescription
   D. Providing patient consultation

3. In most states, when a new prescription is called in to the pharmacy, who can take the prescription over the phone?
   A. Pharmacy clerk
   B. Pharmacy technician
   C. Pharmacist
   D. Pharmacy custodian

4. If a prescription is for a controlled substance, the technician must make sure the prescription includes the physician's:
   A. FDA number
   B. DEA number
   C. HMO number
   D. NABP number

5. Which of the following is *not* an exception to the child-resistant container?
   A. Nitroglycerin
   B. Patient's request
   C. Oral contraceptives
   D. Technician's opinion that the patient looks too weak to open a safety lid

6. Which of the following is *not* printed on a prescription label as required by law?
   A. Address and phone number of prescriber
   B. Prescription number
   C. Drug, strength, and dosage form
   D. Refill information

7. Which of the following is *not* a common auxiliary label for NSAIDs?
   A. May cause drowsiness
   B. May cause sensitivity to light
   C. May cause dizziness
   D. Take with food

8. The pharmacy must maintain all controlled substance invoices for a minimum of:
   A. 6 months
   B. 1 year
   C. 2 years
   D. 5 years

9. Prescriptions that have a red "C" stamped on the lower right side when filed in the pharmacy indicate that the prescription is:
   A. A controlled substance
   B. A cough medication
   C. A drug containing codeine
   D. A cardiac medication

10. Pharmacy technicians must be capable of:
    A. Interpreting and transcribing prescriptions
    B. Filling prescriptions quickly and accurately
    C. Following proper billing practices
    D. All of the above

11. Most boards of pharmacy prefer to allow transfer of prescriptions only _____ time(s).
    A. one
    B. two
    C. three
    D. zero

12. If the medication has to be counted or measured:
    A. Have the pharmacist check measurements
    B. Put medication into a bottle of appropriate size
    C. Place into the refrigerator
    D. None of the above

13. Which of the following is *not* an advantage of e-prescribing?
    A. Linking information from a patient's medical file to a patient's prescription file
    B. Expediting refills
    C. Notifying the prescriber if a drug product is covered by the patient's insurance plan when the order is being generated rather than when it is presented at the pharmacy
    D. Increasing errors associated with illegible handwriting

14. Which of the following is *not* a form of nonverbal communication?
    A. Eye rolling
    B. Smiling at a customer
    C. Saying hello to each customer
    D. Crossing your arms when talking with a customer

15. A purchaser aged 16 years old or older may purchase no more than _____ of ephedrine contacting products in a 30-day period.
   A. 1 g
   B. 3.6 g
   C. 5 g
   D. 9 g

Fill in the Blanks

Answer each question by completing the statement in the space provided.

1. A _____ designates a specific medication and dosage to be administered to a particular patient at a specific time.

2. A patient profile is a tool that can assist in helping _____ medication errors.

3. The _____ symbol represents prescription and the pharmacy.

4. The _____ is responsible for reducing medication errors and drug-related illnesses.

5. Scanning prescriptions is a quality assurance tool used to _____ medication errors.

6. To prevent _____ of tablets and capsules, the counting tray should be wiped clean after each use, as powder from tablets may remain on the tray.

7. A retail pharmacy will have a locked _____ to ensure that Schedule II medications are kept secure at all times.

8. Every patient should be treated with the _____ dignity and respect.

9. Your _____ can have a direct effect on whether a pharmacy customer comes back and can also alter your image as a technician.

10. Often the pharmacy technician will record and _____ information such as diseases states, immunizations, current conditions, providers, and medications.

Matching

Match the pharmacy abbreviations with the correct meaning.

A. ac
B. SQ
C. gtts
D. ut dict
E. qd
F. as
G. tsp
H. ung
I. os
J. qid
K. stat
L. Tbsp

_____ 1. Teaspoonful

_____ 2. Left eye

_____ 3. Subcutaneously

_____ 4. Left ear

_____ 5. Immediately

_____ 6. As directed

_____ 7. Drops

_____ 8. Every day

_____ 9. Ointment

_____ 10. Before meals

_____ 11. Four times a day

_____ 12. Tablespoonful

Match the pharmacy abbreviations with the correct meaning.

A. aa
B. ad
C. prn
D. tid
E. WA
F. po
G. ou
H. bid
I. od
J. au
K. pc
L. hs

_____ 13. Both ears

_____ 14. Three times a day

_____ 15. Both eyes

_____ 16. At bedtime

_____ 17. By mouth

_____ 18. Right ear

_____ 19. As needed

_____ 20. Twice a day

_____ 21. After meals

_____ 22. Right eye

_____ 23. Of each

_____ 24. While awake

Short Answer

Write a short response to each question in the space provided.

1. List the five rights of the patient to medication safety.

   A. _____

   B. _____

   C. _____

   D. _____

   E. _____

2. List the two options for filing filled prescriptions.

   A. _____

   B. _____

3. List four different ways a new prescription can be received in a community pharmacy.

   A. _____

   B. _____

   C. _____

   D. _____

4. List the required information every prescription is required to contain.

   _____

   _____

5. List six advantages of e-prescribing.

   _____

   _____

   _____

   _____

   _____

   _____

6. List the tasks a pharmacy technician can perform to help the pharmacist focus on clinical activities and making an MTM program more sustainable.

   _____

   _____

   _____

   _____

7. Explain the importance of having durable and non-durable supplies and equipment in the community pharmacy. List five examples of durable or non-durable supplies that the community pharmacy would stock.

   _____

   _____

   _____

   _____

Research Activities

Follow the instructions given in each exercise and provide a response.

1. Access the website http://www.mckesson.com/pharmacies/pharmacies/.

   A. List one product/solution available to community pharmacies.

   B. How can this product/solution help the community pharmacy?

2. Access the website https://www.nabp.net/boards-of-pharmacy to access your state board of pharmacy website.

   A. Does your state pharmacy law allow pharmacists to administer immunizations?

   B. If so, which immunizations may a pharmacist administer in a community pharmacy setting?

   C. How can a pharmacy technician be helpful to an immunizing pharmacist in a community pharmacy setting?

3. Access the website https://www.deadiversion.usdoj.gov/21cfr_reports/.

   A. What is DEA Form 106 used for? What is the preferred method to submit this form?

   B. What is DEA Form 41 used for? What is the preferred method to submit this form?

4. Many computer systems have a labeling system. What information is printed on one sheet?

5. When labeling prescription bottles, a technician should remember professionalism. Why is this important?

REFLECT CRITICALLY

Critical Thinking

Reply to each question based on what you have learned in the chapter.

1. When you check the label against the script, for what are you checking?

2. Why would elderly patients want non–child-resistant container on their medications?

3. Why should pharmacy technicians initial any prescriptions that they fill?

6. After filling about 25 prescriptions on a very busy morning in the pharmacy, you realize that you might have made a mistake on the last one. It is time to go to lunch, so you decide to let it go, believing that the pharmacist will catch it. Unfortunately, the pharmacist checks the prescription hurriedly, trusting that you did your job correctly, and the prescription goes home with the patient.

   A. What should you have done to prevent this medication error?

   B. Whose fault is it that the prescription was dispensed as is?

   C. What can you do to remedy the situation before the patient is harmed by your mistake?

RELATE TO PRACTICE

Lab Scenarios
The Patient Profile
Objective: To familiarize the pharmacy technician with the information required for a patient profile

> The patient profile is a full list of patient prescriptions and all related information for the prescriptions including the original date of fill, refill dates, and the prescribing practitioner.
>   A complete patient profile will also include the following information:
>
> - Full name
> - Home address—number, street, city, state, and zip code
> - Telephone numbers—home, mobile, and work
> - Birth date

96

- Gender
- Allergies—drug and food
- Physical and medical conditions
- Generic preference
- Prescription insurance information—group number, member number, and relationship to the cardholder
- Non–child-resistant container preference
- List of over-the-counter medications and herbal supplements being taken

This information is used to develop a patient profile for the patient and should be reviewed for accuracy *each time* a patient fills a prescription at the pharmacy. A thorough and accurate patient profile can help eliminate possible adverse drug events and medication errors.

Lab Activity #8.1: Identify what is missing from the following patient profiles.

Equipment needed:
- Pen

Time needed to complete this activity: 30 minutes

Patient Profile 1

Patient Profile

Name: _____Sandy Smith_____

Address: _____125 N. Main Street_____

City: _____Anywhere_____ State: ____WI___ Zip code _____

Gender: ☐ M   ☒ F   Birthdate: _____

Home Ph: ___212-555-5476_____ Cell Ph: _____

Email: _____

Prescription insurance provider: __Cigna_____

ID Number: __U52428_____ Group Number: __1X854_____

Relationship to Cardholder   ☐ Self   ☒ Spouse   ☐ Child   ☐ Other

Allergies to Medications: __none_____

Medical Conditions: _____

List any OTC products, herbal supplements, or other medications: _____

_____

_____

Would you like child-resistant containers?   ☒ Yes   ☐ No

Would you like generic drugs when available?   ☒ Yes   ☐ No

What I have provided is true and correct. If my medical conditions change or if I have drug or food reaction, I will inform the pharmacy.

Signature: __*Sandy Smith*_____ Date: __*04-23-2X*_____

What is missing from this patient profile?

_____

Patient Profile 2

```
┌─────────────────────────────────────────────────────────────────────────────┐
│                              Patient Profile                                  │
│                                                                               │
│   Name:_____Andrew Rodriguez_____        │
│                                                                               │
│   Address: _____145 S 1st_____     │
│                                                                               │
│   City: _____Austin_____ State: ____TX_____ Zip code __78748___  │
│                                                                               │
│   Gender:     ☒ M        ☐ F                 Birthdate: __7-14-70_____   │
│                                                                               │
│   Home Ph: ___512-555-1154_____ Cell Ph: _____  │
│                                                                               │
│   Email: _____ │
│                                                                               │
│   Prescription insurance provider: _TXBC_____  │
│                                                                               │
│   ID Number: _____ Group Number: _____   │
│                                                                               │
│   Relationship to Cardholder   ☒ Self    ☐ Spouse   ☐ Child   ☐ Other        │
│                                                                               │
│   Allergies to Medications: _____ │
│                                                                               │
│   Medical Conditions: _____High blood pressure_____  │
│                                                                               │
│   List any OTC products, herbal supplements, or other medications: __none____ │
│                                                                               │
│   _____   │
│                                                                               │
│   _____   │
│                                                                               │
│   Would you like child-resistant containers?         ☒ Yes      ☐ No          │
│                                                                               │
│   Would you like generic drugs when available?       ☒ Yes      ☐ No          │
│                                                                               │
│   What I have provided is true and correct. If my medical conditions change   │
│   or if I have drug or food reaction, I will inform the pharmacy.             │
│                                                                               │
│   Signature: _Andrew Rodriguez_____ Date: _2-1-2X_____         │
│                                                                               │
└─────────────────────────────────────────────────────────────────────────────┘
```

What is missing from this patient profile?

_____

Patient Profile 3

Patient Profile

Name: _____

Address: _____55 North Main_____

City: _____Yonder_____ State: ____NM____ Zip code __87004_____

Gender: ☒ M ☐ F Birthdate: __6-1-82_____

Home Ph: _____ Cell Ph: ___215-555-0789_____

Email: _____

Prescription insurance provider: _____

ID Number: _____ Group Number: _____

Relationship to Cardholder ☐ Self ☐ Spouse ☐ Child ☐ Other

Allergies to Medications: ____Penicillin_____

Medical Conditions: ____none_____

List any OTC products, herbal supplements, or other medications: ___none_____

_____

_____

Would you like child-resistant containers? ☐ Yes ☐ No

Would you like generic drugs when available? ☐ Yes ☐ No

What I have provided is true and correct. If my medical conditions change or if I have drug or food reaction, I will inform the pharmacy.

Signature: _____ Date: ___1-4-2X_____

What is missing from this patient profile?

_____

Patient Profile 4

Patient Profile

Name: _____ Megan Morris _____

Address: _____ 8978 West Parkway _____

City: _____ Park _____ State: _____ NY _____ Zip code ___ 17352 _____

Gender: ☐ M   ☒ F   Birthdate: _____

Home Ph: _____ Cell Ph: _____ 212-555-8952 _____

Email: _____

Prescription insurance provider: _____ BCBS _____

ID Number: ____ Y5238 _____ Group Number: ____ 52138 _____

Relationship to Cardholder   ☐ Self   ☐ Spouse   ☒ Child   ☐ Other

Allergies to Medications: _____ none _____

Medical Conditions: _____ none _____

List any OTC products, herbal supplements, or other medications: _____

_____

_____

Would you like child-resistant containers?   ☒ Yes   ☐ No

Would you like generic drugs when available?   ☐ Yes   ☐ No

What I have provided is true and correct. If my medical conditions change or if I have drug or food reaction,
I will inform the pharmacy.

Signature: _Megan Morris_____ Date: _8-14-2X_____

What is missing from this patient profile?

_____

Patient Profile 5

Patient Profile

Name: _____ David Castro _____

Address: _____ 9634 East 29th Ave _____

City: _____ Park City _____ State: ___ UT ___ Zip code __ 84060 _____

Gender: ☒ M ☐ F Birthdate: _____

Home Ph: _____ Cell Ph: _____

Email: _____

Prescription insurance provider: __ BCBS _____

ID Number: _____ Group Number: _____

Relationship to Cardholder ☒ Self ☐ Spouse ☐ Child ☐ Other

Allergies to Medications: ___ Sulfa _____

Medical Conditions: ___ none _____

List any OTC products, herbal supplements, or other medications: _____

_____

_____

Would you like child-resistant containers? ☒ Yes ☐ No

Would you like generic drugs when available? ☒ Yes ☐ No

What I have provided is true and correct. If my medical conditions change or if I have drug or food reaction, I will inform the pharmacy.

Signature: _____ Date: _____

What is missing from this patient profile?

_____

Patient Profile 6

Patient Profile

Name: _____ Minh Nguyen _____

Address: _____ 5247 Train Ave _____

City: _____ Railroad _____ State: ____ OK ____ Zip code ___ 73002 _____

Gender: ☐ M   ☐ F   Birthdate: _____

Home Ph: _____ Cell Ph: ___ 405-555-8474 _____

Email: _____ mnguyen@email.com _____

Prescription insurance provider: ___ Aetna _____

ID Number: ___ T854569 _____ Group Number: ___ 03289 _____

Relationship to Cardholder   ☒ Self   ☒ Spouse   ☐ Child   ☐ Other

Allergies to Medications: ___ Biaxin _____

Medical Conditions: _____

List any OTC products, herbal supplements, or other medications: ___ none _____

_____

_____

Would you like child-resistant containers?   ☒ Yes   ☐ No

Would you like generic drugs when available?   ☒ Yes   ☐ No

What I have provided is true and correct. If my medical conditions change or if I have drug or food reaction, I will inform the pharmacy.

Signature: _____ *Minh Nguyen* _____ Date: _____ 9-19-2X _____

What is missing from this patient profile?

_____

Patient Profile 7

Patient Profile

Name: _____ Brian Navarro _____

Address: _____ 2367 Treetop Drive _____

City: _____ Forrest City _____ State: _____ AR _____ Zip code _____ 72335 _____

Gender: ☐ M ☐ F Birthdate: _____

Home Ph: _____ 870-555-7458 _____ Cell Ph: _____ 870-555-2147 _____

Email: _____ brian.navarro@email.net _____

Prescription insurance provider: _____ Cigna _____

ID Number: _____ U85469 _____ Group Number: _____ 20135 _____

Relationship to Cardholder ☒ Self ☐ Spouse ☐ Child ☐ Other

Allergies to Medications: _____ Codeine _____

Medical Conditions: _____

List any OTC products, herbal supplements, or other medications: _____ St. John's Wort _____

Would you like child-resistant containers? ☒ Yes ☒ No

Would you like generic drugs when available? ☒ Yes ☐ No

What I have provided is true and correct. If my medical conditions change or if I have drug or food reaction, I will inform the pharmacy.

Signature: _____ Brian Navarro _____ Date: _____ 5-2-2X _____

What is missing from this patient profile?

_____

Patient Profile 8

Patient Profile

Name: _____ Danielle Davila _____

Address: _____ 7156 Long Road _____

City: _____ Long Beach _____ State: ____ NY ____ Zip code ___ 11561 _____

Gender: ☐ M ☒ F Birthdate: __ 4-23-85 _____

Home Ph: __ 512-555-5871 _____ Cell Ph: ____ 516-555-1934 _____

Email: _____ d.davila@email.com _____

Prescription insurance provider: ___ Caremark _____

ID Number: ___ X13570 _____ Group Number: ___ 87014 _____

Relationship to Cardholder ☐ Self ☒ Spouse ☐ Child ☐ Other

Allergies to Medications: ___ none _____

Medical Conditions: ___ none _____

List any OTC products, herbal supplements, or other medications: ___ Claritin _____

_____

_____

Would you like child-resistant containers? ☒ Yes ☐ No

Would you like generic drugs when available? ☒ Yes ☐ No

What I have provided is true and correct. If my medical conditions change or if I have drug or food reaction, I will inform the pharmacy.

Signature: ___ *Danielle Davila* _____ Date: _____ 3-18-2X _____

What is missing from this patient profile?

_____

Patient Profile 9

Patient Profile

Name: _____ Mary Nu _____

Address: _____

City: _____ State: _____ Zip code _____

Gender: ☐ M   ☒ F   Birthdate: __11-12-65_____

Home Ph: _____ Cell Ph: ___505-555-0231_____

Email: _____

Prescription insurance provider: ___Express Scripts_____

ID Number: ___T14320_____ Group Number: ___019732_____

Relationship to Cardholder   ☒ Self   ☐ Spouse   ☐ Child   ☐ Other

Allergies to Medications: ___none_____

Medical Conditions: ___diabetes_____

List any OTC products, herbal supplements, or other medications: ___cinnamon capsules_____

_____

_____

Would you like child-resistant containers?   ☒ Yes   ☐ No

Would you like generic drugs when available?   ☒ Yes   ☐ No

What I have provided is true and correct. If my medical conditions change or if I have drug or food reaction, I will inform the pharmacy.

Signature: _Mary Nu_____ Date: ___9-8-2X_____

What is missing from this patient profile?

_____

Patient Profile 10

Patient Profile

Name: _____Nikki_____

Address: _____321 Lane Street_____

City: _____ State: _____ Zip code _____

Gender: ☐ M   ☒ F   Birthdate: __4-21-77_____

Home Ph: _____ Cell Ph: ___854-555-0354_____

Email: _____Nikki30@email.net_____

Prescription insurance provider: ___Meridian Rx_____

ID Number: ___Z46217_____ Group Number: ___013978_____

Relationship to Cardholder   ☐ Self   ☒ Spouse   ☐ Child   ☐ Other

Allergies to Medications: ___Tylenol_____

Medical Conditions: ___none_____

List any OTC products, herbal supplements, or other medications: ___Vitamin D_____

_____

_____

Would you like child-resistant containers?   ☒ Yes   ☐ No

Would you like generic drugs when available?   ☐ Yes   ☒ No

What I have provided is true and correct. If my medical conditions change or if I have drug or food reaction, I will inform the pharmacy.

Signature: ___Nikki_____ Date: ____8-17-2X_____

What is missing from this patient profile?

_____

The Prescription

Objective: To familiarize the pharmacy technician with the information required in a legal prescription

Every day, retail pharmacies receive prescriptions for patients. A prescription is an order for a specific medication prescribed by a physician or other health care professional, such as a physician assistant or a nurse practitioner, who is permitted by state law to prescribe medications. Each prescription must contain specific information if the pharmacy is to fill the order.

Information required on a prescription includes the following:

- Prescriber information: Name, office address, office telephone number, NPI number, and DEA number if the prescription is a controlled substance
- Patient information: Patient's complete name, birth date, and home address. A pharmacy will attempt to obtain a telephone number for the patient.
- Date: The date on which the prescription was written. This date may be different from the date the prescription is filled.
- Rx symbol: A symbol for a Latin word meaning "recipe" or "take this drug"
- Inscription: Medication prescribed, which may be listed under the brand or generic name, and the strength and quantity of the drug to be dispensed
- Subscription: Instructions to the pharmacist on dispensing the medication
- Signa (sig): Directions for the patient to follow
- Additional filling information, such as refills permitted or generic substitution
- Prescriber's signature

Lab Activity #8.2: Identify what is missing from the following prescriptions.

Equipment needed:
- Pencil/pen

Time needed to complete this activity: 30 minutes

1. Rx 1:

```
                    Dr. Stephanie Hernandez
                    1313 Main Blvd, Suite B10
                    Arlington, VA 22209
                    703-936-8087
                    DEA FH4567890

Brian Waters                                    August 3, 202X


Rx      Amoxicillin 500 mg   #30
        1 cap po tid

Ref x 1                        Dr. Stephanie Hernandez
```

What is missing on this prescription?

_____

2. Rx 2:

```
                    Dr. Andrew A. Sheen
                    1313 Main Blvd, Suite B10
                    Arlington, VA 22209
                    703-936-8087
                    DEA FS1234563

Brian Waters                                    July 2, 202X
4433 Simon Blvd, Apt 321, Arlington, VA 22209

Rx      Ibuprofen 400 mg      #30
        1 tab po tid prn back pain

Ref x 2
```

What is missing on this prescription?

_____

3. Rx 3:

```
                    Dr. Stephanie Hernandez
                    1313 Main Blvd, Suite B10
                    Arlington, VA 22209
                    703-936-8087
                    DEA FH4567890

Brian Waters
4433 Simon Blvd, Apt 321, Arlington, VA 22209

Rx      Z-pak  #6
        2 tabs po stat, then 1 tab po qd x 4 days

Ref x 1                        Dr. Stephanie Hernandez
```

What is missing on this prescription?

_____

4. Rx 4:

```
                    Dr. Stephanie Hernandez
                    1313 Main Blvd, Suite B10
                    Arlington, VA 22209
                    703-936-8087
                    DEA FH4567890

Brian Waters                                    May 20, 202X
4433 Simon Blvd, Apt 321, Arlington, VA 22209

Rx      Nizoral Cream
        Apply to the affected rash on arm twice a day

Ref x 1                        Dr. Stephanie Hernandez
```

What is missing on this prescription?

_____

5. Rx 5:

```
              Dr. Andrew A. Sheen
              1313 Main Blvd, Suite B10
              Arlington, VA 22209
              703-936-8087

Brian Waters                                    March 15, 202X
4433 Simon Blvd, Apt 321, Arlington, VA 22209

Rx     Carisoprodol 350 mg        #30
       1 tab po tid prn pain

Ref x 1                            Dr. Andrew Sheen
```

What is missing on this prescription?

_____

6. Rx 6:

```
              Dr. Andrew A. Sheen
              1313 Main Blvd, Suite B10
              Arlington, VA 22209
              703-936-8087
              DEA FS1234563

Brian Waters                                    October 5, 202X
4433 Simon Blvd, Apt 321, Arlington, VA 22209

Rx     Flexeril        #30
       1 tab po tid prn muscle spasms

Ref x 1                            Dr. Andrew Sheen
```

What is missing on this prescription?

_____

7. Rx 7:

```
              Dr. Stephanie Hernandez
              1313 Main Blvd, Suite B10
              Arlington, VA 22209
              703-936-8087
              DEA FH4567890

Brian Waters                                    April 14, 202X
4433 Simon Blvd, Apt 321, Arlington, VA 22209

Rx     Xalantan eye drops    1 bottle
       UD

Ref x 1                            Dr. Stephanie Hernandez
```

What is missing on this prescription?

_____

8. Rx 8:

```
              Dr. Andrew A. Sheen
              1313 Main Blvd, Suite B10
              Arlington, VA 22209
              703-936-8087
              DEA FS1234563

Brian Waters                                    June 23, 202X
4433 Simon Blvd, Apt 321, Arlington, VA 22209

Rx     Synthroid         #30
       1 tab po qd

Ref x 6                            Dr. Andrew Sheen
```

What is missing on this prescription?

_____

9. Rx 9:

```
              Dr. Stephanie Hernandez
              1313 Main Blvd, Suite B10
              Arlington, VA 22209
              703-936-8087
              DEA FH4567890

                                                December 12, 202X
4433 Simon Blvd, Apt 321, Arlington, VA 22209

Rx     Xanax 0.5 mg      #60
       1 tab po tid prn anxiety

Ref x 5                            Dr. Stephanie Hernandez
```

What is missing on this prescription?

_____

10. Rx 10:

```
              Dr. Andrew A. Sheen
              1313 Main Blvd, Suite B10
              Arlington, VA 22209
              703-936-8087
              DEA FS1234563

Brian Waters                                    November 13, 202X
4433 Simon Blvd, Apt 321, Arlington, VA 22209

Rx     Coreg
       1 tab po tid

Ref x 1                            Dr. Andrew Sheen
```

What is missing on this prescription?

_____

Lab Activity #8.3: Review the following DEA numbers and determine whether each is valid. If a number is not a valid DEA number, explain why.

Equipment needed:
- Pencil/pen
- Calculator

Time needed to complete this activity: 15 minutes

1. Dr. Andrew Shedlock   AS123987

_____

2. Dr. William Dagit   BD7643219

_____

3. Dr. Jerry Kraisinger   JK1234563

_____

4. Dr. Richard Kunze   RK5555555

_____

5. Dr. Bruce Fisher   BF1236579

_____

6. Dr. Clark Andersen   FD4596328

_____

Interpreting a Prescription

Objective: To properly identify the specific information that must be entered into a pharmacy's computer for processing and reimbursement for the prescription.

In a community pharmacy setting, the pharmacy technician may be asked to enter the information from the prescription into the pharmacy's computer (information) system. The computer system prompts the technician to enter information in a particular sequence. Although each organization's system is unique, the information requested is the same.

The technician will be asked to enter the quantity of the medication being dispensed in metric terms, unless it is just the number of tablets or capsules. If an ointment or cream is prescribed, it will be dispensed in grams; if a liquid is prescribed, it will be dispensed in milliliters.

The days' supply can be calculated by dividing the quantity dispensed by the total amount taken during the day.

The prescriber must indicate the number of refills permitted on the prescription. If no refills are indicated, the technician would indicate "0." Some physicians may indicate "prn" refills on a prescription. Depending on state board of pharmacy regulations, most states will permit a "prn" refill to be valid for 1 year from the date the prescription is written.

The pharmacy technician will be required to select the appropriate DAW code. Before selecting the DAW code, the pharmacy technician must determine whether the prescriber will permit a generic drug to be dispensed. A pharmacy will dispense a generic medication unless the physician writes in his or her own handwriting one of the following: "Brand Name Medically Necessary," "Dispense as Written," or "DAW." Most state boards of pharmacy no longer recognize the checking of boxes to indicate whether a generic can be dispensed. If in doubt, refer to your state board of pharmacy's regulations involving generic substitution.

The following are approved DAW codes:

DAW 0: no product selection indicated
DAW 1: substitution not allowed by provider
DAW 2: substitution allowed: patient requested product dispensed
DAW 3: substitution allowed: pharmacist selected product dispensed
DAW 4: substitution allowed: generic drug not in stock
DAW 5: substitution allowed: brand drug dispensed as generic
DAW 6: override
DAW 7: substitution not allowed: brand drug mandated by law
DAW 8: substitution allowed: generic drug not available in marketplace
DAW 9: other

If a pharmacy technician selects the incorrect DAW code, the pharmacy may not be properly reimbursed by a third-party provider.

Lab Activity #8.4: Answer the questions based on the prescription orders for each question.

Equipment needed:
- *Physicians' Desk Reference* or *Drug Facts and Comparisons*
- Pencil/pen
- Calculator

Time needed to complete this activity: 45 minutes

1. Rx 1:
   Augmentin 250 mg #30
   1 tab PO tid with yogurt
   Ref ×1

   A. How much will be dispensed?

   _____

   B. How many days will the medication last?

   _____

   C. How many refills are permitted on the prescription?

   _____

   D. What DAW code will be used?

   _____

   E. Write the directions as they would appear on the medication label.

   _____

   _____

   _____

   F. What auxiliary label(s) should be affixed to the medication label?

   _____

   _____

2. Rx 2:
   Cefdinir 250 mg/tsp
   300 mg PO q12h × 10d
   Ref ×0

   A. How much should be dispensed (use metric quantity)?

   _____

   B. How many days will the medication last?

   _____

   C. How many refills are permitted on the prescription?

   _____

   D. What DAW code will be used?

   _____

   E. Write the directions as they would appear on the medication label.

   _____

   _____

   _____

   F. What auxiliary label(s) should be affixed to the medication label?

   _____

   _____

3. Rx 3:
   Zithromax 250 mg #6
   2 caps PO stat, then 1 cap qd × 4 days

   A. How much will be dispensed?

   _____

   B. How many days will the medication last?

   _____

   C. How many refills are permitted on the prescription?

   _____

   D. What DAW code will be used?

   _____

   E. Write the directions as they would appear on the medication label.

   _____

   _____

   _____

110

F. What auxiliary label(s) should be affixed to the medication label?

_____

_____

4. Rx 4:

Vigamox Opth Soln 3 mL
gtt i ou tid × 7 days
Ref × 0

A. How much will be dispensed (use metric quantities)?

_____

B. How many days will the medication last?

_____

C. How many refills are permitted on the prescription?

_____

D. What DAW code will be used?

_____

E. Write the directions as they would appear on the medication label.

_____

_____

_____

F. What auxiliary label(s) should be affixed to the medication label?

_____

_____

5. Rx 5:

Zocor 40 mg, 1-month supply
1 tab PO qd
Ref × 6

A. How much will be dispensed?

_____

B. How many days will the medication last?

_____

C. How many refills are permitted on the prescription?

_____

D. What DAW code will be used?

_____

E. Write the directions as they would appear on the medication label.

_____

_____

_____

F. What auxiliary label(s) should be affixed to the medication label?

_____

_____

6. Rx 6:

Tylenol #3, Dispense 30 tablets (Hint: Controlled Substance Schedule III)
1–2 tab PO q4–6h prn pain
Ref × one

A. How much will be dispensed?

_____

B. How many days will the medication last?

_____

C. How many refills are permitted on the prescription?

_____

D. What DAW code will be used?

_____

E. Write the directions as they would appear on the medication label.

_____

_____

_____

111

F. What auxiliary label(s) should be affixed to the medication label?

_____

_____

7. Rx 7:
   Flonase Nasal Spray, 16 g bottle (120 sprays)
   2 spr to each nost bid
   Ref × 6

   A. How much will be dispensed (use metric quantities)?

   _____

   B. How many days will the medication last?

   _____

   C. How many refills are permitted on the prescription?

   _____

   D. What DAW code will be used?

   _____

   E. Write the directions as they would appear on the medication label.

   _____

   _____

   _____

   F. What auxiliary label(s) should be affixed to the medication label?

   _____

   _____

8. Rx 8:
   Viscous Xylocaine 100 mL
   1 tsp PO swish and spit qid

   A. How much will be dispensed (use metric quantities)?

   _____

   B. How many days will the medication last?

   _____

C. How many refills are permitted on the prescription?

_____

D. What DAW code will be used?

_____

E. Write the directions as they would appear on the medication label.

_____

_____

_____

F. What auxiliary label(s) should be affixed to the medication label?

_____

_____

9. Rx 9:
   Lodine 200 mg #14
   1 tab PO bid c food

   A. How much will be dispensed?

   _____

   B. How many days will the medication last?

   _____

   C. How many refills are permitted on the prescription?

   _____

   D. What DAW code will be used?

   _____

   E. Write the directions as they would appear on the medication label.

   _____

   _____

   _____

   F. What auxiliary label(s) should be affixed to the medication label?

   _____

   _____

10. Rx 10:
Prednisone 5 mg
ii tab PO qd × 5 d; i tab qd × 5 d. Take with milk.

A. How much will be dispensed?

_____

B. How many days will the medication last?

_____

C. How many refills are permitted on the prescription?

_____

D. What DAW code will be used?

_____

E. Write the directions as they would appear on the medication label.

_____

_____

_____

F. What auxiliary label(s) should be affixed to the medication label?

_____

_____

11. Rx 11:
Terazol 3 Vag supp 1 box of 3
1 supp pv q hs
Ref ×1

A. How much will be dispensed?

_____

B. How many days will the medication last?

_____

C. How many refills are permitted on the prescription?

_____

D. What DAW code will be used?

_____

E. Write the directions as they would appear on the medication label.

_____

_____

_____

F. What auxiliary label(s) should be affixed to the medication label?

_____

_____

12. Rx 12:
Sporanox 200 mg #7
1 cap PO qd c food for 7 d, skip 21 d and resume
Ref × 6

A. How much will be dispensed?

_____

B. How many days will the medication last?

_____

C. How many refills are permitted on the prescription?

_____

D. What DAW code will be used?

_____

E. Write the directions as they would appear on the medication label.

_____

_____

_____

F. What auxiliary label(s) should be affixed to the medication label?

_____

_____

13. Rx 13:
    Flagyl 250 mg 14-day supply
    1 tab PO qid for patient for 14 days. No alcohol.
    Brand name medically necessary

    A. How much will be dispensed?

    _____

    B. How many days will the medication last?

    _____

    C. How many refills are permitted on the prescription?

    _____

    D. What DAW code will be used?

    _____

    E. Write the directions as they would appear on the medication label.

    _____

    _____

    F. What auxiliary label(s) should be affixed to the medication label?

    _____

    _____

14. Rx 14:
    Xopenex HFA Inhaler (200 sprays) #ii inhalers
    1-2 inhalations q4–6h prn asthma and 15 min before exercise
    Ref × 6

    A. How much will be dispensed?

    _____

    B. How many days will the medication last?

    _____

    C. How many refills are permitted on the prescription?

    _____

    D. What DAW code will be used?

    _____

E. Write the directions as they would appear on the medication label.

    _____

    _____

    _____

F. What auxiliary label(s) should be affixed to the medication label?

    _____

    _____

15. Rx 15:
    Coumadin 5 mg #45
    1 tab PO odd numbered days, 2 tab PO even numbered days
    DAW
    Ref prn

    A. How much will be dispensed?

    _____

    B. How many days will the medication last?

    _____

    C. How many refills are permitted on the prescription?

    _____

    D. What DAW code will be used?

    _____

    E. Write the directions as they would appear on the medication label.

    _____

    _____

    _____

    F. What auxiliary label(s) should be affixed to the medication label?

    _____

    _____

16. Rx 16:
    Dilantin 100 mg #120
    1 cap PO qid ac and hs
    Dispense as written
    Ref × 6

    A. How much will be dispensed?

    _____

    B. How many days will the medication last?

    _____

    C. How many refills are permitted on the prescription?

    _____

    D. What DAW code will be used?

    _____

    E. Write the directions as they would appear on the medication label.

    _____

    _____

    _____

    F. What auxiliary label(s) should be affixed to the medication label?

    _____

    _____

17. Rx 17:
    Synthroid 0.1 mg #30
    1 tab PO qd
    Brand name medically necessary
    Ref × 3

    A. How much will be dispensed?

    _____

    B. How many days will the medication last?

    _____

    C. How many refills are permitted on the prescription?

    _____

    D. What DAW code will be used?

    _____

E. Write the directions as they would appear on the medication label.

    _____

    _____

    _____

F. What auxiliary label(s) should be affixed to the medication label?

    _____

    _____

18. Rx 18:
    Zoloft 100 mg #30
    1 tab PO q am
    Ref × 3

    A. How much will be dispensed?

    _____

    B. How many days will the medication last?

    _____

    C. How many refills are permitted on the prescription?

    _____

    D. What DAW code will be used?

    _____

    E. Write the directions as they would appear on the medication label.

    _____

    _____

    _____

    F. What auxiliary label(s) should be affixed to the medication label?

    _____

    _____

19. Rx 19:
    Zovirax 200 mg #25
    1 cap PO q4h (5 times per day)
    Ref × 2

    A. How much will be dispensed?

    _____

    B. How many days will the medication last?

    _____

    C. How many refills are permitted on the prescription?

    _____

    D. What DAW code will be used?

    _____

    E. Write the directions as they would appear on the medication label.

    _____

    _____

    _____

    F. What auxiliary label(s) should be affixed to the medication label?

    _____

    _____

20. Rx 20:
    Cheratussin AC, Disp 4 floz
    1 tsp PO q6h prn cough
    Ref × 0

    A. How much will be dispensed (use metric quantities)?

    _____

    B. How many days will the medication last?

    _____

    C. How many refills are permitted on the prescription?

    _____

    D. What DAW code will be used?

    _____

E. Write the directions as they would appear on the medication label.

    _____

    _____

F. What auxiliary labels should be affixed to the medication label?

    _____

    _____

Reviewing the Prescription

Objective: To demonstrate the importance of multiple checks during the prescription filling process.

> During the prescription filling process, a pharmacy technician should check the prescription at least three times.

Lab Activity #8.5: Identify the error that appears on the prescription label.

Equipment needed:
- Pencil/pen
- List of pharmacy abbreviations

Time needed to complete this activity: 45 minutes

1. Rx 1:

Dr. Andrew A. Sheen	
1313 Main Blvd, Suite B10	
Arlington, VA 22209	
703-936-8087	
DEA FS1234563	

Brian Waters   January 12, 202X
4433 Simon Blvd, Apt 321, Arlington, VA 22209
DOB 12/2/1956

Rx   Cymbalta 60 mg   #30
        1 cap po qd

Ref x 1   Dr. Andrew Sheen

Prescription label:

Your Friendly Pharmacy
1234 Park Avenue
Arlington, VA 22209
703-243-0036; Fax 703-243-0037

Rx 1001   Date 1/13/202X
Brian Waters   Dr. Hernandez
DOB: 12/2/1956
4433 Simon Blvd, Apt 321, Arlington, VA 22209
Duloxetine 60mg DR Capsule   #30
Take one capsule by mouth four times a day.
Refills: 1

Identify the error on the prescription label and indicate how it should be corrected.

_____

_____

_____

2. Rx 2:

Dr. Andrew A. Sheen
1313 Main Blvd, Suite B10
Arlington, VA 22209
703-936-8087
DEA FS1234563

Brian Waters   January 12, 202X
4433 Simon Blvd, Apt 321, Arlington, VA 22209
DOB: 12/2/1956

Rx   Warfarin   5 mg   #60
        1 tab po bid

Ref x 3   Dr. Andrew Sheen

Prescription label:

Your Friendly Pharmacy
1234 Park Avenue
Arlington, VA 22209
703-243-0036; Fax 703-243-0037

Rx 1002
Brian Waters   Dr. Sheen
DOB: 12/2/1956

4433 Simon Blvd, Apt 321, Arlington, VA 22209
Warfarin   5 mg   #60
Take one tablet by mouth two times a day.
Refills: 0

Identify the error on the prescription label and indicate how it should be corrected.

_____

_____

_____

3. Rx 3:

Dr. Stephanie Hernandez
1313 Main Blvd, Suite B10
Arlington, VA 22209
703-936-8087
DEA FH4567890

Brian Waters   January 12, 202X
4433 Simon Blvd, Apt 321, Arlington, VA 22209
DOB: 12/2/1956

Rx   Lipitor   10 mg   #30
        1 tab po with evening meal

Ref x 5   Dr. Stephanie Hernandez

Prescription label:

Your Friendly Pharmacy
1234 Park Avenue
Arlington, VA 22209
703-243-0036; Fax 703-243-0037

Rx 1003   Date 1/13/202X
Brian Waters   Dr. Sheen
DOB: 12/2/1956

4433 Simon Blvd, Apt 321, Arlington, VA 22209
Atorvastatin   10 mg   #60
Take one tablet by mouth with evening meal

Refills: 3

Identify the error on the prescription label and indicate how it should be corrected.

_____

_____

_____

4. Rx 4:

Dr. Stephanie Hernandez
1313 Main Blvd, Suite B10
Arlington, VA 22209
703-936-8087
DEA FH4567890

Brian Waters   January 12, 202X
4433 Simon Blvd, Apt 321, Arlington, VA 22209
DOB: 12/2/1956

Rx   Lasix   40 mg   #30
        1 tab po q am

Ref x 11   Dr. Stephanie Hernandez

Prescription label:

Your Friendly Pharmacy
1234 Park Avenue
Arlington, VA 22209
703-243-0036; Fax 703-243-0037

Rx 1004   Date 1/13/202X
Brian Waters   Dr. Sheen
DOB: 12/2/1956

4433 Simon Blvd, Apt 321, Arlington, VA 22209
Furosemide 40 mg   #30
Take one tablet by mouth every morning.
Refills: 10

Identify the error on the prescription label and indicate how it should be corrected.

_____

_____

_____

5. Rx 5:

Dr. Andrew A. Sheen
1313 Main Blvd, Suite B10
Arlington, VA 22209
703-936-8087
DEA FS1234563

Brian Waters   January 12, 202X
4433 Simon Blvd, Apt 321, Arlington, VA 22209
DOB: 12/2/56

Rx   Cephalexin   500 mg   #30
        1 cap po tid

Ref x 0   Dr. Andrew Sheen

Prescription label:

Your Friendly Pharmacy
1234 Park Avenue
Arlington, VA 22209
703-243-0036; Fax 703-243-0037

Rx 1005   Date 1/13/202X
Brian Waters   Dr. Hernandez
DOB: 10/18/1990

4433 Simon Blvd, Apt 321, Arlington, VA 22209
Cephalexin   500 mg   #30
Take one capsule by mouth three times a day.
Refills: 1

Identify the error on the prescription label and indicate how it should be corrected.

_____

_____

_____

117

6. Rx 6:

```
                    Dr. Andrew A. Sheen
                   1313 Main Blvd, Suite B10
                    Arlington, VA 22209
                       703-936-8087
                      DEA FS1234563

Brian Waters                                    January 12, 202X
4433 Simon Blvd, Apt 321, Arlington, VA 22209
DOB: 12/2/1956

  Rx    ProAir HFA inhaler    17 g          #1
          1 spray to each nost q 4-6 hr prn asthma

  Ref x 11                              Dr. Andrew Sheen
```

Prescription label:

```
                    Your Friendly Pharmacy
                      1234 Park Avenue
                     Arlington, VA 22209
                703-243-0036; Fax 703-243-0037

Rx 1006                        Date 1/13/202X
Brian Waters                       Dr. Shedlock
DOB: 12/2/1956

4433 Simon Blvd, Apt 321, Arlington, VA 22209
ProAir HFA Inhaler  17 g                    #1
One spray to one nostril every 6-8 hours as needed for asthma.

Refills: 11
```

Identify the error on the prescription label and indicate how it should be corrected.

_____

_____

_____

7. Rx 7:

```
                    Dr. Stephanie Hernandez
                    1313 Main Blvd, Suite B10
                     Arlington, VA 22209
                        703-936-8087
                       DEA FH4567890

Brian Waters                                    January 12, 202X
4433 Simon Blvd, Apt 321, Arlington, VA 22209
DOB: 12/2/1956

  Rx    Hydrocortisone 25mg  Supp          #12
          1 supp pr q 12 hr

  Ref x 1                            Dr. Stephanie Hernandez
```

Prescription label:

```
                    Your Friendly Pharmacy
                      1234 Park Avenue
                     Arlington, VA 22209
                703-243-0036; Fax 703-243-0037

Rx 1007                        Date 1/13/202X
Brian Waters                       Dr. Sheen
DOB: 12/2/1956

4433 Simon Blvd, Apt 321, Arlington, VA 22209
Hydrocortisone 25mg Supp                    #12
Take one suppository by mouth every 12 hours.

Refills: 1
```

Identify the error on the prescription label and indicate how it should be corrected.

_____

_____

_____

8. Rx 8:

```
                    Dr. Andrew A. Sheen
                   1313 Main Blvd, Suite B10
                    Arlington, VA 22209
                       703-936-8087
                      DEA FS1234563

Brian Waters                                    January 12, 202X
4433 Simon Blvd, Apt 321, Arlington, VA 22209
DOB: 12/2/1956

  Rx    Levothyroxine       0.1 mg        #30
          1 tab po q am

  Ref x 5                              Dr. Andrew Sheen
```

Prescription label:

```
                    Your Friendly Pharmacy
                      1234 Park Avenue
                     Arlington, VA 22209
                703-243-0036; Fax 703-243-0037

Rx 1008                        Date 1/13/202X
Brian Waters                       Dr. Shedlock
DOB: 12/2/1956

4433 Simon Blvd, Apt 321, Arlington, VA 22209
Levothyroxine   0.1 mg                      #30
1 tab po q am.

Refills: 5
```

Identify the error on the prescription label and indicate how it should be corrected.

_____

_____

_____

9. Rx 9:

```
                    Dr. Stephanie Hernandez
                    1313 Main Blvd, Suite B10
                     Arlington, VA 22209
                        703-936-8087
                       DEA FH4567890

Brian Waters                                    January 12, 202X
4433 Simon Blvd, Apt 321, Arlington, VA 22209
DOB: 12/2/1956

  Rx    Nitrostat     1/150 gr     #25
          1 tab sl prn angina attack, may repeat every 5 minutes up to 3 doses per attack

  Ref x prn                            Dr. Stephanie Hernandez
```

Prescription label:

```
                    Your Friendly Pharmacy
                      1234 Park Avenue
                     Arlington, VA 22209
                703-243-0036; Fax 703-243-0037

Rx 1009                        12/13/202X
Brian Waters                       Dr. Hernandez
DOB: 12/2/1956

4433 Simon Blvd, Apt 321, Arlington, VA 22209
Nitrostat         1/150               #25
Take one tablet by mouth as needed for angina attack; may repeat every 5 minutes up to 3 doses per attack.

Refills: prn
```

Identify the error on the prescription label and indicate how it should be corrected.

_____

_____

_____

10. Rx 10:

```
                    Dr. Stephanie Hernandez
                      1313 Main Blvd, Suite B10
                         Arlington, VA 22209
                            703-936-8087
                           DEA FH4567890
Brian Waters                                        January 12, 202X
4433 Simon Blvd, Apt 321, Arlington, VA 22209
DOB: 12/2/1956

Rx     Alprazolam 1 mg                #90
          1 tab po q 8 hr prn anxiety

Ref x 2                              Dr. Stephanie Hernandez
```

Prescription label:

```
                    Your Friendly Pharmacy
                       1234 Park Avenue
                       Arlington, VA 22209
                703-243-0036; Fax 703-243-0037

Rx 1010                          Date 8/3/202X
Brian Waters
DOB: 12/2/1956

4433 Simon Blvd, Apt 321, Arlington, VA 22209
Alprazolam      1 mg                #90
Take one tablet by mouth three times a day as needed for anxiety.

Refills: 2
```

Identify the error on the prescription label and indicate how it should be corrected.

_____

_____

_____

Customer Service

Objective: To emphasize the importance of customer service in the practice of pharmacy

The pharmacist and the pharmacy technician assist patients in their treatment. During their interaction with the patient, it is vital that they listen carefully to the patient. They must be able to explain things to the patient in words the patient can understand. In addition to the words that are used, the pharmacist and the pharmacy technician must be aware of their body language and what it conveys to the patient. Empathy should be conveyed to the patient.

Customer service issues occur every day. Many of these issues could have been avoided if the customer had been acknowledged in a timely manner and treated properly. Common complaints by the patient include the wait time for a prescription to be processed, being out of stock of a medication, and issues caused through billing of their prescription to their third-party prescription carrier. A pharmacy technician must be able to assist in finding solutions to problems that arise in the practice of pharmacy.

Lab Activity #8.6: Read each of the following scenarios. Explain how you would resolve the issue and why you made that decision.

Equipment needed:
- Paper
- Pencil/pen

Time needed to complete this activity: 45 minutes

1. Kathy Kraisinger brings her empty prescription bottle of hydrochlorothiazide 5 mg into the pharmacy for a refill on Saturday afternoon at 4 PM. No refills are indicated on the bottle. You call the physician's office for a refill, but the office has closed for the day and will not reopen until Monday morning at 8 AM. What will you do and why?

_____

_____

_____

_____

2. Bill Kunze is picking up his prescription at Preston's Pharmacy. The pharmacy technician notices that a prescription for Bill's wife has been filled and is in the prescription bins. What will you do and why?

_____

_____

_____

_____

3. A patient comes to the pharmacy counter and asks you where they can find a bottle of ibuprofen to purchase. What will you do and why?

_____

_____

_____

_____

4. What will you say when you are answering the pharmacy's telephone?

_____

_____

_____

_____

5. A patient comes to the pharmacy and asks you to recommend an allergy medication. What would you do and why?

_____

_____

_____

_____

6. You are the only pharmacy technician working with the pharmacist today. The pharmacist has asked you to accept patients' prescriptions at the drug counter. A patient approaches the drug counter at the same time the telephone begins to ring. How will you handle this situation?

_____

_____

_____

_____

7. A patient brings in a new prescription to be filled at the pharmacy. When you ask the patient for their address and insurance information, you learn that they do not speak English but speaks Spanish. Neither the pharmacist nor you are able to speak Spanish. How would you handle this situation?

_____

_____

_____

_____

8. It is Friday afternoon at 4 PM and you are ringing up customers' prescriptions at the cash register. A total of 11 people are waiting in line to drop off or pick up their prescriptions. How would you handle the situation? Why?

_____

_____

_____

_____

9. A woman found a prescription for penicillin for her boyfriend from the community's sexually transmitted disease clinic. The prescription was filled at the pharmacy 2 days ago, and she would like to know what it is used to treat. What would you tell her?

_____

_____

_____

_____

10. A mother is dropping off a prescription at the pharmacy with her 12-year old son. As they are waiting for the prescription to be filled, the son asks you what the difference is between prescription and over-the-counter medications. How would you explain this to him?

_____

_____

_____

_____

11. A patient comes to the pharmacy and asks for a box of pseudoephedrine that is kept at the pharmacy. You ask to see their driver's license as a form of identification. The patient becomes extremely upset with your request and states that at other pharmacies they do not have this requirement. How would you handle the situation?

_____

_____

_____

_____

12. A patient appears to be upset as they hand you a prescription for a terminal illness for which they have been diagnosed. Would you demonstrate sympathy or empathy toward the patient? Why?

_____

_____

_____

_____

9 Institutional Pharmacy Practice

Terms and Definitions

Select the correct term from the following list and write the corresponding letter in the blank next to the statement.

A. Aseptic technique
B. Computerized physician order entry (CPOE)
C. Electronic medication administration record (E-MAR)
D. Institutional pharmacy
E. Medication order
F. Protocol
G. Satellite pharmacy
H. The Joint Commission
I. United States Pharmacopeia (USP)

_____ 1. A set of standards and guidelines by which a facility operates

_____ 2. Procedures used in the sterile compounding of hazardous and nonhazardous materials to minimize the introduction of microbes or unwanted debris that could contaminate the preparation

_____ 3. A compendium of drug information, published annually, comprising enforceable guidelines for the safe preparation of sterile products

_____ 4. A pharmacy in facilities where patients receive care on site (eg, hospitals, extended-living homes, long-term care, and hospice facilities); also found in government-supported hospitals run by the Department of Veterans Affairs, Indian Health Service, and the Bureau of Prisons

_____ 5. An independent, nonprofit organization that accredits hospitals and other health care facilities in the United States; the facility must be accredited to receive Medicare and Medicaid payment

_____ 6. A computer program that automatically documents the administration of medication into certified electronic health record (EHR) systems; the report serves as a legal record of medications administered to a patient at a facility by a health care professional

_____ 7. A prescription written for administration in a hospital or institution

_____ 8. A specialty pharmacy located away from the central pharmacy, such as an operating room (OR), emergency department (ED), or a neonatal pharmacy; satellite pharmacies typically are staffed by a pharmacist and a pharmacy technician

_____ 9. Computerized order entry

Select the correct term from the following list and write the corresponding letter in the blank next to the statement.

A. ASAP order
B. Formulary
C. Investigational drug
D. NKA
E. NKDA
F. Nonformulary medications
G. Parenteral medication
H. prn
I. Standing order
J. Stat order

_____ 10. A drug that has not been approved by the US Food and Drug Administration (FDA) for marketing but is in clinical trials; also, an FDA-approved drug seeking a new indication for use

_____ 11. Written procedure for drug or treatment that is to be used in a specific situation

_____ 12. Medication that bypasses the digestive system but is intended for systemic action; most commonly describes medications given by injection such as intravenously or intramuscularly

_____ 13. A list of drugs approved for use in hospitals by the pharmacy and therapeutics committee of the institution that have become the standard stock carried by the pharmacy and other departments

_____ 14. Drugs that are not approved for use within an institution unless specific exceptions are filed and accepted by institutional protocols

_____ 15. From the Latin term *pro re nata,* meaning "as needed"

_____ 16. No known allergies

_____ 17. A medication order that must be filled immediately, as quickly as is safely possible to prepare the dose, usually within 10 to 15 minutes

_____ 18. As soon as possible but not an emergency

_____ 19. No known drug allergy

Select the correct term from the following list and write the corresponding letter in the blank next to the statement.

A. Automated dispensing system (ADS)
B. Crash carts
C. Floor stock
D. Periodic automatic replenishment (PAR)
E. Pyxis
F. SureMed
G. Unit dose (UD)

_____ 20. A set level of certain medications kept on hospital floors

_____ 21. An automated dispensing system often used in hospitals

_____ 22. Drugs not labeled for a specific patient and maintained at a nursing station or other department of the institution (excluding the pharmacy) for the purpose of administration to a patient of the facility

_____ 23. Individualized packaged doses used in institutional practice settings

_____ 24. Computerized cabinets and integrated systems that control inventory on nursing floors, in emergency departments, and in surgical suites and other patient care areas

_____ 25. An automated dispensing system often used in hospitals

_____ 26. Moveable carts containing trays of medications, administration sets, oxygen, and other materials used in life-threatening situations such as cardiac arrest; also known as code carts

True or False

Write T or F next to each statement.

_____ 1. A hospital pharmacy is one of the most challenging areas in which a pharmacy technician can work.

_____ 2. Hospital pharmacies have more job openings than community pharmacies.

_____ 3. Large hospitals may have a central pharmacy and smaller satellite pharmacies throughout the hospital.

_____ 4. The satellite pharmacies fill most of the daily medications for patients on their floors.

_____ 5. All hospitals must meet only state guidelines to be reimbursed for patients who have Medicare or Medicaid.

_____ 6. Technicians must have scheduling flexibility because they will need to work all shifts, including weekends and holidays.

_____ 7. It is not necessary for a hospital pharmacy technician to be able to work in all areas of the pharmacy.

_____ 8. When unit dose medications are prepared, the final check is always done by the lead technician.

_____ 9. The Joint Commission now requires hospitals to make all medications patient-dose specific.

_____ 10. The task of counting and tracking controlled substances is not a critical job in inventory control.

Multiple Choice

Complete each question by circling the best answer.

1. The policies and procedures handbook contains information about:
   A. Mandatory training
   B. Cafeteria menus
   C. Physicians' orders
   D. All the above

2. Factors that differentiate hospitals include:
   A. Outpatient services
   B. Diagnostic capabilities
   C. Surgical procedures
   D. All the above

3. One of the agencies that governs the operation of hospitals is the:
   A. HFC
   B. HCFA
   C. RPH
   D. ICU

4. All necessary information included on a patient's admitting record to ensure that orders are filled correctly is provided by:
   A. A physician
   B. A unit clerk
   C. Nurse
   D. All the above

5. When patients with the same last name end up on the same floor, which auxiliary label should be used?
   A. Take as directed
   B. Name alert
   C. May cause drowsiness
   D. Shake well

Chapter **9 Institutional Pharmacy Practice**

6. Investigational drug logbook must contain which of the following pieces of information:
   A. Drug name and strength
   B. Principle investigator
   C. Stock balance
   D. All the above

7. The technician responsible for stocking the intravenous room with all the supplies needed for the day is the:
   A. IV technician
   B. Satellite technician
   C. Unit dose cart fill technician
   D. Floor stock technician

8. Point-of-entry (POE) systems allow physicians, nurses, and pharmacists to directly communicate with one another, limiting errors of transcription by allowing electronic access to:
   A. Medical and drug information data
   B. Secure entry into the pharmacy
   C. Pyxis machine
   D. Hospital supply room

9. Using the computerized prescriber order entry, a _____ can enter all labs, dietary requirements, medications, and special notes into the computer.
   A. nurse
   B. physician
   C. unit clerk
   D. pharmacy technician

10. Enforceable regulations for IV preparations have been provided by the:
    A. The Joint Commission
    B. Board of Pharmacy
    C. USP <797>
    D. *Physicians' Desk Reference*

Fill in the Blanks

Answer each question by completing the statement in the space provided.

1. _____ are small specialty pharmacies that supply a clinic, such as the emergency department or an entire floor of a hospital.

2. The SOP manual contains the policies and the rules of the facility and the _____ that explain how, when, and/or why the policies are to be executed.

3. Nurses are the pharmacy's _____ customers and should be provided with the highest level of support.

4. All controlled substances are counted two or three times _____ depending on the length of a nursing shift.

5. A pharmacy technician and a _____ must observe the addition or return of controlled substance stock.

6. Only specially trained and properly garbed pharmacy personnel are allowed into the _____ _____.

7. All drugs must be _____ before they leave the pharmacy.

8. All crash cart medications should always be _____ in the tray in the same order.

9. _____ areas of a hospital can include areas that a patient never sees or those areas that are used as temporary patient care areas.

10. The technician who has experience in many different settings and a broad knowledge of pharmacy practices will be in _____ demand.

Matching

Match the following primary unit acronyms with their correct meaning.

A. CCU
B. ED
C. ICU
D. L&D
E. NICU
F. NSY
G. OR
H. ORTHO
I. PACU
J. PED

_____ 1. Neonatal intensive care unit

_____ 2. Post anesthesia care unit

_____ 3. Emergency department

_____ 4. Operating room

_____ 5. Labor and delivery

_____ 6. Intensive care unit

_____ 7. Pediatrics

_____ 8. Nursery

_____ 9. Coronary care unit

_____ 10. Orthopedics unit

Match the following hospital codes with their correct meaning.

A. Code red
B. Code blue
C. Code white
D. Code pink
E. Code purple
F. Code yellow
G. Code gray
H. Code silver
I. Code orange
J. Code triage internal
K. Code triage external

_____ 11. Medical emergency—pediatric

_____ 12. Bomb threat

_____ 13. An external disaster

_____ 14. Medical emergency—adult

_____ 15. Combative person

_____ 16. Child abduction

_____ 17. Hazardous material spill/release

_____ 18. Fire

_____ 19. An internal disaster

_____ 20. Person with a weapon and/or hostage situation

_____ 21. Infant abduction

Short Answer

Write a short response to each question in the space provided.

1. List three main advantages of an automated dispensing system (ADS).

_____

_____

_____

2. What three specialty departments in an institution (hospital) stock many drugs in injectable forms, as well as a variety of oral and injectable controlled substances?

_____

_____

_____

3. List three types of stat trays stocked for code carts by hospital pharmacies.

_____

_____

_____

4. For what are the following governmental agencies responsible?

   A. TJC _____

   B. CMS _____

   C. HHS _____

   D. DPH _____

   E. BOP _____

Research Activities

Follow the instructions given in each exercise and provide a response.

1. Access http://www.nabp.net/boards-of-pharmacy and look up the duties of a hospital technician in your state.

2. Visit or call a local hospital pharmacy and interview the following hospital technicians: IV therapy, chemotherapy, UD fill, and controlled substance technicians. Ask the following questions:

   A. What are your job duties?

   B. What training did you receive?

   C. Does your job require a specialty certification (i.e., IV certification)?

   D. What is the most satisfying part of your job?

REFLECT CRITICALLY

Critical Thinking

Reply to each question based on what you have learned in the chapter.

1. Many pharmacy technicians work in inpatient hospital pharmacies because the pay scale is higher than that found in community pharmacies. What are some other reasons a pharmacy technician might want to work in an inpatient hospital pharmacy?

2. The job descriptions of inpatient pharmacy technicians are changing because of the various automated systems coming into use to fill medication carts. Outline a job description for an automated dispensing technician.

3. The relationship between nursing and pharmacy staffs can be tumultuous at times. How can you, as a pharmacy technician, foster a better relationship between these two groups of professionals?

RELATE TO PRACTICE

Lab Scenarios

Hospital Pharmacy Inventory

Objective: To learn the procedures for maintaining inventory in the institutional pharmacy.

> Automated dispensing systems are used in hospital pharmacies and result in improved patient care. Automation speeds up the dispensing process, resulting in fewer medication errors and improved patient outcomes. Computer dispensing systems allow for improved inventory management by the institution, resulting in fewer dollars invested in the pharmacy's inventory. Many of the tasks previously performed in the pharmacy by an individual were time-consuming and had a high potential for error. Technology enables the role of both the pharmacist and the pharmacy technician to continue to evolve.

Lab Activity #9.1: Order up-to quantity

   Equipment needed:
   ■ Calculator
   ■ Pencil/Pen

   Time needed to complete this activity: 30 minutes

Calculate the number of full bottles of medication you would order to meet the order up-to quantity of each medication.

Medication	Package Size	Quantity on Hand (Bottles)	Desired Quantity (Bottles)	Number of Bottles Ordered
Albuterol inhaler (200 sprays)	1	45	75	
Alprazolam 0.5 mg	1000	1	2.5	
Amitriptyline 50 mg	500	1.75	2	
Amlodipine 10 mg	500	3	2	
Amoxicillin 500 mg	500	2.5	4.25	
Cephalexin 500 mg	500	3.25	3.75	
Citalopram 10 mg	90	3.05	4.25	
Furosemide 40 mg	1000	2.75	4	
Hydrochlorothiazide 50 mg	1000	0.75	3.5	
Hydrocodone 5mg/APAP 325 mg	500	1	2	
Levothyroxine 0.1 mg	1000	2.75	3.25	
Lisinopril 10 mg	1000	0.95	1.8	
Metoprolol 50 mg	1000	0.25	2.75	
Montelukast 10 mg	100	0.75	1.25	
Potassium chloride 8 mEq	500	2	3.5	
Propranolol 40 mg	1000	3	5.5	
Simvastatin 40 mg	1000	1.75	2.8	
Spiriva HandiHaler	1	34	52	
Warfarin 5 mg	1000	3.25	4.5	
Zolpidem 5 mg	500	0.75	1.25	

Lab Activity #9.2: Perpetual inventory of controlled substances

Equipment needed:
- Calculator
- Pencil/pen
- Paper

Time needed to complete this activity: 15 minutes

The hospital pharmacy has received the following orders for alprazolam 0.5 mg to be delivered to the narcotics cart in various parts of the hospital on the following dates:

- February 1, 2021: dispensed 100 tablets to the emergency room

- February 3, 2021: received 1000 tablets from wholesaler on invoice 0202201108
- February 3, 2021: dispensed 50 tablets to ICU
- February 4, 2021: received 10 outdated tablets from crash cart
- February 4, 2021: dispensed 30 tablets to crash cart
- February 5, 2021: dispensed 100 tablets cardiac care unit
- February 6, 2021: dispensed 200 tablets to the emergency room

Based on the above information, complete the following log.

Date	Dispensed	Received	Invoice Number	On-Hand Quantity
January 31, 2021	X	X	X	475

Crash Cart

Objective: To learn the procedures for preparing crash cart trays.

Lab Activity #9.3: Crash Cart Fill

Equipment needed:
- Crash cart
- Medications as listed
- Pen

Time needed to complete this activity: 30 minutes

1. Fill the following medications into the assigned crash cart drawers.
2. List the soonest expiration date for each drug placed in the crash cart.
3. Have pharmacist verify medications, quantity, expiration date, and placement of items.

Item	PAR Level	Drawer #	Expiration Date
Alcohol swabs	6	1	
Amiodarone 150 mg 3 mL vial	2	1	
Atropine 1 mg/10 mL syringe	3	1	
Calcium chloride 1 g/10 mL syringe	2	1	
Dextrose 50% (0.5 mg/mL) 50 mL syringe	1	1	
Dopamine 400 mg/250 mL IV bag	1	1	
Epinephrine 1 mg/10 mL (1:10,000) syringe	6	1	
Lidocaine 100 mg, 5 mL syringes	4	1	
Lidocaine 2 g/250 mL IV bag	1	1	
Povidone-iodide swab stick	2	1	
Sodium bicarbonate 50 mEq/50 mL syringe	3	1	
Sodium chloride 0.9% 10 mL vial	2	1	
Sterile water for injection 20 mL vial	2	1	
Vasopressin 20 units/mL, 1 mL vial	2	2	
Dextrose 5% 250 mL IV bag	2	2	
Sodium chloride 0.9% 100 mL IV bag	2	2	

Item	PAR Level	Drawer #	Expiration Date
Sodium chloride 0.9% 1000 mL IV bag	2	2	
Atropine 0.5 mg/5 mL syringe	3	3	
Sodium bicarbonate 10 mEq/10 mL (8.4%) syringe	4	3	
Saline flush syringes	5	3	
Sodium chloride 0.9% 10 mL flush syringe	5	3	

Task	Yes/No
Pulled the correct medications/items.	
Pulled the correct number of medications/items needed.	
Placed medications/items in the correct drawer.	
Listed the correct expiration date for each medication/item.	

Automated Dispensing System

Objective: To learn the procedures for refilling the automated dispensing machine.
Lab Activity #9.4: Automated Dispensing Machine Fill

Equipment needed:
- Automated dispensing system
- Medications as listed
- Pencil/pen

Time needed to complete this activity: 45 minutes

1. List the quantity of each medication needed to fill the ADS to the indicated PAR level.
2. Pull each of the medications needed to fill the ADS to PAR level.
3. Have the pharmacist verify medications and quantity.
4. Place the medications in the ADS.

ADS	Medication	PAR Level	Quantity Available	Quantity to Fill
Med/Surg #1	Lovastatin 20 mg tab	5	1	
Med/Surg #1	Fluoxetine 20 mg tab	4	0	
Med/Surg #1	Gabapentin 300 mg cap	6	2	
Med/Surg #1	Diltiazem 30 mg tab	4	1	
Med/Surg #1	Atenolol 50 mg tab	6	2	
Med/Surg #2	Benztropine 1 mg tab	4	1	
Med/Surg #2	Acetaminophen 325 mg tab	6	2	
Med/Surg #2	Methotrexate 2.5 mg tab	4	1	
Med/Surg #2	Sertraline 50 mg	4	0	
Med/Surg #2	Glyburide 2.5 mg	4	2	
Med/Surg #2	Amitriptyline 10 mg	4	1	

Continued

ADS	Medication	PAR Level	Quantity Available	Quantity to Fill
ICU	Furosemide 20 mg tab	5	2	
ICU	Digoxin 0.125 mg tab	4	1	
ICU	Aspirin 81 mg	5	2	
ED #1	Cefaclor 250 mg cap	4	1	
ED #1	Metronidazole 500 mg tab	4	0	
ED #1	Aspirin 325 mg	6	2	
ED #1	Diphenhydramine 50 mg tab	5	1	
ED #2	Metoprolol 50 mg	3	1	
ED #2	Acetaminophen 325 mg tab	6	3	
ED #2	Promethazine 25 mg supp	4	1	
ED #2	Famotidine 20 mg tab	3	1	
ED #2	Amoxicillin/Clavulanate 500 mg tab	4	0	
L&D	Ibuprofen 600 mg tab	8	3	
L&D	Acetaminophen 325 mg	6	2	

Narcotic Fill List:
   5. List the quantity of each medication needed to fill the ADS to the indicated PAR level.
   6. Pull each of the medications needed to fill the ADS to PAR level.
   7. Have the pharmacist verify medications and quantity.
   8. With a nurse, verify the current quantity of each controlled substance medication listed in the ADS.
   9. With a nurse, place the controlled substance medications in the ADS.

ADS	Medication	PAR Level	Quantity Available	Quantity to Fill	Nurse's Initials
Med/Surg #1	Alprazolam 0.5 mg tab	4	1		
Med/Surg #1	Diazepam 5 mg tab	4	2		
Med/Surg #2	Lorazepam 2 mg/mL, 1 mL vial	6	2		
Med/Surg #2	Oxycodone 5 mg tab	4	3		
Med/Surg #2	Zolpidem 5 mg tab	5	2		
ICU	Diazepam 5 mg tab	5	1		
ICU	Lorazepam 2 mg/mL, 1 mL vial	8	3		
ICU	Hydromorphone 4 mg tab	4	1		
ED #1	Hydrocodone 5 mg/APAP 325 mg	5	2		
ED #2	Carisoprodol 350 mg tab	5	1		
ED #2	Diazepam 5 mg tab	5	2		
L&D	Hydrocodone 5 mg/APAP 325 mg	8	2		
L&D	Oxycodone 5 mg tab	5	2		

Task	Yes/No
Correctly calculated quantity needed for each medication to fill to PAR level.	
Pulled the correct medication in the correct quantity.	
Had pharmacist verify medication and quantity.	
Placed medication in the correct ADS in the correct quantity.	
Had nurse verify controlled substance medications placed in ADS.	

Medication Cart Fill

Objective: To learn the procedures for preparing daily medication cart fill.

Lab Activity #9.5: 24-Hour Medication Cart Fill

Equipment needed:
- Medication cart
- Medications as listed
- Pencil/pen

Time needed to complete this activity: 30 minutes

1. Fill the medication orders for each patient as listed for a 24-hour period.
2. Pull each of the medications needed for each patient room.
3. Have pharmacist verify medications and quantity.
4. Place the medications in the correct patient drawer.

Patient Room	Medication	Directions	Quantity to Fill for 24 Hours
201	Amoxicillin/Clavulanate 250 mg tab	1 cap po qid	
	Promethazine 25 mg tab	1 po ac & hs	
203	Quinapril 40 mg tab	1 po bid	
	Simvastatin 20 mg tab	1 po qd	
205	Theophylline 450 mg	1 po qd	
206	Verapamil ER 120 mg cap	1 po bid	
	Lovastatin 20 mg tab	1 po qpm	
210	Finasteride 5 mg	1 po qam	
302	Isosorbide dinitrate 40 mg tab	1 po q6h	
304	Benzonatate 100 mg cap	1 po q12h	
	Fexofenadine 60 mg tab	1 po q6h	
305	Glipizide ER 5 mg tab	1 po 30 min ac	
306	Lansoprazole 30 mg cap	1 po bid	
	Potassium chloride 20 mEq tab	1 po q6h	
310	Metoclopramide 10 mg tab	1 po ac & hs	
	Nifedipine 60 mg tab	1 po bid	
401	Ondansetron 8 mg tab	1 po q8h	
402	Gabapentin 800 mg cap	1 po tid	
404	Amoxicillin 875 mg cap	1 po qid	
	Hydroxyzine 25 mg tab	1 po hs	
406	Levofloxacin 500 mg tab	1 po bid	
408	Hydrochlorothiazide 25 mg tab	1 po q6h	
	Enalapril 5 mg	1 po bid	
410	Dicyclomine 20 mg	1 po q8h	
	Famotidine 20 mg	1 po ac & hs	

Task	Yes/No
Correctly calculated quantity needed for each medication to fill.	
Pulled the correct medication in the correct quantity.	
Had pharmacist verify medication and quantity.	
Placed medication in the correct patient drawer in the correct quantity.	

Personnel Cleansing and Garbing Order

Objective: To learn the steps required to cleanse and don PPE to properly prepare compounded sterile preparations.

Lab Activity #9.6: Personnel Cleansing and Garbing Order

Equipment needed:
- Antiseptic hand cleaner
- Nonshedding disposable towels or an electronic hand dryer
- Nailbrush and surgical scrub sponge
- Sink with hot and cold running water
- Waterless alcohol-based hand rub (sterile)
- Face mask
- Foot covering
- Hair covering, facial hair covering
- Sterile gown
- Sterile powder-free gloves

Procedure

1. Remove all cosmetics, jewelry up to the elbows, and remove necklaces and earrings.
2. Remove all outer garments such as coats and hats.
3. All items must be wiped down with aseptic wipes before entering aseptic areas.
4. Wash hands thoroughly with soap and water.
5. Apply sterile alcohol to the palm of one hand and rub hands thoroughly. Allow hands to air dry.
6. Pull shoe cover over the toe of the shoe: first, around the bottom of the shoe and finally over the heel of the shoe. Please note that shoe covers are not designated as left and right but are interchangeable.
7. Apply sterile alcohol to the palm of one hand and rub hands thoroughly. Allow hands to air dry.
8. Pull shoe cover over the toe of the other shoe: first, around the bottom of the shoe and finally over the heel of the shoe.
9. Apply sterile alcohol to the palm of one hand and rub hands thoroughly. Allow hands to air dry.
10. Put on hair cover by gathering loose hair and placing it into the back of the hair cover. Pull front of hair cover over forehead. No hair should be outside of the hair cover.

11. Apply sterile alcohol to the palm of one hand and rub hands thoroughly. Allow hands to air dry.
12. Slip on face mask by situating the top of the mask at the bridge of the nose. Pull the two top ties of the face mask and attach them together. Attach the two lower ties behind the neck. The mask should cover the nose, mouth, and chin.
13. Turn on water faucets with a paper towel if not foot operated.
14. Make sure water temperature is lukewarm.
15. Avoid unnecessary splashing during washing process.
16. Use nail pick to clean under each fingernail.
17. Use a nailbrush to clean cuticle beds and under every fingertip.
18. Apply sufficient disinfecting/cleansing agent to hands; rub in a circular motion, holding the fingertips downward.
19. Clean all four surfaces of each finger and rub well between the fingers.
20. Clean all surfaces of hand, wrist, and arm up to the elbows in a circular motion. Allow cleansing agent to remain in contact with skin for at least 30 seconds.
21. Repeat for other hand, wrist, and arm.
22. Rinse well.
23. Dry hands with nonshedding disposable towel or electronic hand dryer.
24. Do not touch the sink, faucet, or other objects that could contaminate hands.
25. Turn off the water using a nonshedding disposable towel.
26. Discard paper towels in biohazard waste container.
27. Open the package of the sterile gown. The gown should never make contact with any surface.
28. Slip one arm into the sleeve of the sterile gown and pull it up to the shoulder. Repeat this procedure with the other arm. Tie the neck strings behind the neck and repeat with the waist strings.
29. Apply sterile alcohol to the palm of one hand and rub hands thoroughly. Allow hands to air dry.
30. Open package containing sterile powder-free gloves. Remove glove from package and maintain fingers within the cuff of the gown. Place glove on palm of hand with the thumb side of the glove toward the palm. Pull the glove's cuff so that it covers the gown's cuff. Unfold the glove's cuff so that it covers the cuff of the gown. Take hold of the glove and gown at waist level. Pull glove onto the hand and work fingers into the glove. Repeat procedure for the other glove.

*Note, sterile gloves should be donned in the IV room.

Time needed to complete this activity: 15 minutes

Evaluation of Aseptic Hand Washing and Garbing Order	Yes/No
Removed all cosmetics, visible jewelry, watches, and objects up to the elbow.	
Was not wearing acrylic nails or nail polish.	
Applied sterile alcohol to the palm of one hand and rubbed hands thoroughly. Allowed hands to air dry.	
Shoe covers put on.	
Applied sterile alcohol to the palm of one hand and rubbed hands thoroughly. Allowed hands to air dry.	
Hair cover(s) put on properly.	
Applied sterile alcohol to the palm of one hand and rubbed hands thoroughly. Allowed hands to air dry.	
Face mask put on properly.	
Started water and adjusted to the correct temperature.	
Avoided unnecessary splashing during process.	
Used nail pick to clean under each fingernail.	
Used a nailbrush to clean each cuticle bed and under every fingertip.	
Used sufficient disinfecting agent/cleanser.	
Cleaned all four surfaces of each finger.	

Evaluation of Aseptic Hand Washing and Garbing Order	Yes/No
Cleaned all surfaces of hands, wrists, and arms up to the elbows in a circular motion.	
Did not touch the sink, faucet, or other objects that could contaminate the hands.	
Rinsed off all soap residue.	
Rinsed hands, holding them upright and allowing water to drip to the elbow.	
Dried hands with nonshedding disposable towel or electronic hand dryer.	
Did not turn off water until hands were completely dry.	
Turned water off with a clean, dry, nonshedding disposable towel.	
Did not touch the faucet while turning off the water.	
Discarded paper towels in biohazard container.	
Sanitized hands by applying a waterless, alcohol-based hand rub and allowed it to dry completely before putting on remaining PPE.	
Sterile gown put on properly.	
Applied sterile alcohol to the palm of one hand and rubbed hands thoroughly. Allowed hands to air dry.	
Sterile gloves put on properly.	

Additional Pharmacy Practice Settings

ASHP ACCREDITATION STANDARDS FOR PHARMACY TECHNICIAN EDUCATION AND TRAINING PROGRAMS

Standard 1.3: Demonstrate active and engaged listening skills.
Standard 1.4: Communicate clearly and effectively, both verbally and in writing.
Standard 2.3: Describe the pharmacy technician's role, pharmacist's role, and other occupations in the health care environment.
Standard 2.7: Explain the pharmacy technician's role in the medication use process.
Standard 2.10: Describe further knowledge and skills required for achieving advanced competencies.
Standard 4.2: Apply patient- and medication-safety practices in aspects of the pharmacy technician's roles.
Standard 4.7: Explain pharmacist and pharmacy technician roles in medication management services.
Standard 5.10: Describe major trends, issues, goals, and initiatives taking place in the pharmacy profession.

REINFORCE KEY CONCEPTS

Terms and Definitions

Select the correct term from the following list and write the corresponding letter in the blank next to the statement.

A. Interdisciplinary team
B. Managed care
C. Medication reconciliation
D. Pharmacy benefit management (PBM)
E. Pharmacy informatics
F. Telepharmacy

_____ 1. Practice that includes the use of information technology designed to ensure optimal medication use.

_____ 2. Consists of a health care team from different disciplines, including pharmacy technicians, which is designed to provide care for the patient's total needs.

_____ 3. The development and management of broad and cost-efficient prescription drug benefits for a large group of patient populations.

_____ 4. The process of preparing a complete and accurate listing of patient's medications and all related medical information such as allergies.

_____ 5. An organized health care delivery system designed to improve both the quality and accessibility of health care, including pharmaceutical care, while containing costs.

_____ 6. The provision of pharmaceutical care to patients at a distance through the use of telecommunications and information technologies.

True or False

Write T or F next to each statement.

_____ 1. Most pharmacies require the pharmacy purchasing agent to have up to 6 months of experience as a pharmacy technician.

_____ 2. The pharmacy medication reconciliation technician is an essential part of patient safety.

_____ 3. The number of elderly patients has increased because of improved health care and discovery of more effective treatments for medical conditions and diseases.

_____ 4. The purpose of PBMs is to develop and manage broad and costly prescription drug benefits for a large group of patient populations.

_____ 5. A pharmacy technician trainer must have adequate experience in the practice area they are teaching.

_____ 6. It is unnecessary for a pharmacy technician trainee to complete a test proving the technician understands the tasks they are to perform.

_____ 7. Pharmacy technician educators ideally should have retail and hospital pharmacy experience and a bachelor's degree to be competitive.

_____ 8. A pharmaceutical sales representative must have a national pharmacy technician certification.

134

_____ 9. Specialized training is required for everyone handling radioactive material, including the pharmacist and pharmacy technician.

_____ 10. A pharmacy informatics technician must have additional pharmacy education, a bachelor's degree in computer science, and are knowledge in pharmacology.

Multiple Choice

Complete each question by circling the best answer.

1. The expected employment growth rate for pharmacy technician careers between 2018 and 2028 is:
   A. 5%
   B. 7%
   C. 30%
   D. 50%

2. Which of the following is *not* a PAI technician-related initiative promoted by ASHP:
   A. Additional career pathways through advanced certification
   B. Perform traditional preparation and distribution activities
   C. Support to seek non-traditional roles
   D. Allow the pharmacist to determine which advanced certification the pharmacy technician should receive.

3. The process of medication reconciliation has reduced medication errors to less than:
   A. 5%
   B. 9%
   C. 30%
   D. 50%

4. A _____ pharmacy technician requires experience in the pharmacy field and preferably call center experience.
   A. medication reconciliation
   B. managed care
   C. purchasing
   D. nuclear

5. A(n) _____ pharmacy technician is most found working for an accredited college or university, either on campus or online.
   A. educator
   B. medication reconciliation
   C. purchasing
   D. nuclear

6. A pharmacy technician educator must possess a national certification, meet her or his state's regulations for practice, and have, at minimum, _____ of experience in the pharmacy setting.
   A. 6 months
   B. 1 year
   C. 2 years
   D. 3 years

7. A _____ will have important information on hand, including up-to-date knowledge on clinical studies and side effects, as well as the pharmacology knowledge of the medication she or he is trying to sell.
   A. nuclear pharmacy technician
   B. managed care pharmacy technician
   C. pharmaceutical sales representative
   D. pharmacy technician trainer

8. The special class of drugs used in the nuclear pharmacy setting is known as _____.
   A. radioactive prescriptions
   B. radiopharmaceuticals
   C. radiohazards
   D. radiation

9. _____ is an example of radiopharmaceutical medication.
   A. Fluorodeoxyglucose
   B. Diethylenetriamine penta-acetic acid
   C. Pertechnetate
   D. All the above

10. _____ focuses on the use of information technology and drug information to optimize medication use.
    A. Pharmacy informatics
    B. Nuclear pharmacy
    C. Telepharmacy
    D. Medication reconciliation

Matching

Match the following advanced level pharmacy technicians with their correct description.

A. Managed Care Pharmacy Technician
B. Medication Reconciliation Technician
C. Nuclear Pharmacy Technician
D. Pharmaceutical Sales Representative
E. Pharmacy Informatics Technician
F. Pharmacy Inventory and Purchasing Agent
G. Pharmacy Technician Trainer
H. Telepharmacy Technician
I. Pharmacy Technician Educator
J. Prior Approval or Investigational Drug Coordinator
K. Lead Pharmacy Technician
L. Medication Adherence Technician

_____ 1. Provides support for pharmacy information in clinical systems

_____ 2. Provides benefit information to the patient/client; determines the proper usage of benefits

_____ 3. Interviews, identifies, and assesses baseline skill levels of technicians; schedules training and tasks for technicians; has proven leadership skills

_____ 4. Performs on-the-job training for new employees or for technicians in new roles

_____ 5. Teaches pharmacy technician students the knowledge and skills they need to pass an ASHP-approved national certification exam and become certified pharmacy technicians

_____ 6. Recognize roadblocks such as financial hardship, language barriers, or other issues that may lead to nonadherence

_____ 7. Takes specific safety precautions when preparing radioactive products as ordered

_____ 8. Travels to clients' sites and promotes his or her company's assigned medications

_____ 9. Dispenses investigational, prior-approved drugs, or indigent medications that require separate inventory control and documentation, and often uses advanced or specific ordering and return protocols

_____ 10. Performs duties much like those of a technician at a community or hospital setting without a pharmacist physically on site

_____ 11. Interviews patients about their at-home medications including prescription and over-the-counter medications, vitamins, or herbal supplements to help the provider make informed decisions about a patient's medication regimen

_____ 12. Places daily orders to keep the department stocked to fulfill the orders/ prescription requests to satisfy the patient in need and works closely with pharmacy management in implementing cost-saving opportunities

Fill in the Blanks

Answer each question by completing the statement in the space provided.

1. Employers hiring pharmacy technicians in an advanced setting pharmacy setting often seek those individuals who have had previous _____ training and certification.

2. With the increased amount of medications being prescribed, pharmacies need at least one employee to do the _____ for the department.

3. The goal of the medication reconciliation position is to _____ medication errors.

4. Most elderly patients take multiple medications, increasing the need for the management of prescription _____ use.

5. All pharmacy technician programs are moving toward becoming _____ approved, which requires the programs to teach the required goals and objectives of an accredited program.

6. The ultimate goal of a sales rep is to do everything possible to sell specific products, often by persuading the buyer that the products are the _____ on the market.

7. Because of the risks associated with the nuclear pharmacy setting, the pay in this area of pharmacy is most often _____ than that of a traditional pharmacy setting.

8. The pharmacy informatics technician assists in building new systems to be used by the pharmacy staff and must also be available to help _____ if anything needs to be fixed.

9. Multitasking and organizational skills are _____ to a lead pharmacy technician to be able to manage other technicians and projects.

10. _____ is the most important characteristic of any candidate seeking a position in any health care position.

Short Answer

Write a short response to each question in the space provided.

1. List three reasons for the increased need of a highly qualified pharmacy technician.

   _____

   _____

   _____

2. List three responsibilities of the pharmacy purchasing agent.

   _____

   _____

   _____

3. List two responsibilities of a medication reconciliation pharmacy technician.

   _____

   _____

   _____

4. List three responsibilities of a managed care pharmacy technician.

   _____

   _____

5. List two responsibilities of a pharmacy technician trainer.

   _____

   _____

   _____

6. List two responsibilities of a pharmaceutical sales representative.

   _____

   _____

   _____

7. List three competencies a nuclear pharmacy technician must have.

   _____

   _____

   _____

8. List three responsibilities of a telepharmacy pharmacy technician.

   _____

   _____

   _____

9. List three responsibilities of a pharmacy informatics pharmacy technician.

   _____

   _____

   _____

10. List one advanced role for a pharmacy technician and how the role plays a part in patient safety.

_____

_____

_____

Research Activities

Follow the instructions given in each exercise and provide a response.

1. Call or visit a local nuclear pharmacy. Ask the lead pharmacy technician or the pharmacist in charge the following questions:

    A. What is the name and location of the pharmacy?

    B. What qualifications do you require for technicians in your pharmacy?

    C. What duties do your pharmacy technicians perform?

    D. Do you require certification and/or additional training?

    List the name and location of the pharmacy: _____

    _____

2. Access the website https://careers.ptcb.org/. What career opportunities are available for pharmacy technicians?

REFLECT CRITICALLY

Critical Thinking

Reply to each question based on what you have learned in the chapter.

1. What opportunities are available to you in your area at an advanced pharmacy technician level? How could you prepare yourself for that opportunity?

2. Medication reconciliation is becoming more important in a hospital setting. What attributes do you possess that could help you become a medication reconciliation technician? What skills would be necessary?

RELATE TO PRACTICE

Lab Scenarios
Advanced Pharmacy Technician Positions

Objective: To prepare a pharmacy technician student for an advanced pharmacy technician position

As the roles of a pharmacist and pharmacy technician change, it will become important to begin thinking about how well prepared you are to move into an advanced pharmacy technician position. As you work in a pharmacy as a pharmacy technician, you should begin to take stock of your strengths and work toward obtaining skills to highlight those strengths. This will help prepare you for an advanced pharmacy technician position in the future.

Lab Activity #10.1: Preparing for an advanced pharmacy technician position

Equipment needed:
- Computer with Internet access
- Paper
- Pencil/pen

Time needed to complete this activity: 90 minutes

You are a certified pharmacy technician who is looking for an advanced pharmacy technician position. Perform a web search to begin looking for available positions in your area. Based on your web search, answer the following questions:

1. What advanced pharmacy technician positions are available in your area?

   _____

   _____

2. Which advanced pharmacy technician position most interests you?

   _____

   _____

3. What pharmacy technician training can help prepare you for that position?

   _____

   _____

   _____

4. Will you need additional education for your interested position? If so, what education is required?

   _____

   _____

5. Does your interested position require certification? If so, which one(s)?

   _____

   _____

6. Why would you be successful as an advanced pharmacy technician?

   _____

   _____

7. Why do you want to work as an advanced pharmacy technician?

   _____

   _____

8. What in your background prepares you for this advanced pharmacy technician position?

   _____

   _____

9. How will this opportunity contribute to your overall goal of being a pharmacy technician?

   _____

   _____

10. What type of job duties is required for this advanced pharmacy technician position?

    _____

    _____

11. What skills do you need to improve or obtain for this advanced pharmacy technician position?

    _____

    _____

12. What is your greatest strength that could help you with this advanced pharmacy technician position?

    _____

    _____

13. What is your greatest weakness that could hinder you with this advanced pharmacy technician position? How can you overcome this weakness?

    _____

    _____

    _____

Lab Activity #10.2: Access the website https://www.ashp.org/Pharmacy-Technician/About-Pharmacy-Technicians/Advanced-Pharmacy-Technician-Roles and choose one advanced pharmacy technician role to learn more about.

Equipment needed:
- Computer with Internet access
- Paper
- Pencil/pen

Time needed to complete this activity: 60 minutes

After reading the case study or the results of a study, prepare a short presentation to help educate your peers about what you learned and how an advanced role as a pharmacy technician can be a rewarding career.

Maintaining Your Education

Objective: To keep up with advanced pharmacy technician information, roles, and education

---

To maintain your pharmacy technician certification, it will soon be required to complete pharmacy technician–specific continuing education. To keep ahead of the times and to help prepare for an advanced pharmacy technician position, it is in the best interest of pharmacy technicians to seek continuing education programs related to advanced pharmacy technician roles.

Lab Activity #10.3: Participate in pharmacy technician continuing education related to an advanced pharmacy technician role.

Equipment needed:
- Computer with Internet access
- Computer printer
- Paper
- Pencil/pen

Time needed to complete this activity: 90 minutes

Using the Internet, select a pharmacy continuing education article related to an advanced pharmacy technician role from one of the following websites:

- http://www.freece.com/
- https://www.pharmacytimes.org/
- http://www.powerpak.com/

Read the article, take the examination, and print out the continuing education certificate. Provide the certificate to your instructor.

11 Bulk Repackaging and Nonsterile Compounding

ASHP ACCREDITATION STANDARDS FOR PHARMACY TECHNICIAN EDUCATION AND TRAINING PROGRAMS

Standard 2.6: Perform mathematical calculations essential to the duties of pharmacy technicians in a variety of settings.

Standard 3.5: Prepare non–patient-specific medications for distribution.

Standard 3.6: Assist pharmacist in preparing, storing, and distributing medication products including those requiring special handling and documentation.

Standard 3.8: Maintain pharmacy facilities and equipment.

Standard 3.9: Use information from Safety Data Sheets (SDS), National Institute of Occupational Safety and Health (NOSH) Hazardous Drug List, and the United States Pharmacopoeia (USP) to identify, handle, dispense, and safely dispose of hazardous medications and materials.

Standard 3.10: Describe Food and Drug Administration product tracking, tracing, and handling requirements.

Standard 3.15: Describe basic concepts related to preparation for sterile and non-sterile compounding.

Standard 3.16: Prepare simple non-sterile medications per applicable USP chapters (e.g., reconstitution, basic ointments and creams).

Standard 3.17: Assist pharmacists in preparing medications requiring compounding of non-sterile products.

Standard 3.22: Prepare, store, and deliver medication products requiring special handling and documentation.

Standard 3.24: Prepare medications requiring moderate and high level non-sterile compounding as defined by USP (e.g., suppositories, tablets, complex creams).

Standard 5.5: Describe pharmacy compliance with professional standards and relevant legal, regulatory, formulary, contractual, and safety requirements.

Standard 5.6: Describe Occupational Safety and Health Administration (OSHA), National Institute of Occupational Safety and Health (NOSH) Hazardous Drug List, and the United States Pharmacopoeia (USP) requirements for prevention and treatment of exposure to hazardous substances (e.g., risk assessment, personal protective equipment, eyewash, spill kit).

REINFORCE KEY CONCEPTS

Terms and Definitions

Select the correct term from the following list and write the corresponding letter in the blank next to the statement.

A. Bubble pack (blister card)
B. Bulk repackaging
C. Periodic automatic replacement (PAR) levels
D. Unit dose
E. Unit dose packs or strip packs

_____ 1. Minimum set amounts of stock that must be kept on hand

_____ 2. The process by which the pharmacy transfers a medication manually or by means of an automated system from a manufacturer's original container to another type of container

_____ 3. A single dose of a drug

_____ 4. A preformed card with 28-, 30-, and 31-day depressions that can hold medications; the medication is sealed into the pack with a foil card backboard; this type of packaging usually is used for long-term care medications

_____ 5. Strip of heat-sealed packets, each packet holding one tablet or capsule; used in the bulk repackaging process

Select the correct term from the following list and write the corresponding letter in the blank next to the statement.

A. Beyond-use date (BUD)
B. Calibration
C. Compounding
D. Compounded Non-Sterile Preparation (CNSP)
E. Compounding record (CR)
F. Containment Ventilated Enclosure (CVE)
G. FDA
H. Good Manufacturing Practices (GMP)
I. Master Formulation record (MFR)
J. Mortars and pestles
K. Non–sterile compounding
L. Punch method
M. Reconstitution
N. USP 795

_____ 6. Federal guidelines that must be followed by all entities that prepare and package medication or medical devices

_____ 7. Preparation created by combining, admixing, diluting, or reconstituting any way other than how the manufacturer lists in the package insert information

_____ 8. Date after which a compounded preparation should not be used, which is determined from the date the compound was prepared

_____ 9. Manual filling of capsules with powdered medication that has been premixed

_____ 10. A detailed record of procedures used to describe how a CNSP is to be prepared

_____ 11. Acronym for the US Food and Drug Administration

_____ 12. Determining graduations (measurements) on a device such as a scale

_____ 13. The act of mixing, reconstituting, and packaging a drug

_____ 14. The mixing of a liquid and a powder to form a suspension or solution

_____ 15. Often referred to as a "powder hood," this is where weighing, measuring, or any other manipulations with API must occur

_____ 16. Bowls and tools with a rounded knob used to grind substances into fine powder or to mix liquids

_____ 17. General chapter defining practices and guidelines for non-sterile compounding

_____ 18. The compounding of two or more medications in a non-sterile environment (no clean room or hood is required)

_____ 19. The form that documents a non-sterile compounding process

Select the correct term from the following list and write the corresponding letter in the blank next to the statement.

A. API
B. Cream
C. Elixir
D. Emulsion
E. Excipient
F. Hydrophilic
G. Hydrophobic
H. Ointment
I. Oleaginous base
J. Solute
K. Solution
L. Solvent
M. Suspension
N. Syrup
O. Triturate
P. Troches

_____ 20. A hydrophobic product, such as petroleum jelly

_____ 21. The ingredient that is dissolved into a solution

_____ 22. Having a strong affinity for water; any substance that easily mixes in water

_____ 23. Flat, disklike tablets that dissolve between the gum and cheek

_____ 24. An ingredient used in compounding that does not dissolve in water

_____ 25. Active pharmaceutical ingredient

_____ 26. Lacking an affinity for water; any substance that does not mix or dissolve in water

_____ 27. A sugar-based liquid

_____ 28. A mixture of two or more liquids that do not usually blend using a stabilizing agent; the process of making an emulsion is called emulsification

_____ 29. To grind or crush powder, such as a tablet, into fine particles

_____ 30. The greater part of a solution that dissolves a solute

_____ 31. A base solution that is a mixture of alcohol and water

_____ 32. A solution in which the powder does not dissolve into the base; the solution must be shaken before use

_____ 33. A water base in which one or more ingredients are dissolved completely

_____ 34. An inert substance added to a drug to form a suitable consistency for dosing

_____ 35. A hydrophilic base

True or False

Write T or F next to each statement.

_____ 1. Institutional pharmacies often purchase medication in bulk quantities to repackage to a unit dose.

_____ 2. The process of repackaging must take place in a horizontal flow hood.

_____ 3. If a pill tray is used to guide tablets or capsules into their containers, the tray does not need to be washed with alcohol after use.

_____ 4. Keeping track of the products you are repackaging is a major step that must not be overlooked.

_____ 5. Medications in a solid form (e.g., tablets) usually have a shorter shelf life than liquid forms.

_____ 6. Beyond-use dates are calculated by the pharmacy when repackaging or compounding medications.

_____ 7. If the expiration date includes the month and year, the drug expires on the first day of the month.

_____ 8. Daily tasks such as maintenance and cleaning of equipment are a very important part of quality control and patient safety.

_____ 9. A technician who is sick or has any open wounds can compound any products.

_____ 10. You must read the graduated cylinder at the bottom of the meniscus.

Multiple Choice

Complete each question by circling the best answer.

1. Which of the following is *not* an example of Good Manufacturing Practices for repackaging?
   A. Prepare two items at a time.
   B. Packaging is appropriate for the drug.
   C. Equipment is in good condition and clean.
   D. All items repackaged are logged for reference.

2. The dosage form normally repackaged in a pharmacy is the:
   A. Tablet form
   B. Capsule form
   C. Liquid form
   D. All the above

3. The manufacturer expiration date of a drug is 4/22, the drug expires on:
   A. April 1, 2022
   B. April 15, 2022
   C. April 30, 2022
   D. April 31, 2022

4. Compounding pharmacies must follow each state's board of pharmacy regulations, in addition to _____ standards
   A. USP <711>
   B. USP <795>
   C. USP <797>
   D. USP <800>

5. The punch method is used to prepare:
   A. Solutions
   B. Tablets
   C. Capsules
   D. Ointments

6. Which of the following could be used as a base when preparing a compounded ointment?
   A. Aquaphor
   B. Mannitol
   C. Bentonite
   D. Kaolin

7. Which of the following is commonly used as an additive when compounding tablets?
   A. Lanolin
   B. Dextrose
   C. PEG
   D. Plastibase

8. Which of the following would be the most suitable flavoring additive for an antibiotic?
   A. Black currant
   B. Cherry
   C. Root beer
   D. Menthol

9. Documents are kept on the pharmacy premises for no less than _____ from the time the medication was prepared.
   A. 1 year
   B. 2 years
   C. 3 years
   D. 4 years

10. The beyond-use date of a preparation is set from:
    A. The time of compounding
    B. When the compound is dispensed
    C. Six months from when the compound was prescribed
    D. One year from when the compound was prescribed

Matching

Match the following additives with their correct description.

A. Gums
B. Coatings
C. Disintegrants
D. Lubricants
E. Suspending agents
F. Plasticizers
G. Emulsifying agents

_____ 1. Added to a tablet or capsule blend to help break up compacted mass when put into a fluid environment; especially important for rapid-release agents

_____ 2. Have a wide variety of functional properties (retarding drug release) and allow for flexibility in coating

_____ 3. Surrounding layer of polymeric material of a tablet, capsule, or pellet; done to change color; protect active ingredient from moisture, light, pH of stomach; avoid bad taste or odor when taken by mouth

_____ 4. Maintains dispersion of finely divided liquid droplets in a liquid vehicle; made from two or more immiscible liquids, such as water and oil, and can be liquid or semisolid (creams and lotions)

_____ 5. Additive for powder blend to prevent compacted powder mass from sticking to equipment during process of making tablets or capsules

_____ 6. Naturally occurring plant derivatives that are water soluble; provide a variety of properties, including gelling, thickening, and film forming

_____ 7. Insoluble particles that are dispersed in a liquid; act by increasing the viscosity of the liquid vehicle; reduces rate of sedimentation of particles

Match the following dosage forms with their auxiliary labels.

_____ 8. Ophthalmics

_____ 9. Otics

_____ 10. Ointments, creams, lotions

_____ 11. Suppositories

_____ 12. Suspensions

_____ 13. Patches

A. For topical use; external use
B. Apply to skin
C. For rectal use
D. For the eye
E. For the ear
F. Shake well

Fill in the Blanks

Answer each question by completing the statement in the space provided.

1. Only _____ drug product at a time should be prepackaged in a specific work area.

2. It is common practice to use only amber-colored containers to avoid possible _____ of medication.

3. All _____ should be kept clean and in good condition at all times.

4. For maximum accuracy in measuring liquids, use the _____ rule.

5. Pharmacy technicians often prepare compounded products and should be familiar with the _____ of each type of additive and of the final product.

6. Two of the most important techniques of mixing solutions are to measure _____ and _____ thoroughly.

7. A drug's _____ dictates the type of dosage form that must be prepared.

8. Keeping accurate records ensures the _____ of the product dispensed and meets FDA guidelines for quality assurance.

9. Every pharmacy has an _____ binder with information regarding all chemical products and how to handle spillage or contact.

10. _____ _____ is the special use of finishing technique to give the final product a professional look.

Short Answer

Write a short response to each question in the space provided.

1. List five reasons a pharmacy may repackage a medication.

   _____

   _____

   _____

   _____

   _____

2. List six reasons medications may need to be compounded by a pharmacy.

   _____

   _____

   _____

   _____

   _____

3. Why is it necessary to use tweezers to grasp metal weights?

   _____

   _____

4. Why is it necessary to clean counting trays?

   _____

   _____

5. List five dosage forms that can be compounded for animal use?

   _____

   _____

Research Activities

Follow the instructions given in each exercise and provide a response.

1. Access the compounding website http://www.pccarx.com/ to answer the following questions:

   A. What types of services do they provide?

   B. Find an interesting compounding recipe (if published). Print it and share it with the class.

   C. Is membership required to use these sites and to obtain their products?

2. A 0.5% sodium hypochlorite mixture is commonly used in the pharmacy as a disinfectant. Access the website https://chemicalsafety.com/sds-search/ to view the SDS for sodium hypochlorite.

   A. What is the recommended use for sodium hypochlorite?

   B. What are the hazard statements for sodium hypochlorite?

145

C. What first aid measures should be taken if sodium hypochlorite gets in your eyes?

D. How should sodium hypochlorite be stored?

E. What PPE should be worn while working with sodium hypochlorite?

REFLECT CRITICALLY

Critical Thinking

Reply to each question based on what you have learned in the chapter.

1. Pediatric medications sometimes require special compounding. What are some ways the pharmacy staff can accommodate pediatric patients to foster their compliance in taking their medications?

2. Preparing capsules using the punch method can be messy. What techniques for preparing capsules can you develop to minimize the mess?

3. Mrs. Foster has been coming to your pharmacy for years. Lately, she has become hard of hearing and often misinterprets the pharmacist's directions about her medications.

   A. How can you, as a technician, aid in this process?

B. What tools can you develop to help Mrs. Foster understand how to take her medications?

RELATE TO PRACTICE

Lab Scenarios

Pharmacy Equipment Used in Compounding Nonsterile Preparations

Objective: To introduce the pharmacy technician to the equipment used in preparing nonsterile preparations

Lab Activity #11.1: Correctly identify the following pharmacy equipment used in extemporaneous compounding and its purpose.

Equipment needed:
- Beaker
- Compounding record
- Conical graduate
- Counterbalance
- Cylindrical graduate
- Droppers
- Electronic scale
- Erlenmeyer flask
- Filter paper
- Forceps
- Funnel
- Glass funnel
- Glass mortar and pestle
- Glassine paper
- Hot plate
- Latex gloves
- Masks
- Metric weights
- Ointment slab
- Parchment paper
- Pipette
- Porcelain mortar and pestle
- Reconstitution tube
- Rubber spatula
- Safety glass
- Stainless steel spatula
- Stirring rod
- Suppository molds
- Tongs
- Torsion balance
- Wedgewood mortar and pestle
- Weighing boat

Time needed to complete this activity: 30 minutes

Equipment	Correctly Identified (Yes/No)	Purpose
Beaker		
Compounding record		
Conical graduate		
Cylindrical graduate		
Counterbalance		
Dropper		
Electronic scale		
Erlenmeyer flask		
Filter paper		
Forceps		
Funnel		
Glass funnel		
Glass mortar and pestle		
Glassine paper		
Hot plate		
Latex gloves		
Masks		
Metric weights		
Ointment slab		
Parchment papers		
Pipette		
Porcelain mortar and pestle		
Reconstitution tube		
Rubber spatula		

Continued

147

Equipment	Correctly Identified (Yes/No)	Purpose
Safety glasses		
Stainless steel spatula		
Stirring rod		
Suppository molds		
Tongs		
Torsion balance		
Wedgewood mortar and pestle		
Weighing boat		

Lab Activity #11.2: Define the following terms used in non-sterile compounding.

Equipment needed:
- Medical dictionary
- Pencil/pen

Time needed to complete this activity: 15 minutes

1. Blending

_____

2. Comminution

_____

3. Diluent

_____

4. Geometric dilution

_____

5. Inert substance

_____

6. Levigation

_____

7. Pulverization

_____

8. Punch method

_____

9. Sifting

_____

10. Solvent

_____

11. Spatulation

_____

12. Trituration

_____

13. Tumbling

_____

The Class A Scale and Weighing Ingredients

Objective: Demonstrate proper procedures in weighing solids in the practice of pharmacy.

Weighing refers to the determination of a definite weight of a material to be used in the compounding of a prescription or the manufacturing of a dosage form. Weight is measured by means of a balance. Four types of balances are used in pharmacy practice: single beam (equal-arm or unequal), compound lever, torsion, and electronic. All pharmacies are required to have a Class A (III) balance, which can be a torsion balance. An unequal arm balance is used to measure weights greater than 60 g and is commonly used in manufacturing.

A torsion balance must have a maximum sensitivity of 6 mg with no load, and full load to one pan must cause the indicator or the rest point to be shifted not less than one division on the index point. A torsion balance can weigh up to 120 g. An electronic balance has a sensitivity of less than 10 mg and can weigh quantities of a drug more accurately than a torsion balance.

If a pharmacy uses a torsion balance, it must have a set of metric weights that consists of one 50-g, two 20-g, one 10-g, one 5-g, two 2-g, one 1-g, one 500-mg, two 200-mg, one 100-mg, one 50-mg, two 20-mg, and one 10-mg weight. These weights are made of brass, and forceps must be used in placing the weight on the pan.

Lab Activity #11.3: Identify the following components of a Class A prescription balance.

Equipment needed:
- Class A balance

Time needed to complete this activity: 5 minutes

Identifying the Parts of a Class A Balance Evaluation	Yes/No	Purpose
Calibrated dial		
Graduate dial		
Index plate		
Leveling screw feet		
Locking or arrest arm		
Weighing pans		

Lab Activity #11.4: Calibrate a Class A prescription balance.

Equipment needed:
- Class A prescription balance

Time needed to complete this activity: 5 minutes

Procedure

1. Arrest the balance by turning the arrest arm, making sure balance is steady on the work surface.
2. Level the balance from front to back by turning the leveling screw feet. Move leveling screw feet until all four sides of the balance are at the same distance from the surface on which they are resting.
3. Turn the calibrated dial to zero.
4. Level balance from left to right by adjusting the leveling screw feet.

Calibrating a Class A Balance Evaluation	Yes/No
Arrested the balance.	
Leveled the balance.	
Calibrated the balance to zero.	
Leveled the balance.	

Lab Activity #11.5: Use a torsion or electronic balance to weigh the proper quantity of ingredient.

Equipment needed:
- Disinfecting agent/cleanser
- Forceps
- Personal protective equipment (PPE)
- Lint-free paper towels
- Metal spatula
- Metric weights
- Sink with running hot and cold water
- Solid powder such as flour or sugar
- Torsion balance
- Weighing boats or glassine paper

Time needed to complete this activity: 30 minutes

Procedure

1. Wash hands thoroughly and put on PPE.
2. Organize materials on workbench.
3. Calibrate the Class A balance.
4. Lock balance.
5. Place a weighing boat or glassine paper on each pan.
6. Unlock the balance by releasing the arrest knob.
7. Make sure the pointer is resting at the center of the index.
8. Arrest the balance.
9. Place the correct weights on the right pan by using forceps.
10. Place the material to be weighed on the left pan using a spatula.
11. Release the balance.
12. If the pointer moves to the left, there is too much ingredient on the left pan. If the pointer moves to the right, there is not enough ingredient on the left pan.
13. Remove or add ingredient by using the spatula. Arrest the balance each time before material is added or released.
14. Double-check that the amount weighed on the left pan is correct.

149

Weight	Amount Weighed
20 mg	
65 mg	
83 mg	
554 mg	
858 mg	
1.25 g	
10 g	
21.25 g	
28.37 g	
45.3 g	

Procedure	Yes/No
Selected proper equipment and materials.	
Ensured that equipment, supplies, and compounding area were clean/disinfected	
Organized materials.	
Washed hands and put on PPE.	
Calibrated the Class A balance.	
Locked balance.	
Placed a weighing boat or glassine weigh paper on each pan.	
Unlocked the balance by releasing the arrest knob.	
Made sure the pointer was resting at the center of the index.	
Arrested the balance.	
Placed the correct weights on the right pan by using forceps.	
Placed the material to be weighed on the left pan using a spatula.	
Released the balance.	
Used pointer as reference to determine if enough ingredient on the left pan.	

Procedure	Yes/No
Removed or added ingredient by using the spatula. Arrested the balance each time before material was added or released.	
Double-checked that the amount weighed on the left pan was correct.	

Measuring Liquids

Objective: Demonstrate the proper procedures in measuring liquids in the practice of pharmacy.

Measuring refers to the exact determination of a definite volume of liquid. Glass measures are preferred for measuring liquids because they can indicate volume more accurately by the transparency of the glass.

When an aqueous or alcoholic liquid is poured into a graduate, surface forces cause its surface to become concave; the portion in contact with the liquid is drawn upward resulting in the formation of a meniscus. Two types of graduates are available: cylindrical and conical. The conical graduate is suitable for some measurements, but cylindrical graduates are more accurate because of their uniform and smaller average diameter. Pipettes are more accurate and convenient than very small graduates in measuring very small volumes. The very narrow bore permits greater distances between graduations on the apparatus, thus allowing greater accuracy in making the reading.

Lab Activity #11.6: Using a graduated cylinder of correct size, measure the following volumes and indicate the volume of the graduated cylinder that was used and why it was selected.

Equipment needed:
- Disinfecting agent/cleanser
- Personal protective equipment (PPE)
- Lint-free paper towels
- Sink with running hot and cold water
- Various sizes of graduated cylinders from 5 mL to 150 mL
- Water

Time needed to complete this activity: 30 minutes

Procedure

1. Collect the appropriate equipment and supplies for this procedure.
2. Ensure that equipment, supplies, and compounding area are clean and disinfected.
3. Organize materials on workbench.
4. Wash hands thoroughly and put on PPE.
5. Select a graduate of proper size; the selected graduate should not measure less than 20% of the capacity of the graduate.

6. Hold the graduate in the nondominant hand and grasp the original container with the label in such a position that any excess of liquid will not soil the label if it should run down the container.
7. Raise the graduate and hold it at eye level so that the graduation point to be read is level with the eye; measure the liquid.
8. Pour the liquid slowly into the graduate.
9. Remove excess liquid or add additional liquid to measure the proper quantity of liquid.
10. Place the graduated cylinder on a stable surface. Read the graduation point of the meniscus at eye level.

Volume	Amount Measured	Size of Graduate Cylinder Used	Reason for Selection of Graduate
2.5 mL			
5 mL			
9 mL			
10 mL			
24 mL			
30 mL			
38 mL			
48 mL			
66 mL			
88 mL			

Procedure	Yes/No
Selected proper equipment and materials.	
Ensured equipment, supplies, and compounding area were clean/disinfected.	
Organized materials.	
Washed hands and put on latex PPE.	
Selected a graduate of proper size; the selected graduate did not measure less than 20% of the capacity of the graduate.	
Did not soil the label of product being measured while pouring it into the graduated cylinder.	
Raised the graduate and held it at eye level so that the graduation point to be read was level with the eye; measured the liquid.	
Poured the liquid slowly into the graduate.	
Removed excess liquid or added additional liquid to measure the proper quantity of liquid.	
Placed the graduated cylinder on a stable surface to read the graduation point of the meniscus at eye level.	

Lab Activity #11.7: Measuring a liquid using a pipette.

Equipment needed:
- Disinfecting agent/cleanser
- Empty containers (2)
- Personal protective equipment (PPE)
- Lint-free paper towels
- Pipette
- Pipette filler
- Sink with running hot and cold water
- Water

Time needed to complete the activity: 15 minutes

151

Procedure

1. Collect the appropriate equipment and supplies for this procedure.
2. Ensure that equipment, supplies, and compounding area are clean/disinfected.
3. Organize materials on workbench.
4. Wash hands thoroughly and put on PPE.
5. Insert the pipette into the liquid to be withdrawn.
6. Squeeze the pipette bulb slowly.
7. Gently release your grip until the correct amount is withdrawn.
8. Remove the pipette from the liquid and hold above the container to which the liquid is being added.
9. Remove the bulb while holding your finger over the top of the pipette, slowly allowing the correct amount of liquid to flow into the empty container by releasing your finger from the top of the pipette.
10. Verify final measurement of liquid in the pipette.

Measuring a Liquid Using a Pipette Evaluation	Yes/No
¼ of a pipette	
½ of a pipette	
¾ of a pipette	
1 pipette	

Procedure	Yes/No
Selected proper equipment and materials.	
Ensured equipment, supplies, and compounding area were clean/disinfected.	
Organized materials.	
Washed hands and put on PPE.	
Inserted the pipette into the liquid to be withdrawn.	
Squeezed the pipette bulb slowly.	
Gently released grip until the correct amount was withdrawn.	
Removed the pipette from the liquid and held above the container to which the liquid was being added.	
Removed the bulb while holding a finger over the top of the pipette, slowly allowed the correct amount of liquid to flow into the empty container by releasing the finger from the top of the pipette.	

Calculating Beyond-Use Date

Objective: Properly calculate beyond-use date using current USP <795> guidelines.

> If a beyond-use date is not found in literature or is not included on the formulation record, beyond-use date is determined using USP <795> guidelines.

Lab Activity #11.8: Using USP <795> guidelines for beyond-use date, calculate the beyond-use date for the compounded products.

Equipment needed:
- Calculator
- Pen/pencil
- Calendar

Time needed to complete this activity: 30 minutes

1. You compounded 120 mL of simple syrup on May 30, 2021, from the following products:

   - Sucrose
   - Purified water

   What is the beyond-use date? _____

   _____

2. Using the punch method, you prepare 100 acetaminophen 500-mg capsules on July 21, 2021, from the following products:

   - Acetaminophen 500 mg tablets
   - Size 0 gelatin capsules

   What is the beyond-use date? _____

   _____

3. You made 100 mL of 2% ibuprofen gel on July 28, 2021, from the following products:

   - 200 mg ibuprofen tablets
   - PLO gel (pluronic lecithin organogel)

4. You made 100 mL of 5 mg/mL active pharmaceutical ingredient on July 14, 2021, from the following products:

   - Active pharmaceutical ingredient 5-mg tablets
   - Sterile water for injection
   - Artificial banana flavoring
   - Simple syrup

   What is the beyond-use date? _____

   _____

5. You made 120 g of Ointment X on July 23, 2021, from the following products:

   ■ Ointment B
   ■ Ointment D

   What is the beyond-use date? _____

   _____

Preparing Powders and Capsules

Objective: Demonstrate proper techniques in preparing capsules by using the punch method. Complete a compounding log and assign the correct beyond-use date.

A powder is a solid dosage form that can be taken orally or externally, depending on the drug being used. Powders are used in compounding tablets, capsules, and suspensions. A capsule is a solid dosage form in which the drug substance is enclosed in a hard or soft soluble container or shell of a suitable form of gelatin. A hard gelatin capsule, also known as a dry-filled capsule, consists of two sections. These capsules range in size from 000 to 5, measuring from 1000 to 100 mg. A soft elastic capsule is a soft, globular gelatin shell somewhat thicker than a hard gelatin capsule. A capsule dissolves in the stomach after 10 to 30 minutes, and the drug is released. A capsule eliminates objectionable tastes and odors of certain drugs.

A compounding log or mixing record is an official detailed record of the processes and materials used in the compounding process. A compounding log contains the name of the final product; the quantity prepared; a copy of the patient label; the recipe; the names, lot numbers, and quantities of all products and ingredients used; a record of the steps followed to prepare the prescription; the lot number assigned to the final product; and a beyond-use date.

Lab Activity #11.9: Preparing powders.

Equipment needed:
■ Electronic or torsion balance
■ Disinfecting agent/cleanser
■ Label
■ Personal protective equipment (PPE)
■ Lint-free paper towels
■ Mortar and pestle
■ Powder papers
■ Sieve
■ Sink with running hot and cold water
■ Spatula
■ Ointment slab
■ Powder A
■ Powder B
■ Powder C
■ Powder papers
■ Weighing boats

Time to needed complete this activity: 30 minutes

Procedure

1. Collect the appropriate equipment and supplies for this procedure.
2. Ensure that equipment, supplies, and compounding area are clean and disinfected.
3. Organize materials on workbench.
4. Wash hands thoroughly and put on PPE.
5. Triturate (grind) each powder using geometric dilution in the correct mortar and pestle; triturate in a circular motion to reduce the particle size of each powder.
6. Blend (mix) all three powders until the particle size is uniform and the powders are mixed thoroughly.
7. Stir the powder thoroughly using the appropriate spatula.
8. Pour the mixed powders through a sieve onto an ointment slab.
9. Place weighing boats or glassine weigh paper on the balance pan(s), and then tare the balance.
10. Weigh the correct quantity of powder.
11. Empty the ingredients from the weighing boat into a powder paper.
12. Fold powder paper.
13. Complete compounding log.
14. Label product.
15. Clean equipment and compounding area.

153

Pharmacy Compounding Log						
Product Compounded:						
Patient Name:			**Date Prepared:**			
			Date Dispensed:			
MRN or Rx #:			**Pharmacy Lot #:**			
Storage Requirements:			**Beyond-Use Date:**			
Drug Products/Ingredients Used						
Drug Name	**Mfg. Name and NDC**	**Mfg. Lot #**	**Mfg. Exp. Date**	**Quantity Measured**	**Measured By**	**Verified By**

Compounding Powder Evaluation	Yes/No
Selected proper equipment and materials.	
Ensured equipment, supplies, and compounding area were clean/disinfected.	
Organized materials.	
Washed hands thoroughly and put on PPE.	
Properly triturated powders using geometric dilution.	
Added powders in correct order.	
Blended powder properly.	
Stirred powders properly with a spatula.	
Sifted powders properly.	
Weighed the proper quantity of powder for each powder paper.	
Poured powder into papers and folded properly to avoid spillage.	
Observed the finished preparation to ensure it appeared as expected. Investigated any discrepancies and took appropriate actions to rectify before dispensing.	
Assigned correct beyond-use date.	
Properly completed compounding record.	
Properly labeled compounded product.	
Cleaned equipment and compounding area.	

Lab Activity #11.10: Preparing capsules using the punch method.

Equipment needed:
- 10 Acetaminophen 500-mg tablets
- 10 Empty size 0 gelatin capsules
- Clean gauze
- Counting tray
- Disinfecting agent/cleanser
- Electronic or torsion balance
- Label
- Personal protective equipment (PPE)
- Lint-free paper towels
- Metal spatula
- Mortar card
- Ointment slab
- Sink with running hot and cold water
- Soap
- Wedgewood or porcelain mortar and pestle
- Weighing boat or glassine weigh paper

Time to needed complete this activity: 30 minutes

Procedure

1. Gather supplies necessary for this exercise.
2. Ensure that equipment, supplies, and compounding area are clean and disinfected.
3. Organize materials on workbench.
4. Wash hands thoroughly and put on PPE.
5. Count out 10 acetaminophen 500-mg tablets on a counting tray.
6. Pour tablets into a Wedgewood mortar. Triturate with Wedgewood pestle.
7. Pour acetaminophen powder from mortar onto ointment slab.
8. Scrape remaining acetaminophen from mortar with spatula or mortar card onto ointment slab.
9. Using the spatula, form the powder into a "cake."
10. Place weighing boats or glassine weigh paper on the balance pan(s) and then tare the balance.
11. Place an empty capsule in weighing boat or on glassine weigh paper and obtain reading.
12. Tare the balance again to reset the scale to zero.
13. Remove empty capsule from weighing boat or glassine weigh paper.
14. Remove the capsule cap from the capsule body.
15. Hold the body of the capsule, open side down, with thumb and first finger.
16. Punch capsule into acetaminophen powder. After reaching the bottom of the powder on the ointment slab, turn the capsule lightly and pinch the open end of the capsule.
17. Repeat the process with the same capsule until body of capsule is filled.
18. Place the capsule cap on the body of the capsule.
19. Place the filled capsule on the weighing boat or glassine weigh paper and weigh the capsule.
20. If the capsule weighs more than 500 mg, gently remove the cap from the body of the capsule and take out some of the powder from the capsule; reweigh the capsule. If the capsule weighs less than 500 mg, remove the cap from the body of the capsule, add powder from the ointment slab, and reweigh the filled capsule.
21. Wipe off powder from exterior of capsule with a dry piece of gauze.
22. Repeat this process nine additional times and record the weight of each capsule in the table below.
23. Complete the compounding record.
24. Label product.
25. Clean equipment and compounding area.

Capsule #	Desired Weight	Actual Weight	Difference
1	500 mg		
2	500 mg		
3	500 mg		
4	500 mg		
5	500 mg		
6	500 mg		
7	500 mg		
8	500 mg		
9	500 mg		
10	500 mg		

Pharmacy Compounding Log	
Product Compounded:	

Patient Name:	**Date Prepared:**
	Date Dispensed:
MRN or Rx #:	**Pharmacy Lot #:**
Storage Requirements:	**Beyond-Use Date:**

Drug Products/Ingredients Used						
Drug Name	**Mfg. Name and NDC**	**Mfg. Lot #**	**Mfg. Exp. Date**	**Quantity Measured**	**Measured By**	**Verified By**

Evaluation of Capsule Preparation	Yes/No
Selected proper equipment and materials.	
Ensured equipment, supplies, and compounding area were clean/disinfected.	
Organized materials.	
Washed hands properly and put on PPE.	
Counted out proper quantity of acetaminophen tablets.	
Used Wedgewood or porcelain mortar and pestle.	
Triturated tablets to a fine powder.	
Tared balance before and after punching capsule; did not include capsule weight in the final capsule weight.	
Filled capsules properly using punch method.	
Final weight of capsules within 2 mg of desired weight.	
Removed excess powder from exterior of capsule.	
Observed the finished preparation to ensure it appeared as expected. Investigated any discrepancies and took appropriate actions to rectify before dispensing.	
Assigned correct beyond-use date.	
Properly completed compounding log.	
Properly labeled compounded product.	
Cleaned equipment and compounding area.	

Reconstituting a Powder

Objective: Demonstrate the proper steps in reconstituting a powder into a solution.

Reconstitution is the process by which a predetermined quantity of liquid is added to a powder to form a solution or a suspension. The drug manufacturer provides on the drug label the quantity and type of liquid to be added to the powder.

Lab Activity #11.11: Reconstituting a powder.

Equipment needed:
- 6-fl oz amber bottle
- Disinfecting agent/cleanser
- Distilled water
- Electronic or torsion balance
- Label
- Personal protective equipment (PPE)
- Lint-free paper towels
- Reconstitution tube
- "Shake well" label
- Sink with running hot and cold water
- Steel spatula
- Sugar
- Weighing boat/glassine weigh paper

Time needed to complete this activity: 15 minutes

Procedure

1. Gather supplies necessary for this exercise.
2. Ensure that equipment, supplies, and compounding area are clean and disinfected.
3. Organize materials on workbench.
4. Wash hands thoroughly and put on PPE.
5. Measure 2 g of sugar and pour into 6-fl oz amber bottle.
6. Bring amber bottle with sugar to reconstitution area.
7. Make sure the lower clamp on the reconstitution tube is clamped closed by pinching the clamp until it clicks shut.
8. Open the upper clamp on the reconstitution tube by clicking the clamp open.
9. Allow 88 mL of distilled water to flow into the reconstitution tube. When the tube is filled to 88 mL, close the upper clamp by pinching it shut.
10. Shake the amber bottle to loosen the sugar, then remove the bottle top.
11. Place the tip of the lower tube of reconstitution tube into mouth of amber bottle.
12. Open the lower clamp to allow approximately two-thirds of the water (60 mL) to enter the amber bottle slowly. Close the lower clamp.
13. Place bottle top back on amber bottle and shake amber bottle with distilled water-sugar solution until solution is evenly dissolved.
14. Remove bottle top and place the reconstitution tube into the mouth of the amber bottle; add remaining water from reconstitution tube into amber bottle and shake well.
15. Tightly recap the amber bottle and shake thoroughly.
16. Complete the compounding log.
17. Label product.
18. Clean equipment and compounding area.

Pharmacy Compounding Log						
Product Compounded:						
Patient Name:			**Date Prepared:**			
			Date Dispensed:			
MRN or Rx #:			**Pharmacy Lot #:**			
Storage Requirements:			**Beyond-Use Date:**			
Drug Products/Ingredients Used						
Drug Name	**Mfg. Name and NDC**	**Mfg. Lot #**	**Mfg. Exp. Date**	**Quantity Measured**	**Measured By**	**Verified By**

Reconstituting a Solid Powder Evaluation	Yes/No
Selected proper equipment and materials.	
Ensured equipment, supplies, and compounding area were clean/disinfected.	
Organized materials.	
Washed hands properly and put on PPE.	
Tared electronic or torsion balance.	
Weighed 2 g of sugar properly.	
Transferred sugar to amber bottle.	
Measured 88 mL of distilled water properly in reconstitution tube.	
Loosened sugar, then added 2/3 of water from reconstitution tube into amber bottle with sugar.	
Shook amber bottle with distilled water-sugar solution until solution was evenly dissolved.	
Emptied remaining water from reconstitution tube into amber bottle with sugar solution; shook solution thoroughly.	
Observed the finished preparation to ensure it appeared as expected. Investigated any discrepancies and took appropriate actions to rectify before dispensing.	
Affixed "Shake well" label to amber bottle.	
Assigned correct beyond-use date.	
Properly completed compounding log.	
Properly labeled compounded product.	
Cleaned equipment and compounding area.	

Nonsterile Compounding of Syrups and Elixirs

Objective: Demonstrate the proper technique for preparing oral syrup.

A syrup is a concentrated, viscous, aqueous solution of sugar or sugar substitute with or without flavors and medical substances. When purified water alone is used in making the solution of sucrose, the preparation is known as a syrup or simple syrup if the sucrose concentration is 85%. Sometimes alcohol is included in the preparation of syrup as a preservative and a solvent for flavors. A medicated syrup is one that contains a medicinal syrup. A flavored syrup is not usually medicated and is intended as a vehicle or flavor for prescriptions.

Syrups possess the ability to mask the taste of bitter or saline drugs. Disadvantages of syrups include the possibility of producing cavities and gingivitis in individuals. Another concern regarding syrups is the calorie content resulting from sugar.

Syrups can be compounded by using one of the following four techniques: solution with heat, solution by agitation, addition of sucrose to a liquid medication or flavored vehicle, and percolation. Solution with heat can be used if the ingredients are not volatile or can be broken down by heat. Purified water is heated to 80° C to 85° C; it is removed from its source of heat and sucrose is added. Other ingredients can be added at this time, and the solution is able to cool down. Agitation without heat is used when heat would cause the ingredients to break down. During this process, sugar is dissolved in purified water in a container that is larger than the volume being prepared and is shaken vigorously. Addition of sucrose to a liquid medication or a flavored extract is often used with fluid extracts and tinctures. A disadvantage of this process is that a precipitate may develop. Percolation is the process by which purified water is passed slowly over a bed of crystalline sugar, resulting in a syrup.

An elixir is a clear, pleasantly flavored, sweetened hydroalcoholic liquid for oral use. The primary ingredients in an elixir are ethanol and water, but glycerin, sorbitol, propylene glycol, flavoring agents, preservatives, and syrups are also used. An elixir is more fluid than syrup because it contains less sucrose than syrup. An elixir can be used as a vehicle for flavors and medications. An elixir does not mask the taste of saline ingredients. A major disadvantage of elixirs is their many incompatibilities with medications.

Lab Activity #11.12: Compounding Simple Syrup-NF.

Equipment needed:
- 4-oz prescription bottle
- Beaker
- Disinfecting agent/cleanser
- Graduated cylinder
- Label
- Personal protective equipment (PPE)
- Lint-free paper towels
- Metric weights
- Purified water
- Sink with running hot and cold water
- Sucrose
- Torsion or electronic balance

Time needed to complete this activity: 30 minutes

Procedure
1. Gather supplies necessary for this exercise.
2. Ensure that equipment, supplies, and compounding area are clean and disinfected.
3. Organize materials on workbench.
4. Wash hands thoroughly and put on PPE.
5. Place weighing boat on balance.
6. Tare torsion or electronic balance.

7. Weigh 85 g of sucrose and place in a beaker that has a capacity greater than 100 mL.
8. Measure 100 mL of purified water in graduate cylinder.
9. Add purified water to sucrose.
10. Agitate (shake) sucrose solution slowly.
11. Pour sucrose solution into a 4-oz bottle and qs up to 120 mL.
12. Complete the compounding log.
13. Label product.
14. Clean equipment and compounding area.

Pharmacy Compounding Log						
Product Compounded:						
Patient Name:			**Date Prepared:**			
			Date Dispensed:			
MRN or Rx #:			**Pharmacy Lot #:**			
Storage Requirements:			**Beyond-Use Date:**			
Drug Products/Ingredients Used						
Drug Name	**Mfg. Name and NDC**	**Mfg. Lot #**	**Mfg. Exp. Date**	**Quantity Measured**	**Measured By**	**Verified By**

Compounding a Syrup Evaluation	Yes/No
Selected proper equipment and materials.	
Ensured equipment, supplies, and compounding area were clean/disinfected.	
Organized materials.	
Washed hands properly and put on PPE.	
Tared electronic or torsion balance.	
Weighed sucrose properly.	
Measured purified water properly.	
Added ingredients properly.	
Shook sucrose solution thoroughly.	

Continued

Compounding a Syrup Evaluation	Yes/No
Poured sucrose solution into prescription bottle of proper size.	
Syrup qs to 120 mL with purified water.	
Observed the finished preparation to ensure it appeared as expected. Investigated any discrepancies and took appropriate actions to rectify before dispensing.	
Assigned correct beyond-use date.	
Properly completed compounding log.	
Properly labeled compounded product.	
Cleaned equipment and compounding area.	

Lab Activity #11.13: Compounding an elixir.

Prepare 4 fl oz of acetaminophen elixir using the following formula:

Acetaminophen	4 g
Propylene glycol	50 mL
Ethanol	200 mL
Sorbitol solution	600 mL
Saccharin sodium	5 g
Flavor	qs
Purified water	qsad 1000 mL

Equipment needed:
- 4-fl oz prescription bottle
- Acetaminophen tablets
- Calculator
- Disinfecting agent/cleanser
- Ethanol
- Filter paper
- Flavoring
- Funnel
- Graduated cylinders
- Label
- Personal protective equipment (PPE)
- Lint-free paper towels
- Propylene glycol
- Purified water
- Saccharin sodium
- Sink with running hot and cold water
- Sorbitol solution
- Spatula
- Torsion or electronic balance
- Wedgewood or porcelain mortar and pestle
- Weighing boat

Time needed to complete this activity: 30 minutes

Procedure

1. Perform the necessary calculations using a calculator to reduce the formula to 4 fl oz.
2. Gather supplies necessary for this exercise.
3. Ensure that equipment, supplies, and compounding area are clean and disinfected.
4. Organize materials on workbench.
5. Wash hands thoroughly and put on PPE.
6. Count out the correct number of acetaminophen tablets; weigh them on the balance.
7. Triturate acetaminophen tablets.
8. Weigh the triturated acetaminophen in weighing boat on balance.
9. Count out the correct quantity of saccharin sodium tablets.
10. Triturate the saccharin sodium tablets.
11. Weigh the triturated saccharin sodium in weighing boat on balance.
12. Measure the proper volumes of sorbitol solution, ethanol, and purified water in graduated cylinders.
13. Dissolve water-soluble ingredients in part of water.
14. Add and solubilize the sucrose in the aqueous solution.
15. Prepare an alcoholic solution containing the other ingredients.
16. Add the aqueous phase to the alcoholic solution.
17. Fold filter paper and place in funnel on top of graduated cylinder.
18. Filter the elixir.
19. QS the elixir to 120 mL with purified water.
20. Transfer elixir to 4-oz prescription bottle.
21. Complete compounding log.
22. Label product.
23. Clean equipment and compounding area.

Pharmacy Compounding Log						
Product Compounded:						
Patient Name:			**Date Prepared:**			
			Date Dispensed:			
MRN or Rx #:			**Pharmacy Lot #:**			
Storage Requirements:			**Beyond-Use Date:**			
Drug Products/Ingredients Used						
Drug Name	**Mfg. Name and NDC**	**Mfg. Lot #**	**Mfg. Exp. Date**	**Quantity Measured**	**Measured By**	**Verified By**

Compounding an Elixir Evaluation	Yes/No
Reduced formula to 120 mL.	
Selected proper equipment and materials.	
Ensured equipment, supplies, and compounding area were clean/disinfected.	
Organized materials.	
Washed hands properly and put on PPE.	
Measured correct quantities of acetaminophen and saccharin tablets.	
Triturated and weighed acetaminophen.	
Triturated and weighed saccharin.	
Measured liquids properly in correct graduates.	
Dissolved water-soluble ingredients in water.	
Mixed sucrose in aqueous phase.	
Prepared alcoholic solution.	
Added aqueous solution to alcoholic solution.	
Filtered elixir.	

Continued

Chapter **11** **Bulk Repackaging and Nonsterile Compounding**

Compounding an Elixir Evaluation	Yes/No
Transferred elixir to prescription bottle of proper size.	
Observed the finished preparation to ensure it appeared as expected. Investigated any discrepancies and took appropriate actions to rectify before dispensing.	
Assigned correct beyond-use date.	
Properly completed compounding log.	
Properly labeled compounded product.	
Cleaned equipment and compounding area.	

Nonsterile Compounding of Suspensions

Objective: Demonstrate the proper technique in preparing a suspension.

A suspension is a coarse dispersion containing finely divided insoluble material suspended in a liquid. All suspensions require that a suspending agent be used in their preparation. Examples of suspending agents include Avicel, Methocel, Metocel, Tylopur, Culminol, Celocel, Ethicel, Natrasol, Cellocize, Bermacol, Tylose, Carbopol, Povidone, and Kollidon. Sometimes a product can be prepared in dry form and is placed in the form of a suspension, with water added at the time of dispensing. A suspension may be taken orally, injected intramuscularly or subcutaneously, instilled intranasally, inhaled into the lungs, applied as a topical preparation, or used as an ophthalmic or otic agent.

Suspensions offer the following advantages over other dosage forms:

- They offer an alternative oral dosage form for patients who are unable to swallow a tablet or capsule, especially pediatric and geriatric patients.
- Some medications are poorly water soluble and cannot be formulated as solutions.
- Some drugs have an unpleasant taste, and a suspension allows for less interaction with the taste receptors in the mouth.
- Suspensions offer a method to provide sustained release of a drug by parenteral, topical, and oral routes of administration.

It is important to remember the size of the dispersed particles so they do not settle rapidly in their container. However, if the particles do settle in the container, they should be able to be redispersed with minimum effort by the patient. In addition, the suspension should be easy to pour, should have a pleasant taste, and should be resistant to microbial attack.

Lab Activity #11.14: Compounding a suspension.

Equipment needed:
- 120 mL of Syrpalta (or other wetting agent)
- Acetaminophen 500-mg tablets or caplets, 24 tablets
- Class A balance
- Disinfecting agent/cleanser
- Glass mortar and pestle
- Graduate
- Label
- Personal protective equipment (PPE)
- Light-resistant bottle
- Lint-free paper towels
- "Shake well" label
- Sink with running hot and cold water
- Size 100 sieve
- Spatula
- Stirring rod
- Wedgewood or porcelain mortar and pestle

Time to needed complete this activity: 30 minutes

Procedure

1. Gather supplies necessary for this exercise.
2. Ensure that equipment, supplies, and compounding area are clean and disinfected.
3. Organize materials on workbench.
4. Wash hands thoroughly and put on PPE.
5. Weigh the dry ingredients.
6. Triturate all dry ingredients with Wedgewood or porcelain mortar and pestle.
7. Filter a pulverized powder through a size 100 mesh sieve.
8. Measure 120 mL of Syrpalta into a graduate cylinder.
9. Transfer pulverized powder to glass mortar.
10. In the glass mortar, wet the powder with Syrpalta.
11. Using the glass pestle, levigate pulverized powder with Syrpalta until it forms a thick paste.
12. Pour the mixture into a graduate.
13. Add the remaining Syrpalta until the desired volume is obtained.
14. Stir mixture until it is mixed thoroughly.
15. Pour suspension into a container of appropriate size.
16. Complete compounding log.
17. Label product.
18. Clean equipment and compounding area.

Pharmacy Compounding Log

Product Compounded:

Patient Name:		Date Prepared:	
		Date Dispensed:	
MRN or Rx #:		Pharmacy Lot #:	
Storage Requirements:		Beyond-Use Date:	

Drug Products/Ingredients Used

Drug Name	Mfg. Name and NDC	Mfg. Lot #	Mfg. Exp. Date	Quantity Measured	Measured By	Verified By

Compounding a Suspension Evaluation	Yes/No
Selected proper equipment and materials.	
Ensured equipment, supplies, and compounding area were clean/disinfected.	
Washed hands properly and put on PPE.	
Organized materials.	
Counted out the correct quantity of tablets or caplets of acetaminophen.	
Measured Syrpalta correctly.	
Triturated ingredients properly.	
Filtered powder with sieve.	
Levigated pulverized powder properly.	
Pasted qs'd to proper volume.	
Mixed suspension properly.	
Poured suspension into container of proper size.	
Observed the finished preparation to ensure it appeared as expected. Investigated any discrepancies and took appropriate actions to rectify before dispensing.	

Continued

Compounding a Suspension Evaluation	Yes/No
Assigned correct beyond-use date.	
Properly completed compounding log.	
Properly labeled compounded product.	
Cleaned equipment and compounding area.	

Nonsterile Compounding of Emulsions

Objective: Demonstrate the proper technique for preparing an emulsion.

An emulsion is a dispersed system containing at least two immiscible liquid phases. An emulsion consists of at least three components: the dispersed phase, the dispersion medium, and an emulsifying agent. One of the two immiscible liquids is aqueous, and the second is oil. The emulsifying agent used and the quantities of aqueous and oil phases will determine whether the emulsion is oil-in-water (O/W) or water-in-oil (W/O). An oil-in-water emulsion finds oil dispersed as droplets in the aqueous phase. Conversely, when water is dispersed in the oil phase, it is known as a water-in-oil emulsion. Oral emulsions are normally oil-in-water; emulsified lotions may be O/W or W/O, depending on their usage.

Two distinct processes occur in the preparation of an emulsion. Flocculation is the process of clumping together particles or drops. Meanwhile, coalescence occurs when two immiscible liquids are shaken together. An emulsifying agent reduces the possibility that coalescence may occur. An emulsifying agent should:

- Be able to reduce surface tension
- Absorb quickly around the dispersed drops, which will prevent the drops from coalescing
- Provide an electrical potential, so drops repel each other
- Increase the viscosity of the emulsion
- Be effective in low concentration

Emulsifying agents may be classified as synthetic, natural, or finely divided. Examples of emulsifying agents include potassium laureate, triethanolamine stearate, sodium lauryl sulfate, dioctyl sodium sulfosuccinate, acacia, gelatin, lecithin, cholesterol, and Bentonite. In some situations, multiple emulsifying agents may be used in the preparation of an emulsion.

Lab Activity #11.15: Compounding an emulsion using the dry gum method.

Equipment needed:
- Active ingredients
- Class A balance
- Disinfecting agent/cleanser
- Glass mortar and pestle
- Graduate
- Gum acacia
- Label
- Personal protective equipment (PPE)
- Light-resistant container
- Lint-free paper towels
- Oil
- Sink with running hot and cold water
- Spatula
- Water
- Weighing boats

Time to needed complete this activity: 30 minutes

Procedure
1. Gather supplies necessary for this exercise.
2. Ensure that equipment, supplies, and compounding area are clean and disinfected.
3. Organize materials on workbench.
4. Wash hands thoroughly and put on PPE.
5. Measure oil in graduated cylinder and pour the oil into the glass mortar.
6. Place the desired amount of gum acacia into the mortar.
7. Levigate until the acacia is thoroughly wet and smooth.
8. Measure the appropriate amount of water desired for the aqueous phase in a clean graduate.
9. Levigate the mixture with a firm motion and quick movement until the primary emulsion is formed. The emulsion will change from a transparent liquid to a white liquid. The sound associated with the levigation process will change.
10. Add the remaining ingredients until the final volume is reached.
11. Homogenize the emulsion.
12. Pour into a container of appropriate size.
13. Complete compounding log.
14. Label product.
15. Clean equipment and compounding area.

Pharmacy Compounding Log

Product Compounded:

Patient Name:	Date Prepared:
	Date Dispensed:
MRN or Rx #:	Pharmacy Lot #:
Storage Requirements:	Beyond-Use Date:

Drug Products/Ingredients Used

Drug Name	Mfg. Name and NDC	Mfg. Lot #	Mfg. Exp. Date	Quantity Measured	Measured By	Verified By

Compounding an Emulsion (Dry Gum Method) Evaluation	Yes/No
Selected proper equipment and materials.	
Ensured equipment, supplies, and compounding area were clean/disinfected.	
Washed hands properly and put on PPE.	
Organized materials.	
Measured oil properly and poured into the proper mortar.	
Weighed the correct amount of acacia and poured into mortar.	
Levigated acacia properly.	
Measured water properly in the correct graduate.	
Levigated oil-acacia-water mixture properly.	
Mixture qs to proper volume.	
Poured emulsion into bottle of proper size.	
Observed the finished preparation to ensure it appeared as expected. Investigated any discrepancies and took appropriate actions to rectify before dispensing.	
Assigned correct beyond-use date.	

Continued

Compounding an Emulsion (Dry Gum Method) Evaluation	Yes/No
Properly completed compounding log.	
Properly labeled compounded product.	
Cleaned equipment and compounding area.	

Lab Activity #11.16: Compounding an emulsion using the wet gum method.

Equipment needed:
- Active ingredients
- Disinfecting agent/cleanser
- Glass mortar and pestle
- Graduate
- Gum acacia
- Label
- Personal protective equipment (PPE)
- Light-resistant container
- Lint-free paper towels
- Oil
- Sink with running hot and cold water
- Syrup
- Water

Time needed to complete this activity: 30 minutes

Procedure
1. Gather supplies necessary for this exercise.
2. Ensure that equipment, supplies, and compounding area are clean and disinfected.
3. Organize materials on workbench.
4. Wash hands thoroughly and put on PPE.
5. Place the desired amount of gum acacia into a glass mortar.
6. Slowly add the desired amount of water while levigating the mixture.
7. Gradually add the correct volume of oil while levigating the mixture.
8. Measure syrup and weigh active ingredient.
9. Add remaining ingredients to mixture and qs to proper volume.
10. Pour mixture into container of proper size.
11. Complete compounding log.
12. Label product.
13. Clean equipment and compounding area.

Pharmacy Compounding Log						
Product Compounded:						
Patient Name:			**Date Prepared:**			
			Date Dispensed:			
MRN or Rx #:			**Pharmacy Lot #:**			
Storage Requirements:			**Beyond-Use Date:**			
Drug Products/Ingredients Used						
Drug Name	**Mfg. Name and NDC**	**Mfg. Lot #**	**Mfg. Exp. Date**	**Quantity Measured**	**Measured By**	**Verified By**

Compounding an Emulsion (Wet Gum Method) Evaluation	Yes/No
Selected proper equipment and materials.	
Ensured equipment, supplies, and compounding area were clean/disinfected.	
Washed hands properly and put on PPE.	
Organized materials.	
Weighed acacia correctly and poured into correct mortar and pestle.	
Measured water in correct graduate.	
Poured water into mixture and levigated.	
Measured oil, poured into mixture, and levigated.	
Measured syrup correctly.	
Weighed active ingredient properly and incorporated in mixture.	
Poured emulsion into container of proper size.	
Observed the finished preparation to ensure it appeared as expected. Investigated any discrepancies and took appropriate actions to rectify before dispensing.	
Assigned correct beyond-use date.	
Properly completed compounding log.	
Properly labeled compounded product.	
Cleaned equipment and compounding area.	

Nonsterile Compounding of Creams and Ointments

Objective: Demonstrate the proper technique in preparing an ointment.

An ointment is a semisolid preparation intended for external application to the skin or mucous membranes. Normally, it contains a medication. Four different types of bases are used in the preparation of an ointment: hydrocarbon (oleaginous), absorption, water-removable (water washable), and water-soluble bases.

A hydrocarbon base is selected when the ointment will maintain prolonged contact with the skin and produces an emollient effect. An advantage of a hydrocarbon ointment base is that it will retain moisture in the skin. Examples of hydrocarbon bases include white petrolatum USP and white ointment USP.

Absorption bases have the ability to absorb water and are often W/O emulsions. They have the ability to allow aqueous solutions to be incorporated into them and provide an emollient effect. Examples of absorption bases include hydrophilic petrolatum USP and lanolin USP.

Water removable (water washable) bases are O/W emulsions and are the most commonly used type of ointment base. These ointment bases are easily removed from the skin, can be diluted with water, and allow the absorption of discharges from the skin (hydrophilic ointment USP).

A water-soluble ointment base consists of soluble components or may include jelled aqueous solutions. These ointment bases are water washable and leave no water-insoluble residue. Polyethylene glycol ointment NF is an example of a water-soluble base.

An ointment is prepared by dispersing the drug uniformly throughout the vehicle base. The drug material is a fine powder or is present in a solution before it is incorporated into the vehicle base.

A cream is another topical dosage form that may be a viscous liquid or a semisolid emulsion (O/W or W/O). A pharmaceutical cream is classified by the USP as a water removable base. Often creams are used for cosmetic purposes. O/W creams are used as hand and foundation cream; W/O creams include cold and emollient creams.

Lab Activity #11.17: Compounding an ointment.

Prepare 4 oz of the following formula:

Salicylic acid		2%
White petrolatum	qs	4 oz

Equipment needed:
- Calculator
- Disinfecting agent/cleanser
- Label

- Personal protective equipment (PPE)
- Lint-free paper towels
- Ointment jar
- Ointment slab or parchment paper
- Salicylic acid
- Sink with running hot and cold water
- Spatula
- Torsion or electronic balance
- Wedgewood or porcelain mortar and pestle
- Weighing boats
- White petrolatum

Time needed to complete this activity: 30 minutes

Procedure

1. Perform the necessary calculations for the prescription.
2. Gather supplies necessary for this exercise.
3. Ensure that equipment, supplies, and compounding area are clean and disinfected.
4. Organize materials on workbench.
5. Wash hands thoroughly and put on PPE.
6. Weigh proper quantity of salicylic acid in weighing boat on torsion or electronic balance.
7. Transfer salicylic acid to Wedgewood or porcelain mortar and pestle, and triturate.
8. Weigh proper quantity of white petrolatum in a weighing boat on torsion or electronic balance.
9. Transfer white petrolatum to corner of ointment slab or parchment paper.
10. Add salicylic acid to other corner of ointment slab or parchment paper.
11. Add a small amount of the white petrolatum to the salicylic acid and mix thoroughly using an S pattern with the spatula.
12. Continue adding white petrolatum to white petrolatum–salicylic acid compound; mix thoroughly.
13. Ointment should not appear to have a gritty appearance; if it does, continue to mix it until the ointment has a uniform consistency.
14. Transfer ointment to an ointment jar of proper size. The top of the ointment in the ointment jar should be smooth and level.
15. Complete compounding log.
16. Label product.
17. Clean equipment and compounding area.

Pharmacy Compounding Log						
Product Compounded:						
Patient Name:			**Date Prepared:**			
			Date Dispensed:			
MRN or Rx #:			**Pharmacy Lot #:**			
Storage Requirements:			**Beyond-Use Date:**			
Drug Products/Ingredients Used						
Drug Name	**Mfg. Name and NDC**	**Mfg. Lot #**	**Mfg. Exp. Date**	**Quantity Measured**	**Measured By**	**Verified By**

Compounding an Ointment Evaluation	Yes/No
Performed correct calculations.	
Selected proper equipment and materials.	
Ensured equipment, supplies, and compounding area were clean/disinfected.	
Washed hands properly and put on PPE.	
Organized materials.	
Weighed correct quantity of salicylic acid.	
Triturated salicylic acid to a fine powder in Wedgewood or porcelain mortar and pestle.	
Weighed correct quantity of white petrolatum.	
Transferred salicylic acid and white petrolatum to ointment slab or parchment paper.	
Used S motion to incorporate salicylic acid into white petrolatum.	
Texture of salicylic acid-white petrolatum compound is evenly mixed. No visible signs of salicylic acid powder. Ointment is not gritty.	
Transferred salicylic acid-white petrolatum ointment to ointment jar of proper size.	
Final product has a pharmaceutically elegant appearance.	
Observed the finished preparation to ensure it appeared as expected. Investigated any discrepancies and took appropriate actions to rectify before dispensing.	
Assigned correct beyond-use date.	
Properly completed compounding log.	
Properly labeled compounded product.	
Cleaned equipment and compounding area.	

Nonsterile Compounding of Molded Tablets

Objective: To be able to calibrate the mold before making molded tablets and accurately compound pharmaceutically elegant tablets with a mold

Molded tablets, also known as tablet triturates, have a limited use because they disintegrate quickly when exposed to moisture and are limited to substances that require a smaller dose. This dosage form also requires a base and additional additives to the active drug ingredient. Common additives include dextrose, lactose, and sucrose. A wetting agent, typically a hydroalcoholic solution (50% to 80% alcohol), is used to bind the tablet ingredients; alcohol is used to dry the triturate while the water causes sugar to dissolve and bind the tablet. The ingredients are pressed into a tablet mold and allowed to completely dry. Because each tablet mold varies in size, calibrating the mold to the specific strength of each molded tablet compounded is necessary. Therefore, it takes great skill and experience to make molded tablets. For more information about molded tablets and to view a video of calibrating a molded tablet and preparing molded tablets, visit http://pharmlabs.unc.edu/labs/tablets/molded.htm.

Lab Activity #11.18: Calibrating the tablet mold.

Equipment needed:
- 80- to 100-Mesh sieve
- Active drug ingredient
- Calculator
- Disinfecting agent/cleaner
- Glass mortar and pestle
- Glassine weigh paper
- Personal protective equipment (PPE)
- Tablet mold
- Ointment slab
- Powder base
- Sink with running hot and cold water
- Spatula
- Torsion or electronic balance
- Wetting agent (alcohol and water)

Time needed to complete this activity: 30 minutes

Procedure
1. Gather supplies necessary for this exercise.
2. Ensure that equipment, supplies, and compounding area are clean and disinfected.
3. Organize materials on workbench.

169

4. Wash hands thoroughly and put on PPE.
5. Make tablets that contain only a powder base first. Weigh the entire batch and then average the weight per tablet.
6. Determine the average weight of only the active drug; fill a few cavities in the mold and determine the average weight per tablet.
7. Divide the quantity of drug required per tablet in the prescription by the average weight per tablet of the active drug to get the percentage of the cavity that will be active drug.
8. Subtract the percentage in step 7 from 100%; this equals the percentage of the cavity that will be inactive powder base.
9. Use percentages of both the active drug in the cavity and the base in the cavity to calculate the amount of base and drug to weigh.
10. For example, if the mold holds 10 cavities, each holding 100 mg, then 1000 mg of mixture is needed to fill the entire mold. From this calculation, calculate the base and drug to weigh; multiply 1000 mg by the two different percentages from steps 7 and 8.
11. Prepare 5% to 10% excess mixture.
12. Clean equipment and compounding area.

Calibrating the Tablet Mold Evaluation	Yes/No
Selected proper equipment and materials.	
Ensured equipment, supplies, and compounding area were clean/disinfected.	
Organized materials on workbench.	
Washed hands thoroughly and put on PPE.	
Made tablets that contained only a powder base first. Weighed the entire batch and then averaged the weight per tablet.	
Determined the average weight of only the active drug; filled a few cavities in the mold and averaged the weight per tablet.	
Divided the quantity of the total prescription by the average weight of each tablet's active ingredient.	
Subtracted the percentage in step 7 from 100% and determined the volume (%) available for the base.	
Used percentages of both the active drug in the cavity and the base in the cavity to calculate the amount of base and drug to weigh.	
Prepared 5% to 10% excess mixture.	
Cleaned equipment and compounding area.	

Lab Activity #11.19: Using the calculations determined in Lab Activity #11.18, compounding molded tablets.

Equipment needed:
- 80- to 100-Mesh sieve
- Active drug ingredient
- Disinfecting agent/cleaner
- Glass mortar and pestle
- Glassine weigh paper
- Personal protective equipment (PPE)
- Ointment slab
- Powder base
- Sink with running hot and cold water
- Spatula
- Tablet mold
- Torsion or electronic balance
- Wetting agent (alcohol and water)

Time needed to complete this activity: 30 minutes

Procedure
1. Gather supplies necessary for this exercise.
2. Ensure that equipment, supplies, and compounding area are clean and disinfected.
3. Organize materials on workbench.
4. Wash hands thoroughly and put on PPE.
5. Prepare the powder mixture using proper techniques for that specific recipe; sift the mixture through an 80- to 100-mesh sieve.
6. Moisten the powder mixture with the wetting agent (alcohol/water) until it adheres to the pestle.
7. Place the cavity plate on the ointment slab.
8. Take the molded form and press mixture into the cavity plate using a hard rubber spatula.
9. Apply sufficient pressure onto each cavity to make sure all cavities are filled entirely and fully.
10. Inspect the cavity plate to ensure all cavities are filled to capacity; very little mixture should be left unused.
11. Align the cavity plate onto the peg plate and then slowly press down evenly onto the peg plate.
12. The cavity plate will fall, having pushed out the tablets onto the pegs.
13. Allow the tablets to dry in the pegs, approximately 1 to 2 hours.
14. Invert the plate and press the tablets off.
15. Complete compounding log.
16. Package and label product.
17. Clean equipment and compounding area.

Pharmacy Compounding Log

Product Compounded:

Patient Name:	Date Prepared:
	Date Dispensed:
MRN or Rx #:	Pharmacy Lot #:
Storage Requirements:	Beyond-Use Date:

Drug Products/Ingredients Used

Drug Name	Mfg. Name and NDC	Mfg. Lot #	Mfg. Exp. Date	Quantity Measured	Measured By	Verified By

Compounding Molded Tablets Evaluation	Yes/No
Selected proper equipment and materials.	
Ensured equipment, supplies, and compounding area were clean/disinfected.	
Organized materials on workbench.	
Washed hands thoroughly and put on PPE.	
Prepared the powder mixture using proper techniques for the specific recipe; sifted the mixture through an 80- to 100-mesh sieve.	
Moistened the powder mixture with the wetting agent (alcohol/water) until it adhered to the pestle.	
Placed the cavity plate on the ointment slab.	
Used the molded form and pressed mixture into the cavity plate using a spatula. Chose correct spatula for the tablets being prepared.	
Applied sufficient pressure onto each cavity to make sure all cavities were filled entirely and fully.	
Inspected the cavity plate to ensure all cavities were filled to capacity; very little mixture was left unused.	
Aligned the cavity plate onto the peg plate and slowly pressed down evenly onto the peg plate.	

Continued

171

Compounding Molded Tablets Evaluation	Yes/No
Pushed out the tablets onto the pegs.	
Allowed the tablets to dry in the pegs.	
Inverted the plate and pressed the tablets off.	
Observed the finished preparation to ensure it appeared as expected. Investigated any discrepancies and took appropriate actions to rectify before dispensing.	
Assigned correct beyond-use date.	
Properly completed compounding log.	
Packaged and labeled product.	
Cleaned equipment and compounding area.	

Repackaging Bulk Medications

Objective: To be able to use good manufacturing practices when packaging a unit dose or single dose container, properly label each unit dose and properly document repackaging

Pharmacies will often repackage bulk medications into single (unit) doses. This is done to help lower pharmacy cost and decrease dosing errors. When repackaging, good manufacturing practices must be followed, each unit dose must be labeled appropriately, and the procedure must be documented.

Lab Activity #11.20: Repacking bulk medications.

Equipment needed:
- Alcohol prep pads
- Counting tray and spatula
- Personal protective equipment (PPE)
- Sink with running hot and cold water

- Unit dose packing of choice—plastic cups/oral syringes, blister packs/ADS supplies
- Various medications as assigned

Time needed to complete this activity: 60 minutes

Procedure
1. Gather supplies necessary for this exercise.
2. Ensure that equipment, supplies, and compounding area are clean and disinfected.
3. Organize materials on workbench.
4. Wash hands thoroughly and put on PPE.
5. Repackage the medications as listed by your instructor using good manufacturing practices and proper labeling.
6. Document each medication repackaged in the Unit Dose Log.
7. Have pharmacist verify unit doses/single doses and Unit Dose Log.
8. Clean equipment and work area.
9. Store unit doses in proper place in the pharmacy.

	Date	Drug	Strength	Dosage Form	Amount	Mfg.	Mfg. Lot #	Mfg. Exp. Date	Pharmacy Exp. Date	Pharmacy Lot #	Tech	RPh
1												
2												
3												
4												
5												

	Date	Drug	Strength	Dosage Form	Amount	Mfg.	Mfg. Lot #	Mfg. Exp. Date	Pharmacy Exp. Date	Pharmacy Lot #	Tech	RPh
6												
7												
8												
9												
10												
11												
12												
13												
14												
15												
16												
17												
18												
19												
20												
21												
22												
23												
24												
25												

Chapter **11** **Bulk Repackaging and Nonsterile Compounding**

Repacking Bulk Medications Evaluation	Yes/No
Selected proper equipment and materials.	
Ensured equipment, supplies, and compounding area were clean/disinfected.	
Organized materials on workbench.	
Washed hands thoroughly and put on PPE.	
Repackaged the medications as listed in the table using good manufacturing practices.	
Properly labeled each unit/single dose.	
Documented each medication repackaged in the Unit Dose Log.	
Assigned correct expiration date.	
Had pharmacist verify unit doses/single doses and verify the Unit Dose Log.	
Cleaned equipment and work area.	
Placed unit doses in proper storage area in the pharmacy.	

12 Aseptic Technique and Sterile Compounding

Standard 2.6: Perform mathematical calculations essential to the duties of pharmacy technicians in a variety of settings.

Standard 2.7: Explain the pharmacy technician's role in the medication use process.

Standard 2.8: Practice and adhere to effective infection control procedures.

Standard 3.2: Receive, process, and prepare prescriptions/medication orders for completeness, accuracy, and authenticity to ensure safety.

Standard 3.5: Prepare non–patient-specific medications for distribution.

Standard 3.6: Assist pharmacist in preparing, storing, and distributing medication products including those requiring special handling and documentation.

Standard 3.8: Maintain pharmacy facilities and equipment.

Standard 3.9: Use information from Safety Data Sheets (SDS), National Institute of Occupational Safety and Health (NOSH) Hazardous Drug List, and the United States Pharmacopoeia (USP) to identify, handle, dispense, and safely dispose of hazardous medications and materials.

Standard 3.13: Use current technology to ensure the safety and accuracy of medication dispensing.

Standard 3.15: Describe basic concepts related to preparation for sterile and non-sterile compounding.

Standard 3.22: Prepare, store, and deliver medication products requiring special handling and documentation.

Standard 3.28: Apply accepted procedures in inventory control of medications, equipment, and devices.

Standard 3.23: Prepare compounded sterile preparations per applicable, current USP Chapters.

Standard 3.25: Prepare or simulate chemotherapy/hazardous drug preparations per applicable, current USP Chapters.

Standard 3.31: Manage drug product inventory stored in equipment or devices used to ensure the safety and accuracy of medication dispensing.

Standard 4.2: Apply patient- and medication-safety practices in aspects of the pharmacy technician's roles.

Standard 4.7: Explain pharmacist and pharmacy technician roles in medication management services.

Standard 4.8: Describe best practices regarding quality assurance measures according to leading quality organizations.

Standard 5.1: Describe and apply state and federal laws pertaining to processing, handling, and dispensing of medications including controlled substances.

Standard 5.2: Describe state and federal laws and regulations pertaining to pharmacy technicians.

Standard 5.3: Explain that differences exist between states regarding state regulations, pertaining to pharmacy technicians, and the processing, handling, and dispensing of medications.

Standard 5.5: Describe pharmacy compliance with professional standards and relevant legal, regulatory, formulary, contractual, and safety requirements.

Standard 5.6: Describe Occupational Safety and Health Administration (OSHA), National Institute of Occupational Safety and Health (NOSH) Hazardous Drug List, and the United States Pharmacopoeia (USP) requirements for prevention and treatment of exposure to hazardous substances (e.g., risk assessment, personal protective equipment, eyewash, spill kit).

Standard 5.7: Describe OSHA requirements for prevention and response to blood-borne pathogen exposure (e.g., accidental needle stick, post-exposure prophylaxis).

Standard 5.9: Participate in pharmacy compliance with professional standards and relevant legal, regulatory, formulary, contractual, safety requirements.

Standard 5.10: Describe major trends, issues, goals, and initiatives taking place in the pharmacy profession.

Terms and Definitions

Select the correct term from the following list and write the corresponding letter in the blank next to the statement.

A. Anteroom
B. Aseptic technique
C. Clean room
D. Health care–associated infection (HAI)
E. Infection control
F. Standard operating procedures (SOPs)
G. Standard Precautions (Universal Precautions)
H. Sterile preparation
I. *United States Pharmacopeia <797>* (USP <797>)
J. *United States Pharmacopeia <800>* (USP <800>)

_____ 1. A preparation that contains no living microorganisms

_____ 2. The procedures used to eliminate the possibility of a drug becoming contaminated with microbes or particles

_____ 3. Pharmaceutical Compounding—Sterile Preparations, of the *USP National Formulary*; contains a set of enforceable sterile compounding standards; describes the guidelines, procedures, and compliance requirements for compounding sterile preparations; and sets the standards that apply to all settings in which sterile preparations are compounded

_____ 4. The room adjacent to the "clean room" used for donning all personal protective equipment (PPE) and wiping down all supplies that will be used in the compounding area

_____ 5. Written guidelines and criteria that list specific steps for various competencies

_____ 6. In pharmacy, a contained and controlled environment in the pharmacy that has a low level of environmental pollutants (eg, dust, airborne microbes, aerosol particles, and chemical vapors); the clean room is used for preparing sterile medication products

_____ 7. General chapter created to identify the requirements for receipt, storage, mixing, preparing, compounding, dispensing, and administration of hazardous drugs to protect the patient, health care personnel, and environment

_____ 8. Policies and procedures put in place to minimize the risk of spreading infections in hospitals or other health care facilities

_____ 9. An infection that patients acquire during the course of receiving treatments for other conditions in an institutional setting

_____ 10. A set of standards that reduces the possibility of contamination and the risk of transmission of infectious disease; these standards are used throughout a health care facility, including to prepare medications

Select the correct term from the following list and write the corresponding letter in the blank next to the statement.

A. Biological safety cabinet (BSC)
B. Compounding aseptic containment isolator (CACI)
C. Horizontal laminar flow hood
D. Laminar airflow work-bench (LAFW)
E. Primary engineering control (PEC)
F. Vertical laminar flow hood

_____ 11. An environment for the preparation of compounded sterile preparations in which air originating from the back of the hood moves forward across the hood and into the room

_____ 12. An environment for the preparation of chemotherapeutic and other hazardous agents in which air originating from the roof of the hood moves downward (over the agent) and is captured in a vent on the floor of the hood

_____ 13. A device or zone that provides Class 5 environment for sterile compounding (ie, hoods)

_____ 14. A vertical flow hood that should be used for making hazardous sterile preparations in the clean room

_____ 15. An environment for the preparation of sterile products

_____ 16. ISO Class 5 compounding area used to prepare hazardous drugs

Select the correct term from the following list and write the corresponding letter in the blank next to the statement.

A. Beyond-use date (BUD)
B. Compounded sterile preparations (CSPs)
C. Critical site
D. Gauges
E. First air
F. Hazardous waste

_____ 17. Any surface or area exposed to first air, which is exposed or at risk for touch, or direct air (ie, vial tops, open ampules, needle hubs, or injection ports)

_____ 18. Defined by USP <797> as the date or time after which a compounded sterile preparation (CSP) shall not be administered, stored, or transported; it is determined from the date the preparation is compounded

_____ 19. The sizes of needle openings

_____ 20. Any waste that meets the Resource Conservation and Recovery Act (RCRA) criteria of ignitability, corrosiveness, reactivity, or toxicity

_____ 21. Air exiting the HEPA filter in a unidirectional air stream

_____ 22. Preparations prepared in a sterile environment using non-sterile ingredients or devices that must be sterilized before administration

Select the correct term from the following list and write the corresponding letter in the blank next to the statement.

A. Hazardous drug
B. Hyperalimentation
C. Parenteral medications
D. Peripheral parenteral
E. Peripheral parenteral nutrition (PPN)
F. Precipitate
G. Reconstituted
H. Total parenteral nutrition (TPN)

_____ 23. Parenteral nutrition for individuals who are unable to eat solids or liquids

_____ 24. Large volume intravenous nutrition administered through a central vein (eg, subclavian vein), which allows for a higher concentration of solutions

_____ 25. A substance that has had a diluent (eg, saline or sterile water) added to a powder

_____ 26. Any drug that has been proven to have dangerous effects during animal or human testing; it may cause cancer or may harm certain organs or pregnant women

_____ 27. Injection of a medication into the veins on the periphery of the body instead of into a central vein or artery

_____ 28. To separate from solution or suspension; a solid that emerges from a liquid solution

_____ 29. Medications that bypass the digestive system but are intended for systemic action; the term *parenteral* most commonly describes medications given by injection, such as intravenously or intramuscularly

_____ 30. Intravenous nutrition administered through veins on the periphery of the body rather than through a central vein or artery

True or False

Write T or F next to each statement.

_____ 1. One of the most trivial responsibilities that a hospital pharmacy technician can have is the proper preparation of parenteral medications.

_____ 2. Medication refrigerators and freezers may hold only medications and should not be used to store food or drink.

_____ 3. Some medications should never be filtered because filtering would remove active drug from the solution.

_____ 4. Supply items do not need to be wiped down with an appropriate cleaning solution before they are brought into the clean room.

_____ 5. Nosocomial infections are infections that originate in a hospital.

_____ 6. For an urgent-use CSP, the compounding process can take no longer than 1 hour and be administered within 12 hours of compounding the CSP.

_____ 7. All donning of PPE occurs in the anteroom.

_____ 8. The pharmacy technician must work at least 2 inches from the sides and front of the hood.

_____ 9. A BSC must be turned on at least 10 minutes before use.

177

_____ 10. Sharps containers are to be replaced when three-quarters full and must be picked up or delivered to an approved "red bag" or medical waste treatment site.

Multiple Choice

Complete each question by circling the best answer.

1. Amiodarone should go in _____.
   A. ½NS
   B. D$_5$W
   C. NS
   D. D$_5$NS

2. Category 1 risk level CSPs can be stored at refrigerated temperature for _____ after compounding.
   A. 12 hours or less
   B. 24 hours or less
   C. 7 days
   D. 3 days

3. Category 2 risk level CSPs can be stored at room temperature for _____ after compounding.
   A. 12 hours or greater
   B. 24 hours or greater
   C. 30 hours
   D. 48 hours

4. Nitroglycerin must be put only into _____.
   A. glass containers
   B. small-volume drips
   C. syringe pumps
   D. Viaflex bags

5. All flow hoods are recertified every _____ by an independent contractor or when the hood is moved.
   A. month
   B. 3 months
   C. 6 months
   D. year

6. A chunk of rubber from the vial stopper is dislodged and falls into the vial, which is known as _____
   A. filtering
   B. beveling
   C. coring
   D. piggybacking

7. When aseptic technique is used, what should *not* be worn?
   A. Gloves
   B. Artificial nails
   C. Hair ties
   D. Prescription glasses

8. For proper hand washing technique, you should wash which areas for 30 seconds?
   A. Hands, nails, face, and forearms
   B. Hands, nails, wrists, and forearms
   C. Fingernails, wrists, and underarms
   D. Fingernails, hands, and face

9. To clean the hood, you should use _____
   A. soap and water
   B. antimicrobial soap and hot water
   C. 70% isopropyl alcohol
   D. hydrogen peroxide

10. The horizontal flow hood (LAFW) must be turned on at least _____ before use.
    A. 30 minutes
    B. 60 minutes
    C. 2 hours
    D. 8 hours

11. The laminar flow hood should be cleaned and disinfected _____
    A. monthly
    B. weekly
    C. daily
    D. at the start of each shift

12. Walls, ceilings, and storage shelves in the clean room should be disinfected _____
    A. monthly
    B. weekly
    C. daily
    D. at the start of each shift

13. Counters and work surfaces in the clean room should be cleaned and disinfected _____
    A. monthly
    B. weekly
    C. daily
    D. at the start of each shift

14. Ciprofloxacin must be put in a(n) _____
    A. glass container
    B. amber bag to protect from light
    C. multiple dose vial
    D. CADD pump

15. While continuous compounding is taking place, the biological safety hood should be cleaned every _____
    A. day
    B. shift
    C. 12 hours
    D. 30 minutes

Fill in the Blanks

Answer each question by completing the statement in the space provided.

1. All parenteral medications should be prepared in a manner that reduces the possibility of _____.

2. To prevent the dissemination of highly contagious diseases, hospitals usually require an employee to receive both tuberculosis (TB) testing and an immunization against influenza _____.

3. A tension-type syringe cannot be used when preparing doses of _____ drugs.

4. A quarterly _____ test must be done for each person compounding products in the hood.

5. A medication that contains any _____ or unwanted debris can cause a dangerous infection, or even death, when administered to a patient.

6. Regardless of the type of hood used, the placement of the _____ is one of the most important aspects to consider when preparing sterile medications.

7. When an MDV solution is used, the _____ the vial was opened must be written on the label, along with the _____ of the person who opened the vial.

8. When a diluent is added to a powder, an equal amount of air must be removed from the vial or _____ pressure is created.

9. Pharmacy technicians should always follow _____ guidelines and should be trained in proper disposal of hazardous substances.

10. Pharmacy technicians and pharmacists must be instructed on all _____ if they are to prepare all types of compounded sterile preparations.

Matching

Match the following abbreviations with their meanings.

A. Amp
B. MDV
C. SDV
D. D_5NS
E. $D_{10}NS$
F. NS
G. ½NS
H. LR
I. ¼NS
J. D_5½NS
K. SWFI
L. D_5W
M. $D_{10}W$
N. NPO
O. Preop
P. Postop

_____ 1. 10% dextrose in normal saline

_____ 2. Lactated Ringer's solution

_____ 3. Single dose vial

_____ 4. 10% dextrose in water

_____ 5. Sterile water for injection

_____ 6. One-half (0.45%) normal saline

_____ 7. Medication to be given before surgery (e.g., sedative or antiemetic)

_____ 8. Ampule

_____ 9. Normal saline (0.9%)

_____ 10. 5% dextrose in water

_____ 11. Multidose vial

_____ 12. Nothing by mouth

_____ 13. One-quarter (0.225%) normal saline

_____ 14. 5% dextrose in normal saline

_____ 15. 5% dextrose in one-half (0.45%) normal saline

_____ 16. Medication to be given after surgery (e.g., pain control or antiemetic)

Match the following USP <797> air standards with the proper area of the pharmacy.

A. ISO Class 8
B. ISO Class 7
C. ISO Class 6
D. ISO Class 5

_____ 17. IV hood

_____ 18. Nonhazardous room

_____ 19. Anteroom

_____ 20. Clean room (i.e., buffer room and anteroom)

Short Answer

Write a short response to each question in the space provided.

1. Name two types of hyperalimentation.

_____

_____

2. List the common needle sizes used for preparing IV medications.

_____

_____

3. What two items can be used to draw up medications from an ampule?

_____

_____

4. How are chemotherapy wastes disposed?

_____

_____

_____

5. Why are dextrose, amino acids, and lipids used in TPNs?

_____

_____

6. Why are syringes not reused when a change is made from one drug to another?

_____

_____

7. Why is the placement of the hands so important when sterile products are prepared?

_____

_____

Research Activities

Follow the instructions given in each exercise and provide a response.

1. Access the website *http://www.usp.org/usp-healthcare-professionals/compounding/compounding-general-chapters/usp-general-chapter-hazardous-drugs-handling-healthcare-se* to answer the following questions:

   A. When was the USP General Chapter <800> Hazardous Drugs first published?

   B. When did USP <800> become official?

2. Access the website *https://www.ptcb.org/credentials/certified-compounded-sterile-preparation-technician* to answer the following questions:

   A. List the requirements to become a Certified Compounded Sterile Preparation Technician.

   B. Would you want to earn this additional certificate as pharmacy technician, why or why not?

Critical Thinking

Reply to each question based on what you have learned in the chapter.

1. You have been preparing injections in the IV room and suddenly stick your finger with a needle. What went wrong? What mistake did you make that caused you to stick your finger?

2. If you stick your finger with a sterile needle, is it necessary to go to the emergency department for treatment?

3. You have been assigned to work in the IV preparation room for your shift. What are the first items you need to take care of when you walk into the IV room? What aseptic technique requirements need to be followed before you begin preparation of IVs?

4. What should you do at the end of your shift to ensure a smooth workflow when your replacement technician comes to relieve you?

5. Use the following drug label and IV order to answer the questions:

Main Hospital
123 Main Street
Anywhere, USA 12345

Name: Martin Perez
MRN: 95478

Room: 2201

Azithromycin 500 mg in
NS 250 mL

Administer IV daily
Infuse over 1 hour

Prepared by: _____ Exp: _____   Checked by: _____

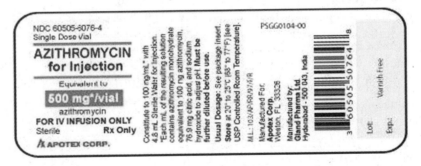

A. What is the name of the medication?

B. What is the route for this medication?

C. The label reads to add 4.8 mL of SWFI to reconstitute. After reconstitution, what will be the concentration of the solution?

181

D. How many milliliters of the reconstituted solution will you need to draw up to make the IV order?

E. What will be the concentration of the IV bag after you add the medication?

F. What auxiliary labels should go on the IV bag?

G. What is the risk level for this CSP?

H. How many milliliters per minute will the patient receive if it is infused over the course of 1 hour?

RELATE TO PRACTICE

Lab Scenarios
Pharmacy Equipment Used in Preparation of Sterile Compounds

Objective: To familiarize the pharmacy technician with equipment used in the preparation of sterile compounds.

Parenteral dosage forms differ from all other drug dosage forms because they are injected directly into body tissues through the skin and mucous membranes. Some of the many routes by which parenteral medications are injected into the body include intravenous, intramuscular, subcutaneous, and intradermal. Parenteral dosage forms differ from other pharmaceutical dosage forms for the following reasons:

- All products must be sterile.
- All products must be free from pyrogenic contamination.
- Injectable solutions must be free from visible particulate matter.
- Parenteral products should be isotonic; however, the degree of isotonicity will vary according to the route of administration of the medication.
- All parenteral products must be stable chemically, physically, and microbiologically.

- These products must be compatible with IV diluents, delivery systems, and other drug products that are co-administered.

Pharmacy technicians need to be familiar with various solutions that serve as vehicles for parenteral drugs. In addition, the technician must be familiar with equipment used in sterile compounding and its purpose.

Lab Activity #12.1: Correctly identify equipment used in the preparation of sterile compounds and its purpose.

Equipment needed:
- Administration set
- Alcohol pads (sterile)
- Ampule
- Ampule breaker
- Depth filter
- Disinfecting cleaning solution
- Filter needle
- Filter straw
- Gloves (powder free)
- Gown
- Hair cover
- Hypodermic needle
- Hypodermic syringe
- In-line filter
- Insulin syringe
- Intravenous piggyback
- Large-volume parenteral
- Mask
- Membrane filter
- Minispike
- Multidose vial
- Nonvented administration set
- Port adapters
- Scrubs
- Sharps container
- Shoe covers
- Single-dose vial
- Small-volume parenteral
- Sterile gauze swabs
- Syringe caps
- Transfer needle
- Tuberculin syringe
- Vented administration set

Time needed to complete this activity: 30 minutes

Equipment	Correctly Identified (Yes/No)	Purpose
Administration set		
Alcohol pads (sterile)		
Ampule		
Ampule breaker		
Depth filter		
Disinfecting cleaning solutions		
Filter needle		
Filter straw		
Gloves		
Gown		
Hair cover		
Hypodermic needle		
Hypodermic syringe		
In-line filter		
Insulin syringe		
Intravenous piggyback		
Large-volume parenteral (LVP)		
Mask		
Membrane filter		
Minispike		
Multidose vial		
Nonvented administration set		

Continued

Chapter **12** **Aseptic Technique and Sterile Compounding**

Equipment	Correctly Identified (Yes/No)	Purpose
Port adapters		
Scrubs		
Sharps container		
Shoe covers		
Single-dose vial		
Small-volume parenteral (SVP)		
Sterile gauze swabs		
Syringe caps		
Transfer needle		
Tuberculin syringe		
Vented administration set		

Lab Activity #12.2: Correctly identify parts of a needle.

Equipment needed:

■ Pen/pencil

Time needed to complete this activity: 5 minutes

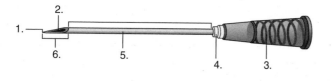

1. _____

2. _____

3. _____

4. _____

5. _____

6. _____

Lab Activity #12.3: Correctly identify parts of a syringe.

Equipment needed:

■ Pen/pencil

Time needed to complete this activity: 5 minutes

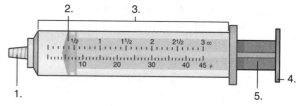

1. _____

2. _____

3. _____

4. _____

5. _____

Calculations, Compatibility, and Storage for Sterile Compounds

Objective: To become familiar with calculations, compatible solutions, and storage when preparing CSPs.

Lab Activity #12.4: Answer the following questions to prepare the following CSPs.

Equipment needed:

- Calculator
- *Handbook on Injectable Drugs*
- Pencil/pen
- Paper

Time to complete this activity: 45 minutes

1. Cefepime HCl is available as a 1-g vial for reconstitution.

   A. How many milliliters of diluent would need to be added to reconstitute to a concentration of 100 mg/mL?

   _____

   B. For intravenous injection, which diluents would be compatible for reconstitution?

   _____

   C. After reconstitution, how long will this reconstitution be stable at room temperature? In the refrigerator?

   _____

2. You receive an order to prepare an IV bag for ampicillin 1000 mg in 50 mL NS q6h. Ampicillin sodium is available in 125-mg, 250-mg, 500-mg, 1-g, or 2-g vials for reconstitution.

   A. Which vial would you choose to make this IV bag?

   _____

   B. Which diluents would be compatible for reconstitution? How many milliliters would you need to draw up to reconstitute this product?

   _____

   C. If you prepare the IV bag at 11:30 on a Monday, what expiration date and time would you need to put on the IV bag label?

   _____

3. You receive an order to prepare an IV bag of furosemide 100 mg in 100 mL D_5W. Furosemide is available in 2-mL, 4-mL, and 10-mL vials with a concentration of 10 mg/mL.

   A. How many milliliters of furosemide will you need to make this IV bag?

   _____

   B. Which vial should you choose? How many vials would you need?

   _____

   C. How long would this IV bag be stable at room temperature? How long would this IV bag be stable if refrigerated?

   _____

4. You need to prepare cefazolin IV bags for 5 different patients as follows:

   - Patient 1—cefazolin 1500 mg in 250 mL NS q6h
   - Patient 2—cefazolin 1000 mg in 100 mL NS q8h
   - Patient 3—cefazolin 750 mg in 100 mL NS q8h
   - Patient 4—cefazolin 500 mg in 100 mL NS q8h
   - Patient 5—cefazolin 1000 mg in 100 mL NS q6h

Cefazolin is available in 500-mg, 1-g, and 10-g vials for reconstitution.

   A. How many IV bags will you need to make for a 24-hour period for each patient?

   _____

   B. Which vial would you choose to make these IV bags? How many vials would you need?

   _____

   C. Which diluents would be compatible for reconstitution? How many milliliters would you need to draw up to reconstitute this product?

   _____

   D. After reconstitution, how many milliliters of cefazolin would you need to draw up to make each IV bag?

   _____

E. How long would each IV bag be stable at room temperature? How long would each IV bag be stable if refrigerated?

_____

5. You receive an order to prepare an IV bag for famotidine 20 mg in 100 mL D$_5$W. Famotidine is available in 2-mL single dose vials, and 4-mL and 20-mL multidose vials with a concentration of 10 mg/mL.

A. How many milliliters of famotidine will you need to make this IV bag?

_____

B. Which vial should you choose? How many vials would you need?

_____

C. How long would this IV bag be stable at room temperature? How long would this IV bag be stable if refrigerated?

_____

6. You need to prepare 4 vancomycin IV bags—750 mg, 1250 mg, and 2 bags with 1500 mg each. Vancomycin is available in 500-mg, 1-g, 5-g, and 10-g vials for reconstitution.

A. Which vial would you choose to make these IV bags? How many vials would you need?

_____

B. Which diluents would be compatible for reconstitution?

_____

C. How many milliliters of diluent would you need to draw up to reconstitute this product to a concentration of 100 mg/mL?

_____

D. After reconstitution, how many milliliters of vancomycin would you need to draw up to make each IV bag?

_____

E. How long would each IV bag be stable at room temperature? How long would each IV bag be stable if refrigerated?

_____

7. You receive an order to prepare an IV bag for tobramycin 110 mg in 100 mL NS. Tobramycin is available in 2-mL and 30-mL vials with a concentration of 40 mg/mL.

A. How many milliliters of tobramycin will you need to make this IV bag?

_____

B. Which vial should you choose? How many vials will you need?

_____

C. How long would this IV bag be stable at room temperature? How long would this IV bag be stable if refrigerated?

_____

8. You receive an order to prepare an IV bag for pantoprazole sodium 40 mg in 100 mL NS. Pantoprazole sodium is available as a 40-mg vial for reconstitution.

A. Which diluents would be compatible for reconstitution?

_____

B. How many milliliters of diluent would you need to draw up to reconstitute this product to a concentration of 4 mg/mL?

_____

C. After reconstitution, how many milliliters of pantoprazole sodium would you need to draw up to make the IV bag?

_____

D. How long would the IV bag be stable at room temperature? How long would the IV bag be stable if refrigerated?

_____

9. You need to prepare 10 PCA syringes with a concentration of 0.1% hydromorphone, 30 mL each for an opioid-tolerant patient. Hydromorphone is available in a 20-mL multidose vial with a concentration of 2 mg/mL.

A. How many milliliters of hydromorphone 2 mg/mL will you need to make one 30-mL PCA syringe with a concentration of 0.1% hydromorphone?

_____

B. The syringes are to be qs'd with NS to 30 mL. How much NS will you need to add to each syringe?

_____

C. How many milliliters of hydromorphone 2 mg/mL will you need to make 10 PCA syringes with a concentration of 0.1% hydromorphone? How many vials will you need?

_____

D. How long can these PCA syringes be stored at room temperature?

_____

10. You receive an order to prepare an IV bag for acyclovir 340 mg in 50 mL NS q8h. Acyclovir sodium is available in 500-mg or 1-g vials for reconstitution.

A. Which vial would you choose to make this IV bag? How many vials would you need?

_____

B. Which diluents would be compatible for reconstitution? How many milliliters would you need to draw up to reconstitute this product?

_____

C. After reconstitution, how many milliliters of acyclovir sodium would you need to draw up to make this IV bag?

_____

D. How long would the IV bag be stable at room temperature? How long would the IV bag be stable if refrigerated?

_____

Personal Protective Equipment (PPEs)

Objective: Identify PPE, explain its purpose in sterile compounding, and demonstrate proper techniques in donning personal protective equipment in the correct sequence.

The Occupational Safety and Health Administration requires the use of PPE to reduce the exposure of employees to hazards. In the practice of pharmacy, PPEs are worn in the compounding of sterile products. These PPEs include foot and hair covers, face masks, gowns, and sterile powder-free gloves.

Gowns are worn to protect the skin and to prevent soiling of clothing during procedures that are likely to generate splashes. Masks, eye protection, and face shields are worn to protect the mucous membranes of the eyes, nose, and mouth during procedures that are likely to produce splashes. In addition, masks prevent moisture from being forced out from the mouth and nose during normal activities such as breathing or talking. Gloves are worn to prevent the spread of disease and to avoid possible contamination. However, the individual who wears gloves must still wash his or her hands before gloving. A pharmacy technician should never wash their hands with gloves on because hand washing may damage the glove's pores, allowing microorganisms to enter the glove.

Lab Activity #12.5: Identify the following PPE worn in the practice of sterile compounding and state its purpose.

Equipment needed:

- Face mask
- Foot coverings
- Goggles
- Hair covering
- Facial hair covering
- Sterile gown
- Sterile powder-free gloves

Time needed to complete this activity: 5 minutes

Personal Protective Equipment	Purpose
Face mask	
Foot coverings	
Goggles	
Hair covering, facial hair covering	
Sterile gown	
Sterile powder-free gloves	

Lab Activity #12.6: Donning personal protective equipment.

Equipment needed:
- Antiseptic hand cleanser
- Face mask
- Waterless alcohol-based hand rub (sterile)
- Foot covering
- Hair covering, facial hair covering
- Nonshedding disposable towel
- Nailbrush
- Sink with hot and cold running water
- Sterile gown
- Sterile powder-free gloves

Procedure

1. Remove all cosmetics, jewelry up to the elbows, and remove necklaces and earrings.
2. Remove all outer garments such as coats and hats.
3. All items must be wiped down with aseptic wipes before entering aseptic areas.
4. Wash hands thoroughly with soap and water.
5. Apply sterile alcohol to the palm of one hand and rub hands thoroughly. Allow hands to air dry.
6. Pull shoe cover over the toe of the shoe: first around the bottom of the shoe and finally over the heel of the shoe. Please note that shoe covers are not designated as left and right but are interchangeable.
7. Apply sterile alcohol to the palm of one hand and rub hands thoroughly. Allow hands to air dry.
8. Pull shoe cover over the toe of the other shoe: first around the bottom of the shoe and finally over the heel of the shoe.
9. Apply sterile alcohol to the palm of one hand and rub hands thoroughly. Allow hands to air dry.
10. Put on hair cover by gathering loose hair and placing it into the back of the hair cover. Pull front of hair cover over forehead. No hair should be outside of the hair cover.
11. Apply sterile alcohol to the palm of one hand and rub hands thoroughly. Allow hands to air dry.
12. Slip on face mask by situating the top of the mask at the bridge of the nose. Pull the two top ties of the face mask and attach them together. Attach the two lower ties behind the neck. The mask should cover the nose, mouth, and chin.
13. Wash hands using aseptic technique.
14. Open the package of the sterile gown. The gown should never make contact with any surface.
15. Slip one arm into the sleeve of the sterile gown and pull it up to the shoulder. Repeat this procedure with the other arm. Tie the neck strings behind the neck and repeat with the waist strings.
16. Apply sterile alcohol to the palm of one hand and rub hands thoroughly. Allow hands to air dry.
17. Open package containing sterile powder-free gloves. Remove glove from package and maintain fingers within the cuff of the gown. Place glove on palm of hand with the thumb side of the glove toward the palm. Pull the glove's cuff so that it covers the gown's cuff. Unfold the glove's cuff so that it covers

the cuff of the gown. Take hold of the glove and gown at waist level. Pull glove onto the hand and work fingers into the glove. Repeat procedure for the other glove.

*Note, sterile gloves should be donned in the IV room.

Time needed to complete this activity: 15 minutes

Evaluation of Donning Personal Protective Equipment	Yes/No
Removed cosmetics and jewelry; was not wearing acrylic nails or nail polish.	
Washed hands properly before donning PPE.	
Applied sterile alcohol to the palm of one hand and rubbed hands thoroughly. Allowed hands to air dry.	
Properly put on shoe covers.	
Applied sterile alcohol to the palm of one hand and rubbed hands thoroughly. Allowed hands to air dry.	
Put on hair cover(s) properly.	
Applied sterile alcohol to the palm of one hand and rubbed hands thoroughly. Allowed hands to air dry.	
Put on face mask properly.	
Properly performed aseptic hand washing.	
Put on sterile gown properly.	
Applied sterile alcohol to the palm of one hand and rubbed hands thoroughly. Allowed hands to air dry.	
Put on sterile gloves properly.	

Lab Activity #12.7: Removal of personal protective equipment.

Equipment needed:
- Hair covering
- Sterile gown
- Sterile powder-free gloves
- Face mask
- Foot covering
- Biohazard container

Procedure

1. Use your dominant hand to grasp the glove of the opposite hand near the palm.
2. Pull glove inside out until you reach your fingers.
3. Place your thumb of the non-gloved hand inside the cuff of the other glove. Pull glove inside out until you reach your fingers and pull over the first removed glove.
4. Dispose of gloves in biohazard container.
5. Remove gown.
6. Remove face mask.

7. Remove hair cover.
8. Remove shoe covers.
9. Dispose of gown, face mask, hair cover, and shoe covers in biohazard container.

Time needed to complete this activity: 5 minutes

Evaluation of Personal Protective Equipment Removal	Yes/No
Gloves removed and disposed of properly.	
Gown removed correctly.	
Face mask removed properly.	
Hair cover removed correctly.	
Shoe covers removed properly.	
Personal protective equipment disposed of appropriately.	

Proper Hand Washing in Aseptic Compounding

Objective: To perform a complete hand washing procedure as necessary before sterile compounding.

The United States Pharmacopeia (USP) is a nongovernmental, official public standards-setting authority for prescription and over-the-counter medicines and other health care products manufactured in the United States. The USP establishes standards for the quality, purity, strength, and consistency of these products. The United States Pharmacopeia publishes the USP-NF, which is the official compendium for the United States. Chapter 797 of the USP addresses sterile compounding and is designed to cut down on infections transmitted to patients through pharmaceutical products. USP 797 addresses appropriate hand washing before preparation of compounded sterile products.

Lab Activity #12.8: Aseptic hand washing.

Equipment needed:
- Biohazard waste container
- Antiseptic hand cleanser
- Nonshedding disposable towels or an electronic hand dryer
- Nailbrush or scrub sponge
- Sink with hot and cold running water
- Waterless alcohol-based hand rub (sterile)

Procedure

1. Remove all cosmetics, visible jewelry, watches, and objects up to the elbow.
2. Turn on water faucets with a paper towel if not foot operated.
3. Make sure water temperature is lukewarm.
4. Avoid unnecessary splashing during washing process.
5. Use nail pick to clean under each fingernail.
6. Use a nailbrush to clean cuticle beds and every fingertip.
7. Apply sufficient disinfecting/cleansing agent to hands and rub in a circular motion, holding the fingertips downward.

8. Clean all four surfaces of each finger and rub well between the fingers.
9. Clean all surfaces of hand, wrist, and arm up to the elbows in a circular motion. Allow cleansing agent to remain in contact with skin for at least 30 seconds.
10. Repeat for other hand, wrist, and arm.
11. Rinse well.
12. Dry hands with nonshedding disposable towel or electronic hand dryer.
13. Do not touch the sink, faucet, or other objects that could contaminate hands.
14. Turn off the water using a nonshedding disposable towel.
15. Discard paper towels in biohazard waste container.
16. Sanitize hands by applying a waterless, alcohol-based hand rub and allow it to dry completely before putting on PPE.

Time needed to complete this activity: 15 minutes

Evaluation of Hand Washing	Yes/No
Removed all cosmetics, visible jewelry, watches, and objects up to the elbow.	
Was not wearing acrylic nails or nail polish.	
Started water and adjusted to the correct temperature.	
Avoided unnecessary splashing during process.	
Used nail pick to clean under each fingernail.	
Used a nailbrush to clean each cuticle bed and every fingertip.	
Used sufficient disinfecting agent/cleanser.	
Cleaned all four surfaces of each finger.	
Cleaned all surfaces of hands, wrists, and arms up to the elbows in a circular motion.	
Did not touch the sink, faucet, or other objects that could contaminate the hands.	
Rinsed off all soap residue.	
Rinsed hands, holding them upright and allowing water to drip to the elbow.	
Dried hands with nonshedding disposable towel or electronic hand dryer.	
Did not turn off water until hands were completely dry.	
Turned water off with a clean, dry, nonshedding disposable towel.	
Did not touch the faucet while turning off the water.	
Discarded paper towels in biohazard container.	
Sanitized hands by applying a waterless, alcohol-based hand rub and allowed it to dry completely before putting on PPE.	

189

Laminar Airflow Workbench

Objective: Demonstrate the proper cleaning of a horizontal laminar airflow workbench.

A laminar airflow workbench is used in the compounding of sterile products. Laminar airflow workbenches are used to filter bacteria and other particulate matter from the air and to maintain constant airflow to prevent contamination. Several types of laminar airflow workbenches are available, including vertical (biological safety cabinet) and horizontal laminar airflow cabinets. Both types of flow hoods are built to allow the flow of sterile air across a work surface. Air particles are removed using a high-efficiency particulate air (HEPA) filter. HEPA filters should be tested every 6 months.

The vertical or biological safety cabinet (BSC) is used in the preparation of chemotherapeutic agents and antineoplastic agents. The vertical airflow workbench filters air from the top down to the workbench and can remove particles 0.3 microns and larger. Horizontal laminar flow workbenches are the most common type used in the preparation of sterile products; they are capable of filtering particulate matter of 0.2 microns or larger. They blow air from the back of the hood to the front of the hood. Horizontal laminar flow workbenches are less likely to wash organisms into the sterility test media. Unfortunately, any airborne particulate matter generated in the unit is blown toward the pharmacy personnel and into the room. Regardless of the type of laminar flow workbench used, the pharmacist or pharmacy technician must be trained properly on its uses and proper maintenance. A laminar airflow workbench must be turned on for at least 30 minutes before it is used.

Lab Activity #12.9: Cleaning a horizontal laminar airflow hood.

Equipment needed:
- Antiseptic hand cleanser
- Horizontal laminar airflow hood
- Isopropyl alcohol 70% (sterile)
- Aseptic cleaning wipes
- Nonshedding disposable towels
- PPEs (foot covers, head cover, mask, gown, and sterile powder-free gloves)
- Sink with running hot and cold water
- Sterile water
- Sterile gauze pads

Procedure

1. Turn horizontal laminar airflow workbench on for at least 30 minutes.
2. All items must be wiped down with aseptic cleaning wipes before entering the IV room.
3. Don PPEs in proper sequence and wash hands using aseptic technique.
4. Remove any items from within the hood.
5. Inspect all surfaces for any crystallized solutions. Clean those with sterile water before continuing.
6. Deposit sterile, lint-free cleaning pads 6 inches inside laminar workflow.
7. Lightly moisten sterile gauze pads with sterile water.
8. Take moist gauze pads and begin to clean the back inside corner of laminar workbench, beginning with the ceiling. Cleaning should be performed using overlapping side-to-side motions, from left to right working from back to front. After ceiling has been cleaned, discard gauze pads.
9. Use moist gauze pads to wipe the horizontal IV poles and any hooks or brackets using a smooth motion from left to right. After IV pole, hooks, and brackets have been cleaned, discard gauze pads.
10. Use moist gauze pads to clean the right-side section with overlapping up-down motion beginning in the back corner and move forward to front of laminar airflow workbench; discard used gauze pads.
11. Repeat process on the left-side section of laminar airflow workbench, beginning in the back corner, with overlapping up-down motion; move forward; discard used gauze pads.
12. Repeat process on the work surface of the workbench. Begin in the back corner, going side-to-side with overlapping motion. Clean to the outer edge of the laminar airflow workbench.
13. Repeat steps 6 through 12 in the same order, using 70% isopropyl alcohol instead of sterile water.
14. Allow 70% alcohol to remain on surfaces to be disinfected for at least 30 seconds before CSPs are prepared in the hood.
15. Record initials, date, and time on the cleaning log.

Time needed to complete this activity: 20 minutes

Evaluation of Cleaning a Horizontal Laminar Airflow Hood	Yes/No
Removed cosmetics and jewelry; was not wearing acrylic nails or nail polish.	
Wiped down all items with aseptic cleaning wipes before entering the IV room.	
Donned personal protective equipment in proper sequence.	
Followed proper aseptic hand washing procedure.	
Turned on laminar airflow workbench for at least 30 minutes.	
Removed items from within the hood.	
Used clean, sterile gauze/sponge and disinfectant to clean the hood.	
Inspected all surfaces for any crystallized solutions. Cleaned with sterile water before moving on.	
Cleaned ceiling using sterile water and proper techniques.	
Cleaned IV pole, hooks, and brackets using sterile water and proper techniques.	
Cleaned the right side of the hood using sterile water with the appropriate motions. Started at the top and worked from side to side with overlapping strokes.	
Cleaned left side of hood using sterile water with correct motions. Started at the top and worked from side to side with overlapping strokes.	
Cleaned the work surface last using sterile water and appropriate strokes. Started at the back and worked from side to side with overlapping strokes.	
Cleaned ceiling with 70% isopropyl alcohol and proper technique.	
Cleaned IV pole, hooks, and brackets with 70% isopropyl alcohol and proper techniques.	
Cleaned right side with 70% isopropyl alcohol with appropriate motions. Started at the top and worked from side to side with overlapping strokes.	
Cleaned left side of hood using 70% isopropyl alcohol with correct motions. Started at the top and worked from side to side with overlapping strokes.	
Cleaned the work surface last using 70% isopropyl alcohol and water with appropriate strokes. Started at the back and worked from side to side with overlapping strokes.	
Did not contaminate the laminar airflow hood.	
Did not at any time block airflow from HEPA filter or air intake grills.	
Completed cleaning log.	

Cleaning Log		
Date of Laminar Airflow Cleaning	Time of Cleaning	Initials of Person Completing the Cleaning

1. What is the difference between a vertical and a horizontal laminar airflow hood? When should they be used?

_____

_____

_____

_____

_____

2. In what direction does air flow in a horizontal airflow workbench?

_____

3. In what direction does air flow in a vertical airflow workbench?

_____

4. How often should the HEPA filter be checked?

_____

Sterile Compounding

Objective: Demonstrate the proper sterile compounding techniques in performing a straight draw, reconstituting a powdered vial, and withdrawing a medication from an ampule.

Lab Activity #12.10: Performing a straight draw.

Equipment needed:
- Alcohol swabs (sterile)
- Biohazard container
- Antiseptic hand cleanser
- Laminar airflow hood
- Isopropyl alcohol 70% (sterile)
- Nonshedding disposable towels
- Aseptic cleaning wipes
- PPE (foot covers, head cover, mask, gown, and sterile powder-free gloves)
- Sharps container
- Single or multidose vial
- Sink with running hot and cold water
- Sterile gauze pad
- Sterile water
- Syringe with needle

Procedure

1. Gather all materials needed for manipulation.
2. All items must be wiped down with aseptic cleaning wipes before entering the IV room.
3. Wash hands using proper aseptic technique.
4. Don PPEs in the proper sequence.
5. Properly clean laminar airflow workbench and document.
6. Check the expiration of the single or multidose vial.
7. Select syringe of proper size. (Note: The syringe should not exceed five times the volume of the drug to be withdrawn into the syringe.)
8. Place all necessary materials in the laminar flow hood.
9. Swab the rubber top with alcohol. Allow the alcohol to dry.
10. Make sure the needle is firmly attached to the syringe.
11. Pull the plunger back on the syringe to slightly less than the amount needed to be withdrawn.
12. Hold the syringe with the thumb and the index and middle fingers.
13. Remove cap from needle. Place cap onto the alcohol swab with the opening pointing toward the HEPA filter of the hood.
14. Insert the needle at a 45-degree angle into the rubber stopper of the vial with beveled part of the needle facing upward.
15. Hold the vial with the hand that is opposite the hand holding the syringe.
16. Push the plunger, forcing the air in the syringe into the vial, and release, gently allowing the fluid to be drawn into the syringe.
17. Withdraw the correct amount.
18. Tap the syringe to force air bubbles out of it.
19. Withdraw the needle and carefully recap.
20. Discard syringe in sharps container.
21. Remove PPEs in the proper sequence and discard.
22. Record initials, date, and time on the cleaning log.

Time needed to complete this activity: 30 minutes

Evaluation of a Straight Draw	Yes/No
Gathered all materials needed.	
Removed cosmetics and jewelry; was not wearing acrylic nails or nail polish.	
Wiped down all items down with aseptic cleaning wipes before entering the IV room.	
Washed hands using proper aseptic technique.	
Donned PPEs properly and in correct sequence.	
Turned on laminar airflow workbench for at least 30 minutes.	
Cleaned laminar airflow workbench properly.	
Checked expiration dates of medications.	
Performed all necessary calculations correctly prior to drug preparation.	
Brought the correct drugs and concentrations into the hood for preparation.	
Inspected all products for particulate matter/contamination prior to use.	
Brought the correct supplies into the hood prior to preparation.	
Cleaned rubber top of vial with alcohol swab.	
Selected syringe of proper size.	
Pulled plunger back to slightly half of amount to be withdrawn.	
Removed needle cap.	
Inserted needle into rubber stopper of vial.	
Pushed air from plunger into vial.	
Withdrew correct volume of medication.	
Tapped air bubbles out of syringe.	
Withdrew needle and recapped.	
Discarded syringe/needle in sharps container.	
Did not contaminate the needle or syringe during preparation.	
Did not contaminate the laminar airflow hood.	
Did not at any time block airflow from HEPA filter or air intake grills.	
Did not utilize the outer 6 inches of the hood opening.	
Did not core or puncture rubber stopper on vial.	
Properly discarded waste, including sharps.	
Removed PPEs in proper sequence.	
Discarded PPEs in appropriate container.	
Completed the cleaning log.	

Cleaning Log		
Date of Laminar Airflow Cleaning	**Time of Cleaning**	**Initials of Person Completing the Cleaning**

Lab Activity #12.11: Using a syringe and needle of proper size, remove the following volumes from a multidose vial within a laminar flow workbench.

Equipment needed:
- Alcohol swabs (sterile)
- Aseptic cleaning wipes
- Laminar airflow workbench
- Multidose vial
- Syringes of multiple sizes with needle
- PPEs (foot covers, head cover, mask, gown, and sterile powder-free gloves)
- Sharps container
- 70% isopropyl alcohol (sterile)

Prescribed Volume	Measured Volume
0.25 mL	
0.5 mL	
0.75 mL	
1.2 mL	
1.5 mL	

Lab Activity #12.12: Reconstituting a powdered vial.

Equipment needed:
- Alcohol swabs (sterile)
- 70% isopropyl alcohol (sterile)
- Horizontal laminar airflow hood
- Aseptic cleaning wipes
- Nonshedding disposable towels
- PPEs (foot covers, head cover, mask, gown, and sterile powder-free gloves)
- Sharps container
- Single or multidose vial
- Diluent for reconstitution
- Sink with running hot and cold water
- Syringe with needle
- Vented needle

Procedure

1. Gather all materials needed for manipulation.
2. All compounding calculations should be performed and checked by instructor.
3. All items must be wiped down with aseptic cleaning wipes before entering the IV room.
4. Wash hands using proper aseptic technique.
5. Don PPEs in the proper sequence.
6. Properly clean laminar airflow workbench.
7. Check the expiration date on the powdered vial and diluent.
8. Select syringe of proper size. (Note: The syringe should not exceed five times the volume of the drug to be withdrawn into the syringe.)
9. Place all necessary materials in the laminar flow hood.
10. Swab the rubber top with alcohol. Allow the alcohol to dry.
11. Make sure the needle is firmly attached to the syringe.
12. Prepare the syringe by adding the amount of air that will be equal to the amount of diluent to be withdrawn into the syringe.
13. Hold the syringe with the thumb and the index and middle fingers.
14. Remove cap from needle. Place cap onto the alcohol swab with the opening pointing toward the HEPA filter of the hood.
15. Insert the needle at a 45-degree angle into the rubber stopper of the vial with beveled part of the needle facing upward.
16. Hold the vial with the hand that is opposite the hand holding the syringe.
17. Push the plunger, forcing the air in the syringe into the vial, and release, gently allowing the fluid to be drawn into the syringe.
18. Tap the syringe to force air bubbles out of it.
19. Draw up the correct amount of diluent needed for reconstitution.
20. Pull the back on the plunger to clear the neck of the syringe. Remove the needle and replace with a vented needle.
21. Remove all excess air from syringe.
22. Swab the top of the powdered vial with an alcohol swab.

23. Insert vented needle of the syringe at a 45-degree angle into the rubber top of the powdered vial and push the diluent into the vial.
24. Gently shake or swirl to dissolve. The powder must dissolve completely.

25. Place needle and syringe into the sharps container.
26. Remove PPEs in the proper sequence and discard.
27. Record initials, date, and time on the cleaning log.

Time needed to complete this activity: 30 minutes

Cleaning Log		
Date of Laminar Airflow Cleaning	**Time of Cleaning**	**Initials of Person Completing the Cleaning**

Lab Activity #12.13: Ampule preparation.

Equipment needed:
- Alcohol swabs (sterile)
- 70% isopropyl alcohol (sterile)
- Ampule
- Filter needle
- Laminar airflow hood
- Aseptic cleaning wipes
- Nonshedding disposable towels
- PPEs (foot covers, head cover, mask, gown, and sterile powder-free gloves)
- Sharps container
- Sink with running hot and cold water
- Syringe with needle
- IV bag

Procedure

1. Gather all materials needed for manipulation.
2. All compounding calculations should be performed and checked by instructor.
3. All items must be wiped down with aseptic cleaning wipes before entering the IV room.
4. Wash hands using proper aseptic technique.
5. Don PPEs in the proper sequence.
6. Properly clean laminar airflow workbench.
7. Check the expiration date of the ampule.
8. Select syringe of proper size. (Note: The syringe should not exceed five times the volume of the drug to be withdrawn into the syringe.)
9. Place all necessary materials in the laminar flow hood.
10. Tap the top of the ampule, forcing all liquid at the top and neck of the ampule to fall into the body of the ampule.
11. Clean the neck of the ampule with an alcohol swab.
12. Hold the body of the ampule with your thumb and index finger.
13. Using your stronger hand, place the thumb and forefinger over the top of the ampule.

14. Apply pressure to the neck of the ampule with a sudden motion of the wrist.
15. Place the head of the ampule into the sharps container and place the ampule on the work surface of the laminar flow workbench.
16. Attach filter needle to syringe.
17. Hold the barrel of the syringe with the hand and remove the cap of the needle.
18. Place cap onto the alcohol swab with the opening pointing toward the HEPA filter of the hood.
19. Hold barrel of syringe so the needle is pointing downward.
20. Cautiously insert the needle into the ampule so the needle enters into the fluid of the ampule.
21. Pull the plunger of the syringe until the syringe contains more than the desired volume.
22. Hold ampule with your other hand as the first hand holds the barrel of the syringe and releases the plunger.
23. Remove the syringe from the ampule, invert the syringe upward, and recap.
24. Remove air bubbles from the syringe by tapping it.
25. Pull plunger downward, causing fluid from the ampule to enter into the syringe.
26. Push remaining air from the syringe by releasing the plunger.
27. Remove the filter needle and attach a new needle to the syringe.
28. Remove excess air and cap syringe.
29. Clean port of IV bag with alcohol swab.
30. Inject drug into IV bag.
31. Properly seal additive port of IV bag.
32. Discard syringe into sharps container.
33. Remove PPEs in the proper sequence and discard.
34. Record initials, date, and time on the cleaning log.

Time needed to complete this activity: 30 minutes

Evaluation of Ampule Preparation	Yes/No
Gathered all materials needed.	
Removed cosmetics and jewelry; was not wearing acrylic nails or nail polish.	
Wiped down all items with aseptic cleaning wipes before entering the IV room.	
Washed hands using aseptic technique.	
Donned PPEs in proper sequence.	
Turned on laminar airflow workbench for at least 30 minutes.	
Cleaned laminar airflow workbench.	
Checked expiration dates of medications.	
Performed all necessary calculations correctly prior to drug preparation.	
Brought the correct drugs and concentrations into the hood for preparation.	
Inspected all products for particulate matter/contamination prior to use.	
Brought the correct supplies into the hood prior to preparation.	
Cleaned ampule neck correctly before breaking.	
Wrapped ampule neck correctly before breaking.	
Broke ampule correctly.	
Attached filter device to syringe correctly.	
Drew up ampule correctly without spilling contents.	
Removed filter needle and replaced it with new needle before injecting into final container.	
Drew up correct amount of drug and checked measurement before injecting into container.	
Cleaned additive port on final container before injecting drug.	
Did not core or puncture side of additive port when adding drug to the final container.	
Properly mixed contents of container and inspected for incompatibilities or particulate matter.	
Properly sealed additive port of container.	
Did not contaminate the needle or syringe during preparation.	
Did not contaminate the laminar airflow hood.	
Did not at any time block airflow from HEPA filter or air intake grills.	
Did not utilize the outer 6 inches of the hood opening.	
Properly discarded waste, including sharps.	
Removed PPEs in proper sequence.	
Discarded PPEs in appropriate container.	
Completed the cleaning log.	

Cleaning Log		
Date of Laminar Airflow Cleaning	**Time of Cleaning**	**Initials of Person Completing the Cleaning**

Preparing Small- and Large-Volume Parenterals

Objective: To introduce the pharmacy technician to the preparation of small- and large-volume parenterals.

The most common type of sterile product prepared by a pharmacy technician is an intravenous (IV) bag that contains a medication. Intravenous bags are classified as small-volume or large-volume. Small-volume IV bags are 250 mL or less, including 50, 100, 150, and 250 mL sizes. Large-volume IV bags include 500 mL, 1 L, 2 L, and 3 L sizes. Some of the medications found in IV bags include antibiotics, antiviral agents, antineoplastics, and analgesics. During the preparation of IV bags, it is extremely important that aseptic techniques are followed.

Lab Activity #12.14: Prepare an intravenous compound.

Equipment needed:
- Alcohol swabs (sterile)
- 70% isopropyl alcohol (sterile)
- Diluent
- Laminar airflow hood
- Aseptic cleaning wipes
- Nonshedding disposable towels
- Large-volume parenteral (LVP) or small-volume parenteral (SVP)
- PPEs (foot covers, head cover, mask, gown, and sterile powder-free gloves)
- Sharps container
- Single-dose vial (SDV) or multidose vial
- Sink with running hot and cold water
- Syringe with needle
- IV bag

Procedure

1. Gather all materials needed for activity.
2. All compounding calculations should be performed and checked by instructor.
3. All items must be wiped down with aseptic cleaning wipes before entering the IV room.
4. Wash hands properly using aseptic technique.
5. Don PPEs in the proper sequence.
6. Clean laminar flow workbench in the proper manner, using the correct supplies and techniques.
7. Collect the medication to be compounded.
8. Check expiration dates on both the vial and the parenteral IV bag.
9. Place all necessary materials in the laminar flow hood.
10. Swab the rubber top with alcohol. Allow the alcohol to dry.
11. Make sure the needle is firmly attached to the syringe.
12. Prepare the syringe by adding the amount of air that will be equal to the amount of medication to be withdrawn into the syringe.
13. Hold the syringe with the thumb and the index and middle fingers.
14. Remove cap from needle. Place cap onto the alcohol swab with the opening pointing toward the HEPA filter of the hood.
15. Insert the needle at a 45-degree angle into the rubber stopper of the vial with beveled part of the needle facing upward.
16. Hold the vial with the hand opposite the hand that is holding the syringe.
17. Invert the vial and pull back on the plunger.
18. Push the plunger, forcing the air in the syringe into the vial, and release gently, allowing the fluid to be drawn into the syringe.
19. Tap the syringe to force air bubbles out of it.
20. Withdraw the correct amount of medication.
21. Remove excess air and cap syringe.
22. Clean port of IV bag with alcohol swab.
23. Inject drug into IV bag.
24. Properly seal additive port of IV bag.
25. Discard syringe into sharps container.
26. Remove PPEs in the proper sequence and discard.
27. Record initials, date, and time on the cleaning log.

Time needed to complete this activity: 30 minutes

Evaluation of Intravenous Bag Preparation	Yes/No
Gathered all materials needed.	
Removed cosmetics and jewelry; was not wearing acrylic nails or nail polish.	
Wiped down all items with aseptic cleaning wipes before entering the IV room.	
Washed hands using aseptic technique.	
Donned PPEs in proper sequence.	
Turned on laminar airflow workbench for at least 30 minutes.	
Followed proper procedure and technique in cleaning the hood.	
Performed all necessary calculations correctly prior to drug preparation.	
Brought the correct drugs and concentrations into the hood for preparation.	
Checked expiration dates of medications.	
Brought the correct supplies into the hood prior to preparation.	
Inspected all products for particulate matter/contamination prior to use.	
Withdrew correct amount of drug and checked measurement before injecting into container.	
Cleaned additive port on final container before injecting drug.	
Did not core or puncture side of additive port when adding drug to the final container.	
Properly mixed contents of container and inspected for incompatibilities or particulate matter.	
Properly sealed additive port of container.	
Did not contaminate the needle or syringe during preparation.	
Did not contaminate the laminar airflow hood.	
Did not at any time block airflow from HEPA filter or air intake grills.	
Did not utilize the outer 6 inches of the hood opening.	
Properly discarded waste, including sharps.	
Removed PPEs in proper sequence.	
Discarded PPEs in appropriate container.	
Completed cleaning log.	

Cleaning Log		
Date of Laminar Airflow Cleaning	Time of Cleaning	Initials of Person Completing the Cleaning

Preparing Cytotoxic Parenterals

Objective: To introduce the pharmacy technician to proper techniques in compounding cytotoxic parenteral medications and disposing of hazardous waste

---

A pharmacy technician may be required to prepare an antineoplastic or cytotoxic medication for a patient diagnosed with a form of cancer. These agents are used to kill a specific type or form of cancer cell found in a patient. Although these agents have many benefits for the patient, they are unable to distinguish a cancer cell from a healthy cell. Therefore, special measures must be taken to protect the pharmacist or pharmacy technician from being exposed to these agents accidentally.

Compounding cytotoxic medications is very similar to compounding sterile medications, with a few exceptions. First, cytotoxic compounds are prepared in biological safety cabinets (vertical laminar airflow workbenches), which are similar to horizontal laminar airflow workbenches except that the air is blown from the top of the hood vertically to prevent fumes inside the hood. Also, biological safety cabinets (BSCs) may take the form of a glove box isolator, wherein the pharmacist or pharmacy technician slips his or her hands into a glove-like component contained in the cabinet.

Many of the policies and procedures used in preparing a sterile compound are applied when cytotoxic agents are prepared.

Lab Activity #12.15: Cleaning a biological safety cabinet (BSC).

Equipment needed:
- 70% isopropyl alcohol (sterile)
- Biological safety cabinet (a laminar airflow workbench in the absence of a biological safety cabinet)
- Biological safety cabinet cleaner
- Deionized water
- Sterile water
- Germicidal cleanser
- Goggles
- Nonshedding disposable towels
- PPE (chemotherapy safety protection)
- Sink with running hot and cold water
- Hazardous waste container

Procedure

1. Gather all materials needed for activity.
2. All items must be wiped down with aseptic cleaning wipes before entering the IV room.
3. Don PPEs in the proper sequence.
4. Wash hands properly using aseptic technique.
5. **MAKE SURE THE BLOWER IS ON!**
6. Remove any items from within the hood.
7. Using the nonshedding disposable towels and sterile water, begin cleaning the bar at the top of the hood and any hooks or brackets using a smooth motion from left to right.
8. Using the nonshedding disposable towels and sterile water, clean each side panel next, going from the top of the panel to the bottom of the panel using overlapping strokes.
9. Using the nonshedding disposable towels and sterile water, clean the back panel of the hood; clean the top of the panel in a side-to-side motion, moving toward the bottom.
10. Using the nonshedding disposable towels and sterile water, wipe the inside of the front shield using a side-to-side motion from left to right, beginning at the top and working down to the bottom.
11. Using the nonshedding disposable towels and sterile water, clean the base of the workbench, moving from the rear forward using a sideward motion.
12. Scrub from top to bottom of the workbench, using the cleaner.
13. Inspect all surfaces for any crystallized solutions. Clean with sterile water before continuing.
14. Rinse cabinet with deionized water.
15. Repeat process with 70% isopropyl alcohol.
16. Allow the 70% alcohol to remain on surfaces for 30 seconds to be disinfected before preparing CSPs.
17. Discard cleaning cloths in a hazardous waste container.
18. Record initials, date, and time on the cleaning log.

Time needed to complete this activity: 15 minutes

Evaluation of Cleaning a Biological Safety Cabinet	Yes/No
Gathered all materials needed.	
Removed cosmetics and jewelry; was not wearing acrylic nails or nail polish.	
Wiped down all items down with aseptic cleaning wipes before entering the IV room.	
Washed hands using aseptic technique.	
Donned PPEs in proper sequence; goggles worn.	
Made sure biological safety cabinet blower was on.	
Removed items from the hood.	
Used nonshedding disposable towels.	
Cleaned inside of biological safety cabinet in proper sequence.	
Used biological safety cabinet cleaner inside of cabinet.	
Rinsed inside of biological cabinet with deionized water.	
Used 70% isopropyl alcohol to clean inside of biological safety cabinet.	
Did not contaminate the BSC.	
Did not at any time block airflow from HEPA filter or air intake grills.	
Discarded cleaning cloths in hazardous waste container.	
Completed the cleaning log.	

Cleaning Log		
Date of Laminar Airflow Cleaning	Time of Cleaning	Initials of Person Completing the Cleaning

If a laminar airflow workbench is used, remember that, in a hospital pharmacy, cytotoxic compounds are prepared in a biological safety cabinet.

Lab Activity #12.16: Vial preparation—hazardous drugs.

Equipment needed:
- 70% isopropyl alcohol (sterile)
- Biohazardous waste bag
- Biological safety cabinet (a laminar airflow workbench in the absence of a biological safety cabinet)
- Biological safety cabinet cleaner
- Calculator
- Chemo mat
- Chemo spill kit
- Deionized water
- Eyewash station
- Gauze
- Germicidal cleanser
- Goggles
- Hazardous waste container
- Large-volume or small-volume parenteral IV bag
- Luer-Lock syringe with needle
- 0.2-micron filter
- Non-shedding disposable towels
- Personal protective equipment (chemotherapy safety protection)

- Sharps container
- Sink with running hot and cold water
- Vial
- Zip seal bag

Procedure

1. Gather all materials needed for activity.
2. All compounding calculations should be performed and checked by instructor.
3. All items must be down with aseptic cleaning wipes before entering the IV room.
4. Wash hands properly using aseptic technique.
5. Don PPEs in the proper sequence.
6. **MAKE SURE THE BLOWER IS ON!**
7. Clean biological safety cabinet.
8. Place chemo mat inside of biological safety cabinet.
9. Check all ingredients for particulate matter and possible contamination.
10. Clean the top of the vial with alcohol swab.
11. Pull the plunger of the Luer-Lock syringe halfway back for the amount of drug to be drawn into the syringe.
12. Take off the cap from the needle.
13. Insert the needle into the center of the vial with the beveled tip of the needle up.
14. Hold vial so that air is being blown onto the syringe and the stopper of the vial.
15. Holding the syringe from the bottom, gradually push the air from the syringe into the vial.
16. Withdraw the correct amount of medication from the vial by slowly pulling the syringe's plunger back.
17. Remove the needle from the vial once the correct amount of drug has been measured.
18. Remove air bubbles from syringe.
19. Recap the syringe.
20. Clean medication port with alcohol swab.
21. Inject medication into IV bag.
22. Thoroughly mix the medication that has been injected into the IV bag.
23. Check for any particulate matter.
24. Clean the outside of the IV bag with moist gauze, as well as all IV ports.
25. Properly seal additive port of IV bag.
26. Label final product and place inside zip seal bag.
27. Place used syringe and needle into sharps container.
28. Properly discard materials used in biohazard bag or sharps container.
29. Remove PPEs in proper sequence and place in a hazardous waste container.
30. Record initials, date, and time on the cleaning log.

Time needed to complete this activity: 20 minutes

Evaluation of Preparing a Hazardous Drug From a Vial	Yes/No
Gathered all materials needed.	
Made sure biological safety cabinet blower was on.	
Eyewash station in compounding area.	
Chemo spill kit in compounding area.	
Had compounding calculations checked by instructor.	
Removed cosmetics and jewelry; was not wearing acrylic nails or nail polish.	
Wiped down all items with aseptic cleaning wipes before entering the IV room.	
Washed hands using proper aseptic technique.	
Donned PPEs in proper sequence.	
Cleaned biological safety cabinet properly using correct tools and in proper sequence.	
Placed chemo mat in biological safety cabinet.	
Performed all necessary calculations correctly prior to drug preparation.	
Brought the correct drugs and concentrations into the hood for preparation.	
Checked expiration dates of medications.	
Brought the correct supplies into the hood prior to preparation.	
Inspected all products for particulate matter/contamination prior to use.	

Continued

Evaluation of Preparing a Hazardous Drug From a Vial	Yes/No
Cleaned vial top with alcohol.	
Inserted needle into vial properly to prevent possible coring.	
Used a venting device that had a 0.2-micron hydrophobic filter.	
Removed air bubbles from syringe before removal of the syringe from the vial.	
Removed needle from syringe, resulting in no spillage.	
Drew up correct amount of drug and checked measurement before injecting into container.	
Cleaned medication port of IV bag before injecting medication into IV bag.	
Mixed IV bag thoroughly, with no visible signs of particulate matter.	
Labeled final product and placed in zip seal bag.	
Placed syringe in sharps container.	
Properly discarded materials used in biohazard bag or sharps container.	
Removed PPEs and goggles in proper sequence.	
Discarded PPEs in hazardous waste container.	
Completed the cleaning log.	

Cleaning Log		
Date of Laminar Airflow Cleaning	Time of Cleaning	Initials of Person Completing the Cleaning

13 Pharmacy Billing and Inventory Management

ASHP ACCREDITATION STANDARDS FOR PHARMACY TECHNICIAN EDUCATION AND TRAINING PROGRAMS

Standard 1.2: Present an image appropriate for the profession of pharmacy in appearance and behavior.
Standard 1.3: Demonstrate active and engaged listening skills.
Standard 1.4: Communicate clearly and effectively, both verbally and in writing.
Standard 1.5: Demonstrate a respectful and professional attitude when interacting with diverse patient populations, colleagues, and professionals.
Standard 1.7: Apply interpersonal skills, including negotiation skills, conflict resolution, customer service, and teamwork.
Standard 1.8: Demonstrate problem solving skills.
Standard 1.10: Apply critical thinking skills, creativity, and innovation.
Standard 1.12: Demonstrate the ability to effectively and professionally communicate with other health care professionals, payors and other individuals necessary to serve the needs of patients and practice.
Standard 3.12: Explain procedures and communication channels to use in the event of a product recall or shortage, a medication error, or identification of another problem.
Standard 3.18: Explain accepted procedures in purchasing pharmaceuticals, devices, and supplies.
Standard 3.19: Explain accepted procedures utilized in inventory control of medications, equipment, and devices.
Standard 3.20: Explain accepted procedures utilized in identifying and disposing of expired medications.

REINFORCE KEY CONCEPTS

Terms and Definitions

Select the correct term from the following list and write the corresponding letter in the blank next to the statement.

A. Civilian Health and Medical Program of the Department of Veterans Affairs (CHAMPVA)
B. Health Maintenance Organization (HMO)
C. Medicaid
D. Medicare
E. Medicare Modernization Act (MMA)
F. Medigap plan
G. Preferred provider organization (PPO)
H. Treatment authorization request (TAR)
I. Workers' compensation

_____ 1. A government-managed insurance program composed of several coverage plans for health care services and supplies funded by both federal and state entities; individuals must be 65 years or older, be younger than 65 with long-term disabilities, or suffer from end-stage renal disease

_____ 2. The process used by Medicare and Medicaid for authorization of assistive technology devices costing more than $100, similar to a preauthorization form

_____ 3. A government-managed insurance program that provides health care services to low-income children, the elderly, blind, and those with disabilities

_____ 4. Supplemental insurance provided through private insurance companies to help cover costs not reimbursed by the Medicare plan, such as coinsurance, copays, and deductibles

_____ 5. Government-required and government-enforced medical coverage for workers injured on the job, paid for by the employer; the programs are managed by each state in accordance with the state's workers' compensation laws

_____ 6. A program for veterans with permanent service-related disabilities and their dependents and for the spouses and children of veterans who died of service-connected disability; also known as the Veterans Health Administration (VHA)

_____ 7. The enactment of prescription drug coverage provided for individuals covered under Medicare

_____ 8. An insurance plan in which patients choose a provider from a specified list, resulting in reduced costs for medical services

_____ 9. An insurance plan that allows coverage for in-network only physicians and services and uses the primary care physician (or provider) as the "gatekeeper" for the patient's health care; patients often have copays to defray the costs of medical care and prescription drugs

Select the correct term from the following list and write the corresponding letter in the blank next to the statement.

A. Adjudication
B. Closed formulary
C. Coinsurance
D. Copayment
E. Deductible
F. Drug utilization evaluation (DUE) or review (DUR)
G. Formulary
H. Health Insurance Portability and Accountability Act (HIPAA)
I. Medicare Modernization Act (MMA)
J. National Provider Identifier (NPI)
K. Open formulary
L. Patient profile
M. Pharmacy and therapeutics committee (P&T committee)
N. Prior authorization

_____ 10. A list of preapproved medications that are covered under a prescription plan or within an institution

_____ 11. Medical staff composed of physicians, pharmacists, pharmacy technicians, nurses, and dieticians who provide necessary information and advice to the institution or insurer on whether a drug should be added to a formulary

_____ 12. A document listing necessary patient personal and health information, including comprehensive information on the medications the patient is taking, disease states, and any food or drug allergies the person might have

_____ 13. A type of insurance in which the policyholder pays a share of the payment made against a claim

_____ 14. An ongoing review by a pharmacist of the prescribing, dispensing, and use of medications, based on predetermined criteria, to decide whether changes need to be made in a patient's drug therapy

_____ 15. A formulary list that is essentially unrestricted in the types of drug choices offered or that can be prescribed and reimbursed under the health provider plan or pharmacy benefit plan

_____ 16. Federal guidelines for the protection of a patient's personal health information

_____ 17. Electronic insurance billing for medication payment

_____ 18. Insurance-required approval for a restricted, nonformulary, or non-covered medication before a prescription medication can be filled

_____ 19. The portion of the prescription bill that the patient is responsible for paying

_____ 20. The enactment of prescription drug coverage provided for individuals covered under Medicare

_____ 21. Tight restriction of medication use to the medications included on the formulary list; medications that are not listed as preapproved drugs per the health plan provider or pharmacy benefits manager are not reimbursed except under extenuating circumstances and with proper documentation

_____ 22. The amount paid by a policyholder out of pocket before the insurance company pays a claim

_____ 23. A number assigned to any health care provider that is used for the purpose of standardizing health data transmissions

Select the correct term from the following list and write the corresponding letter in the blank next to the statement.

A. Average wholesale price (AWP)
B. Direct manufacturer ordering
C. Inventory
D. Just-in-time ordering
E. National Drug Code (NDC)
F. Periodic automatic replenishment (PAR)
G. Point of sale (POS)
H. Prime vendor
I. Safety Data Sheets (SDSs)
J. Trade, brand, or proprietary drug name
K. Wholesalers

_____ 24. A system that allows inventory to be tracked as it is used

_____ 25. Information sheets supplied to the pharmacy from the manufacturer of chemical products; the SDS lists the hazards of the product and procedures to follow if a person is exposed to that product

_____ 26. Pharmacies may join a group purchasing organization (GPO) and contract directly with the manufacturer to obtain better pricing

_____ 27. A large distributor of medications and retail products that contracts with the pharmacy to deliver the bulk of their medications in exchange for lower prices

_____ 28. The name a company assigns for marketing and identification purposes to a commercial drug product; most brand names are trademarked and belong to originator products; the named products are often protected for a time by patents

_____ 29. A system that orders a product just before it is used

_____ 30. The PAR of stock levels to a certain number of allowed units

_____ 31. The average price at which a drug is sold; the data are compiled from information provided by manufacturers, distributors, and pharmacies; often used in calculations related to medication reimbursement

_____ 32. Companies that stock a variety of drug manufacturers' medications and normally have a "just-in-time" turnaround for ordered drugs; this means that drugs ordered today arrive the next day

_____ 33. A 10-digit number given to all drugs for identification purposes; in health and drug databases, it is represented as an 11-digit number, in which placeholder zeros are inserted in the proper order in the code for the purpose of standardizing data transmissions

_____ 34. The amount of product a pharmacy has for sale

True or False

Write T or F next to each statement.

_____ 1. Pharmacy technicians help manage the third-party billing process.

_____ 2. Formularies are the same at all institutional pharmacies or for all health plans.

_____ 3. Many formulary drugs are generic versions of proprietary products.

_____ 4. Generic drugs are less expensive because they are less effective than brand name drugs.

_____ 5. In a PPO, the patient must select a primary physician to coordinate all of the patient's medical needs.

_____ 6. A PPO plan usually has a higher copayment than an HMO.

_____ 7. Each insurance plan has specific guidelines that must be followed for reimbursement.

_____ 8. The cost of prescriptions is the same from pharmacy to pharmacy.

_____ 9. If the cardholder's information does not match the processor's information, the patient does not have coverage.

_____ 10. When an inventory shipment arrives, all included medications and supplies must be verified against the inventory list.

_____ 11. Timing is the least important aspect of keeping inventory at a constant level.

_____ 12. Storing medications in the proper location is the responsibility of everyone working in the pharmacy.

_____ 13. Recall notices arrive by voice mail.

_____ 14. Medications taken out of the pharmacy by a patient can be returned to stock.

_____ 15. Investigational drugs typically have documentation that must be completed and returned to the manufacturer each time a medication is dispensed.

Multiple Choice

Complete the question by circling the best answer.

1. Who is responsible for maintaining the inventory stock in the pharmacy?
   A. Pharmacist
   B. Technician
   C. Inventory technician
   D. All the above

2. The types of drugs typically included in a formulary are:
   A. New drugs
   B. Generic drugs and common branded drugs for which no generic is available in the drug class
   C. Uncommon drugs
   D. Extremely expensive drugs

3. In third-party billing, the third party is the:
   A. Pharmacy
   B. Patient
   C. Insurance company
   D. All the above

4. Which of the following is *not* a type of health insurance plan in use today?
   A. POS
   B. HMO
   C. PPO
   D. Medicare

5. Which of the following is *not* a special feature of an HMO?
   A. Primary care physician
   B. Independent physicians' association
   C. Copayment
   D. Workers' compensation

6. Which of the following is *not* a difference between HMOs and PPOs?
   A. A PPO plan has no requirements for a PCP
   B. PPO plans have a copayment
   C. PPO plans have a deductible
   D. All the above are differences

7. Which of the following is *not* a government-run insurance program?
   A. Medicare
   B. Medicaid
   C. Long-term disability
   D. Workers' compensation

8. Which group is *not* covered by Medicare?
   A. Healthy infants
   B. Disabled patients
   C. Seniors
   D. Dialysis patients

9. Which of the following is *not* a reason for the insurance company to reject a claim?
   A. Coverage has expired
   B. Use of a generic drug
   C. Refill too soon
   D. NDC not covered

10. Sometimes insurance companies refill medications early because:
    A. The patient lost the medication
    B. The patient is going on a vacation
    C. The physician told the patient to increase the dosage
    D. All the above

11. Which of the following is *not* an example of an inventory system that can keep a running inventory of medications, as well as order them?
    A. SOC system
    B. POS system
    C. Order card system
    D. Handheld computer inventory system

12. Which of the following is *not* a reason to return medications to the warehouse or manufacturer?
    A. Drug recalled
    B. Drug damaged during delivery
    C. Drug incorrectly reconstituted
    D. Drug expired

13. Manufacturers are required by law to recall any product that has been found to have which of the following guideline violations?
    A. Labeling is wrong
    B. Product was not packaged or produced properly
    C. Drug batch was contaminated
    D. All the above

14. Drug utilization evaluation (DUE) is an important process used to screen the medication order for:
    A. Duplicate therapy
    B. Possible errors
    C. Drug-drug interactions
    D. All the above

15. A zero for a DAW code means _____
    A. no refills
    B. dispense order as written
    C. generic substitution authorized
    D. patient would like brand name only

16. A one for DAW code means _____
    A. no refills
    B. dispense order as written
    C. generic substitution authorized
    D. patient would like brand name only

17. Point-of-sale billing allows the insurance company to

    _____
    A. price a claim
    B. verify eligibility
    C. identify covered drugs
    D. all the above

18. Reasons for obtaining a prior authorization may

    include _____
    A. patient is demanding the drug
    B. drug of choice not formulary
    C. physician is requesting
    D. none of the above

19. What is the copay for a prescription for brand name Celexa 20 mg #30 if there is no "brand necessary" written on the prescription, but the patient wants to pay the difference pricing for the brand name? The copay amount is $20, the cost of the Celexa 20 mg #30 is $296.52 and the cost of the generic is $76.65.
    A. $20
    B. $316.52
    C. $239.87
    D. $96.65

20. How much will the pharmacy be reimbursed for a prescription if the third-party contract states the pharmacy will be reimbursed at AWP + 5% + $3.50 dispensing fee and if the AWP for the prescription is $33.68?
    A. $38.86
    B. $42.18
    C. $28.50
    D. $37.18

Fill in the Blanks

Answer each question by completing the statement in the space provided.

1. Maintaining inventory is an essential part of the

   _____ tasks of pharmacy staff.

2. For medications to become part of a _____, they must meet certain requirements, such as effectiveness and cost.

3. _____ is a method of payment in which the doctor receives a fixed amount for each member patient regardless of how many times the patient visits the physician.

4. If the patient must self-bill the insurance company for reimbursement, then the patient will need the _____ to submit to the insurance company.

5. A percentage of each _____ budget is applied toward Medicaid.

6. Regardless of the patient's type of insurance, you should always treat people with _____.

7. It is customary for the pharmacy to _____ the insurance company on behalf of the patient.

8. Falsely billing charges for medication that was not dispensed is a _____.

9. Inventory _____ focuses on ordering stock, proper storage of medication and supplies, repackaging, disposal of used and unused pharmaceutical products, and distribution systems.

10. Scanning a _____ _____ can identify the drug, strength, dosage form, quantity, cost, package size, and any other information necessary to a medication or device.

Matching

Match the types of Medicare insurance coverage with its corresponding description.

A. Medicare Part A
B. Medicare Part B
C. Medicare Part C
D. Medicare Part D

_____ 1. Helps pay for physicians' services, outpatient care, durable medical equipment (DME), and even physical and occupational therapists when deemed medically necessary; coverage is optional, and most people pay a monthly premium.

_____ 2. Provides people who are eligible for Medicare a voluntary prescription drug plan.

_____ 3. Helps cover inpatient care in hospitals, skilled nursing facilities, critical care hospitals, hospice, and some home health care; patients who are eligible for Social Security benefits are automatically enrolled.

_____ 4. Allows participants in Medicare Parts A and B to obtain additional insurance through private HMOs or PPOs.

207

Match the classes of recalls with its corresponding description.

A. Class I Recall

B. Class II Recall

C. Class III Recall

_____ 5. Recalls for drugs that violate FDA regulations concerning container defects or have a strange taste or color

_____ 6. Recalls for drugs that may pose a serious threat to users' health or even death

_____ 7. Recalls for drugs that may cause a temporary health problem and have a low risk of creating a serious problem

Match the types of special storage containers with its corresponding description.

A. Yellow waste container

B. Black waste container

C. Purple waste container

D. Blue and white waste container

_____ 8. Non-hazardous intravenous agents waste

_____ 9. Pharmaceutical waste including live vaccines

_____ 10. Hazardous drug waste including nitroglycerin

_____ 11. Chemotherapy waste

Short Answer

Write a short response to each question in the space provided.

1. When billing an insurance company for a patient's medication, what is the minimum information you will need to process the claim?

_____

_____

_____

2. When a pharmacy is billing for medication, what is the minimum information the insurance company requires?

_____

_____

_____

3. List four common reasons a prescription may not be covered.

_____

_____

_____

_____

4. One of the most common problems resulting in a claim rejection is a non-ID match. What patient information should be double-checked in these cases?

_____

_____

_____

5. Why do many pharmacies have a policy of pulling any medication off the shelves that will expire in 3 months or sooner?

_____

_____

_____

6. What are the three main responsibilities of automated return companies?

A. _____

B. _____

C. _____

7. List the medication storage temperature requirements for each of the following:

A. Freezer _____

B. Refrigerator _____

C. Room temperature _____

Research Activities

Follow the instructions given in each exercise and provide a response.

1. Access the website https://chemicalsafety.com/sds-search/ and find a safety data sheet for 70% alcohol.

A. What is the recommend use for 70% alcohol.

B. List the hazard statements for 70% alcohol.

C. How should 70% alcohol be handled and stored?

D. List the PPE that should be worn in handling 70% alcohol.

E. Describe other information that is found in the safety data sheet.

2. Access the website *http://www.deadiversion.usdoj.gov/ drug_disposal/takeback/* for the DEA National Take-Back Initiative.

A. What is the goal of the Take-Back Initiative?

B. When is the next scheduled National Take-Back Initiative day scheduled?

C. What DEA Form must be used to dispose of controlled substances?

REFLECT CRITICALLY

Critical Thinking

Reply to each question based on what you have learned in the chapter.

1. Should Medicare cover all medical and prescription costs for elderly patients? Give three pros and three cons for this issue.

2. Many Canadian pharmacies are offering prescription drugs at vastly reduced prices compared with US prices. Is there any reason not to "go across the border" for your medications?

3. Choosing an insurance health plan can be overwhelming. What type of coverage would best meet your needs? Outline all items you would need to have total health coverage.

209

RELATE TO PRACTICE

Lab Scenarios

Purchase of Pharmaceuticals

Objective: To follow the legal requirements of ordering and receiving Schedule II medications and to become familiar with various types of medication recalls

Lab Activity #13.1: Completion of a DEA Form 222.

Equipment needed:
- Sample DEA Form 222
- Internet access
- *Physicians' Desk Reference* or *Drug Facts and Comparisons*
- *Drug Topics Red Book* or *FDA National Drug Code Directory*
- Black ink pen

Time needed to complete this activity: 15 minutes

See Reverse of PURCHASER'S Copy for Instructions		No order form may be issued for Schedule I and II substances unless a completed application form has been received, (21 CFR 1305.04).		OMB APPROVAL No. 1117-0010

TO: *(Name of Supplier)* — STREET ADDRESS

CITY and STATE — DATE — **TO BE FILLED IN BY SUPPLIER** / SUPPLIERS DEA REGISTRATION No.

TO BE FILLED IN BY PURCHASER

LINE No.	No. of Packages	Size of Package	Name of Item	National Drug Code	Packages Shipped	Date Shipped
1						
2						
3						
4						
5						
6						
7						
8						
9						
10						

◄ **LAST LINE COMPLETED** *(MUST BE 10 OR LESS)* — SIGNATURE OF PURCHASER OR ATTORNEY OR AGENT

Date Issued	DEA Registration No.	Name and Address of Registrant
20010101	DEAREGNO	VOID VOID VOID
Schedules		VOID VOID VOID
XXXXXXXXXXXXX		VOID VOID VOID
Registered as a	No. of this Order Form	VOID VOID VOID
XXXXXXXXXXXXX	000000005	VOID VOID VOID

DEA Form -222 (Oct. 2004)

U.S. OFFICIAL ORDER FORMS - SCHEDULES I & II
DRUG ENFORCEMENT ADMINISTRATION
SUPPLIER'S Copy 1

107051797

Procedure

1. Using a black ink pen, enter the name of the supplier; the supplier's street address, city, and state; and the date the DEA Form 222 is being completed.
2. Enter the number of packages, the bottle size, and the name of the medication on the DEA Form 222.
3. Using the *Drug Topics Red Book* or *FDA National Drug Code Directory*, enter on the DEA Form 222 the NDC number of medications being ordered.
4. Sign the document.

You have been asked to order the following quantities of Schedule II substances for the pharmacy:

- 5 bottles of 100 tablets of Roxicet-5 (oxycodone 5 mg/APAP 325 mg)
- 1 bottle of 100 tablets of Percodan (oxycodone 5 mg/ASA 325 mg)
- 2 boxes of Fentanyl-50
- 4 bottles of 100 tablets of methylphenidate 10 mg
- 5 bottles of 100 tablets of methylphenidate 5 mg
- 1 bottle of 100 tablets of methylphenidate 20 mg
- 2 bottles of 100 capsules Adderall XR 10 mg
- 3 bottles of 100 tablets of OxyContin 10 mg
- 1 bottle of 100 tablets of hydromorphone 2 mg

1. What would you do with a DEA Form 222 if you made an error filling it out?

_____

_____

2. How long must the pharmacy retain a completed DEA Form 222?

_____

_____

Lab Activity #13.2: Receiving a Schedule II order from a wholesaler.

Equipment needed:
- Sample DEA Form 222
- Blue ink pen

Time needed to complete this activity: 15 minutes

Procedure

The pharmacy has received its order of Schedule II medications that were ordered during the previous activity. The pharmacy has received all the medications ordered, but received only three bottles of methylphenidate 10 mg. Using the DEA Form 222 from the previous activity and a blue pen, complete the remainder of the DEA form.

1. How would you handle the shortage of methylphenidate 10 mg?

_____

_____

2. Where does a pharmacy keep its Schedule II medications?

_____

_____

3. Describe how you would place the medication into stock.

_____

_____

_____

_____

Procedure	Yes/No
Had the appropriate invoice to accurately check in the order.	
Accounted for all boxes/items.	
Inspected all boxes/items for storage requirements; stored items needing refrigeration or freezing ASAP.	
Checked all information against the invoice including drug name, strength, dosage form, quantity, and that the expiration date is not too soon.	
Compared the invoice with the order form to ensure that only the items requested were received.	
Signed and dated the invoice and forwarded it for processing per pharmacy protocol.	
Placed the stock in the correct location per pharmacy protocol, placing new stock behind existing stock with the most current expiration dates in the front.	
Returned inventory cards to the medication box for future use.	
Filed invoice per pharmacy protocol.	

Lab Activity #13.3: Medication recall.

Equipment needed:
- Computer with Internet connection
- Paper
- Pen

Time needed to complete this activity: 30 minutes

Procedure

1. Using the Internet, go to *http://www.fda.gov/*.
2. Click on Recalls, Market Withdrawals, & Safety Alerts information.
3. Choose one prescription medication that has been recalled within the last year.
4. Answer the questions regarding your chosen recalled medication:

A. What medication was recalled? Include name of the medication, strength, and dosage form.

_____

_____

B. What date was the medication recalled?

_____

_____

211

C. What was the reason the medication was recalled?

_____

_____

_____

_____

D. List all NDCs, Lot Numbers, and Expiration date of the recalled medication.

_____

_____

_____

_____

E. What advice is given to patients who may be taking this medication?

_____

_____

_____

_____

F. Who can patients call if they have questions about the recall?

_____

_____

_____

_____

G. Who can patients contact if they experience any problems or adverse reactions because of this medication?

_____

_____

_____

_____

Pharmacy Third-Party Billing

Objective: To become familiar with various third-party formularies and requirements, how to handle various third-party and inventory issues in the pharmacy, and communicating information about a prior authorization to the prescriber's office and the patient.

Lab Activity #13.4: Third-party formulary and requirements.

Equipment needed:
- Internet access
- Pencil/pen

Time needed to complete this activity: 45 minutes

1. Access the website *http://www.caremark.com/*. Click on the link named *For Pharmacists and Medical Professionals*, then click on the link named *Drug List*, and look up the *Performance Drug List* to answer the following questions:

   A. What are the therapeutic categories of the formulary?

   B. Which calcium channel blockers are covered?

   C. Which SNRIs are covered?

   D. What are the preferred alternatives to Lantus?

   E. What are the preferred alternatives to Simponi?

2. Access the website *http://www.bcbstx.com/*. Click on the link named *Member Services* and look up *Prescription Drug Lists* for *Prescription Drug Lists for Metallic Individual Plans* to answer the following questions under the 5-tier plan:

   A. What are the therapeutic categories of the formulary for the current year?

   B. Is Gabitril 2-mg tablet a preferred or nonpreferred drug on the formulary?

   C. Is Azopt 1% suspension a preferred or nonpreferred drug on the formulary?

   D. Is divalproex sodium delayed release 500-mg tablet a preferred or nonpreferred drug on the formulary?

   E. Is clopidogrel bisulfate 75-mg tablet a preferred or nonpreferred drug on the formulary?

   F. List three drugs that require step therapy.

   G. List three drugs that require prior authorization.

3. Access the website *http://www.cigna.com/*. Click on the link named *See Prescription Drug List* on the Cigna home page then choose *Advantage Three Tier Plan* to answer the following questions:

   A. List three drugs that would require prior authorization.

   B. List three drugs that require step therapy.

   C. List three drugs that have quantity limits.

Lab Activity #13.5: Communicating information to a patient.

   Equipment needed:
   ■ Pencil/pen

   Time needed to complete this activity: 45 minutes

Read each scenario and develop a response for the situation. With a partner, role play communicating your response to a patient.

1. You are entering a patient's prescription into your computer system and have submitted the prescription to the patient's prescription provider. The prescription is rejected by the prescription provider with the following explanation "INVALID ID NUMBER/INVALID GROUP NUMBER." How would you handle the situation?

   _____

   _____

   _____

   _____

2. Tom Dagit brings in a prescription for Dilaudid 2 mg #30. The pharmacy technician checks for the amount of Dilaudid 2 mg on hand and notices that the pharmacy is temporarily out of stock. What will you do and why?

_____

_____

_____

_____

3. You are processing a prescription for a patient, and the prescription is rejected by the prescription provider with the following explanation "REFILL TOO SOON." You inform the patient of the situation, and he tells you he is leaving on vacation tomorrow for 3 weeks. How would you handle this situation?

_____

_____

_____

_____

4. You are filling a prescription for a patient and receive the following rejection message from the prescription provider: "DRUG NOT ON FORMULARY." How would you handle the situation?

_____

_____

_____

_____

5. You are refilling a prescription for hypertension and receive the following rejection message from the prescription provider: "REFILL TOO SOON." You review the patient's prescription profile and notice he had the medication filled 2 weeks ago. You inform the patient of the situation, and he tells you the doctor has changed the dose from once daily to twice daily. How would you handle this situation?

_____

_____

_____

_____

_____

6. You are filling a new prescription for a patient and receive the following rejection message from the prescription provider: "PRIOR AUTHORIZATION NECESSARY." How would you handle the situation? Ensure you explain what prior authorization is, what the pharmacy technician's responsibility concerning prior authorization is, and how would you explain this to a patient. Additionally, role play initiating the prior authorization by contacting the prescriber.

_____

_____

_____

_____

14 Medication Safety and Error Prevention

Standard 1.10: Apply critical thinking skills, creativity, and innovation.

Standard 2.1: Explain the importance of maintaining competency through continuing education and continuing professional development.

Standard 2.3: Describe the pharmacy technician's role, pharmacist's role, and other occupations in the health care environment.

Standard 2.5: Demonstrate basic knowledge of anatomy, physiology and pharmacology, and medical terminology relevant to pharmacy technician's role.

Standard 2.10: Describe further knowledge and skills required for achieving advanced competencies.

Standard 4.5: Assist pharmacist in the medication reconciliation process.

Standard 4.8: Describe best practices regarding quality assurance measures according to leading quality organizations.

Standard 4.11: Participate in the operations of medication management services.

Standard 4.12: Participate in technical and operational activities to support the *Pharmacists' Patient Care Process* as assigned.

Standard 5.9: Participate in pharmacy compliance with professional standards and relevant legal, regulatory, formulary, contractual, and safety requirements.

Standard 5.10: Describe major trends, issues, goals, and initiatives taking place in the pharmacy profession

REINFORCE KEY CONCEPTS

Terms and Definitions

Select the correct term from the following list and write the corresponding letter in the blank next to the statement.

A. American Society of Health-System Pharmacists (ASHP)
B. Automated dispensing system (ADS)
C. Institute for Healthcare Improvement (IHI)
D. Institute of Medicine (IOM)
E. Institute for Safe Medication Practices (ISMP)
F. Medication error
G. Medication error prevention
H. MedMARx
I. MedWatch
J. National Coordinating Council for Medication Error Reporting and Prevention (NCCMERP)
K. Pharmacy Technician Certification Board (PTCB)
L. Risk evaluation and mitigation strategy (REMS)
M. Society for the Education of Pharmacy Technicians (SEPhT)
N. United States Pharmacopeial (USP) Convention

_____ 1. Founded by the United States Pharmacopeia, this is an independent council of more than 25 organizations gathered to address interdisciplinary causes of medication errors and strategies for prevention

_____ 2. Any preventable event that may cause or lead to inappropriate medication use or patient harm

_____ 3. A nonprofit organization committed to the improvement of health care by promoting promising concepts through safety, efficiency, and other patient-centered goals

_____ 4. A program established by the US Food and Drug Administration (FDA) for reporting drug and medical product safety alerts and label changes; the program also provides a voluntary adverse event reporting system for medications, medical products, and devices

_____ 5. An independent organization that strives to ensure the quality, safety, and benefit of medicines and dietary supplements by setting standards and certification processes

_____ 6. A nonprofit organization devoted entirely to promoting safe medication use and preventing medication errors; it gathers information on drug errors and suggests new, safer standards to avoid such errors

_____ 7. A national pharmacy technician organization that promotes the education and training of pharmacy technicians; it provides links to medication safety and quality practices for technicians

_____ 8. An association of pharmacists, pharmacy students, and technicians practicing in hospitals and health care systems, including home health care

215

_____ 9. A national Internet-accessible database that hospitals and health care systems use to track adverse drug reactions and medication errors

_____ 10. An organization that offers national certification for pharmacy technicians in the United States

_____ 11. Established under the National Academies and a part of the National Academy of Sciences, this nonprofit organization provides scientifically informed analysis and guidance regarding health and health policy; projects include studies of drug safety systems in the United States and recommendations for patient safety

_____ 12. A strategy for managing a known or potential serious risk associated with a drug or biological product

_____ 13. Electronic system used to dispense medications

_____ 14. Methods used by pharmacy, medicine, nursing, and other allied health professionals to prevent medication errors

True or False
Write T or F next to each statement.

_____ 1. Errors are always caught before they can possibly hurt someone.

_____ 2. Pharmacy technicians are at the forefront in the effort to prevent drug errors.

_____ 3. Combined sources suggest that more than 400,000 people per year suffer some type of preventable adverse event while in the hospital that contributes to their death.

_____ 4. All drug errors cause harm to the patient.

_____ 5. Patients themselves cause many drug errors when taking their own medications at home.

_____ 6. Medication errors only occur in hospital settings.

_____ 7. Even the most highly skilled person will make errors at one time or another.

_____ 8. One of the most serious types of errors is with parenteral medications.

_____ 9. A delayed-release drug may be substituted for an extended-release drug.

_____ 10. Many physicians use e-prescribing or computerized physician order entry to circumvent pharmacies having to decipher poor handwriting.

_____ 11. The most important aspect of dealing with errors is the reporting process.

_____ 12. A drug error cannot be reported anonymously.

_____ 13. Misinterpreted abbreviations have resulted in drug errors and are an area of concern.

_____ 14. You should never be afraid to report an error for fear of punishment.

_____ 15. It is imperative that every health care worker view drug error prevention as a priority.

Multiple Choice
Complete each question by circling the best answer.

1. According to a Health and Human Services report, bad hospital care contributes to the deaths of _____ patients on Medicare in a given year.
   A. 440,000
   B. 210,000
   C. 180,000
   D. 7000

2. The Institute for Safe Medication Practices (ISMP) estimates that around _____ deaths per year are linked to actual medication errors.
   A. 440,000
   B. 210,000
   C. 180,000
   D. 7000

3. Which drug is _not_ an example of an ISMP high-alert medication?
   A. Amoxicillin
   B. Warfarin
   C. Methotrexate
   D. Potassium chloride

4. Most reported medication errors are made in this type of setting:
   A. Hospital pharmacies
   B. Mail order pharmacies
   C. Retail pharmacies
   D. Both A and C

216

5. Which of the following is *not* an example of the daily obstructions encountered by pharmacy personnel?
   A. Stress
   B. When their lunch hour is
   C. Hard to read labels because of small print
   D. Medication names that sound alike

6. Anticoagulants such as warfarin have the potential for many interactions with:
   A. Dietary/herbal supplements
   B. Food
   C. Other drugs
   D. All the above

7. Which of the following drugs is of great concern as a cause of error because it is commonly used to flush IV lines?
   A. Heparin
   B. Saline
   C. Potassium
   D. Dextrose

8. Which of the following is a category the USP defines for a modified release formulation?
   A. Sustained release
   B. Delayed release
   C. Controlled release
   D. Long release

9. Receiving care in the home also carries the risk of:
   A. Improper dosing
   B. Contamination of IV sets
   C. High costs
   D. Only A and B

10. Life expectancy in the United States has risen in the past century because of:
    A. Improved health care
    B. Increased activity
    C. Better dietary intake
    D. All the above

11. Pharmacy technicians should always check each

    prescription ＿＿＿＿＿＿＿ throughout the filling process.
    A. once
    B. twice
    C. three times
    D. none of the above

12. Many pharmacies fill upward of:
    A. 200 to 300 prescriptions per day
    B. 300 to 400 prescriptions per day
    C. 400 to 500 prescriptions per day
    D. 500 to 600 prescriptions per day

13. The Institute for Healthcare Improvement has re-

    ported that more than ＿＿＿＿＿＿＿ of all errors in hospitals are caused by poor communication of medication orders.
    A. 50%
    B. 45%
    C. 60%
    D. 75%

14. When completing the medication reconciliation report, which of the following should be included:
    A. OTC medications
    B. Herbals
    C. Prescription medications
    D. All the above

15. The ability to catch mistakes before they occur will always be the responsibility of the personnel involved

    in the prescribing, ＿＿＿＿＿＿＿, and dosing of medications.
    A. reading
    B. writing
    C. filling
    D. filing

Fill in the Blanks

Answer each question by completing the statement in the space provided.

1. An ＿＿＿＿＿＿＿ is any type of preventable event that may cause or lead to inappropriate medication use or patient harm.

2. The first response to an error is normally to

   ＿＿＿＿＿＿＿ rather than to explain the reasons behind such an occurrence.

3. It is human nature to make errors; humans are not

   ＿＿＿＿＿＿＿

4. Multitasking can ＿＿＿＿＿＿＿ the chance of making mistakes and hinder problem solving and creativity.

5. Remember to always ＿＿＿＿＿＿＿ one task before going on to the next task.

6. Pharmacy technicians can identify medications

   requiring ＿＿＿＿＿＿＿ by looking for the indication in bold lettering on the stock bottle or box or by looking for a red or yellow symbol.

7. Tall man lettering uses mixed case letters to draw attention to the ＿＿＿＿＿＿＿ in look-alike drug names.

217

8. The goal is to reduce errors as much as possible through the _____ of how they occur.

9. Pictograms and the use of plain language have been shown to _____ the possibility of parents dosing their children inappropriately.

10. The primary reasons for allergy-related prescribing errors included workload and failure to _____ the patient's drug history and profile.

11. When reporting incidents, questions concerning how the error was discovered and recommendations for preventing _____ of the error are included in the MERP report.

12. The ISMP launched the National Vaccine Error Reporting Program (ISMP VERP) to capture the _____ causes and consequences of vaccine-related errors.

13. Each pharmacy should develop a system designed to _____ its medication management practices and help reduce the number of preventable medication errors.

14. Medication safety is the _____ of all pharmacy personnel.

15. One of the best ways to _____ errors is through training and education.

Matching

Match the type of medication error with its correct description.

A. Prescribing error
B. Omission error
C. Wrong time error
D. Unauthorized drug error
E. Improper dose error
F. Wrong dosage form error
G. Wrong drug preparation error
H. Wrong administration
I. Deteriorated drug
J. Monitoring error
K. Compliance error

_____ 1. Failure to administer an ordered dose to a patient before the next dose is due, without an apparent reason or appropriate documentation

_____ 2. Medication administered in a dosage form other than what was ordered

_____ 3. Failure to review a prescribed medication for proper regimen, appropriateness, and dosage, or failure in using laboratory results to correctly adjust dose

_____ 4. Patient administered a dose that is greater or less than prescribed amount

_____ 5. Drug is given using wrong procedure or technique

_____ 6. Medication administered outside scheduled time frame

_____ 7. Drug is incorrectly formulated or manipulated, and medication is administered to patient

_____ 8. Prescriber orders a medication that is incorrect or is selected incorrectly based on indications or contraindications, and medication reaches patient

_____ 9. Medication is administered that has expired or integrity of ingredients has been compromised

_____ 10. Patient does not adhere to prescribed medication regimen

_____ 11. Medication administered to a patient from an unauthorized prescriber; physician not licensed in that state or not an authorized prescriber

Short Answer

Write a short response to each question in the space provided.

1. List the five basic rights involving medication safety.

_____

_____

2. Why would a patient try to use medical supplies intended for single use more than once, and what risks are associated with this practice?

_____

_____

_____

_____

_____

3. The FDA has recommended new labeling on certain over-the-counter (OTC) medications for young children. What does the new label say?

_____

_____

_____

_____

4. List the five guidelines used to share information with health care professionals about potentially dangerous events.

_____

_____

_____

_____

5. List three forms of identification provided by barcodes.

_____

_____

_____

6. List five safety standards outlined by the Joint Commission to improve patient quality and safety.

_____

_____

_____

_____

_____

7. List six strategies a pharmacy technician can use to help reduce errors.

_____

_____

_____

_____

_____

8. List 10 quality assurance measures than can be performed as good practices and essential to prevent errors.

_____

_____

_____

_____

_____

219

Research Activities

Follow the instructions given in each exercise and provide a response.

1. Access the website http://www.ismp.org/NAN/default.asp. List two special error alerts from ISMP. How could you help your pharmacy not make the mistakes listed in the alert?

2. Use the website http://www.fda.gov/Drugs/DrugSafety/DrugSafetyPodcasts/default.htm to listen to the FDA Drug Safety Podcasts. Listen to one podcast, list the name of the podcast, and summarize what you have learned.

3. Access the website https://www.ptcb.org/credentials/medication-history-certificate. List the requirements to earn the Medication History certificate for pharmacy technicians. Would you want to earn this additional certificate as pharmacy technician, why or why not?

REFLECT CRITICALLY

Critical Thinking

Reply to each question based on what you have learned in the chapter.

1. Everyone reacts differently to medications. Metabolism changes occur over time. A technician should pay special attention to the preparation and administration of drugs for the older adult. List three factors that could lead to serious cumulative effects with medications in the elderly. Briefly explain the results of each.

2. Meticulous care should be taken in the preparation and administration of medications to reduce the chance of error. However, if a mistake is made, how should the technician handle the situation?

RELATE TO PRACTICE

Lab Scenarios
Pharmacy Abbreviations

Objective: To introduce the pharmacy technician to the many abbreviations encountered in the practice of pharmacy, regardless of the pharmacy setting

The pharmacy technician encounters abbreviations when reviewing a prescription/medication order and in pharmacy-related literature. Some of these abbreviations may indicate dosage forms, routes of administration, quantities to be taken, frequency of administration, compounding instructions, and even disease states.

If a pharmacy technician is not familiar with a particular abbreviation, they should always ask the pharmacist for clarification of the abbreviations. The technician should never guess the meaning of an abbreviation. Guessing incorrectly will lead to a medication error and will possibly affect the patient's outcome.

Throughout the years, numerous errors have been associated with misinterpreting abbreviations. As a result of these errors, the Institute of Safe Medication Practices formulated a list of error-prone abbreviations, symbols, and dose designations. Many health care organizations have adopted this list, and practitioners within the organization are not to use these abbreviations. However, pharmacy technicians may continue to see them in the community pharmacy setting.

Lab Activity #14.1: Write the meaning of the following pharmaceutical abbreviations.

Equipment needed
- Pencil/pen

Time needed to complete this activity: 20 minutes

Part 1

1. aa _____

2. dtd _____

3. pm _____

4. L _____

5. mcg _____

6. PO _____

7. qh _____

8. supp _____

9. tbsp _____

10. mOsmol _____

11. inj _____

12. gr _____

Part 2

1. ac _____
2. cc _____
3. elix _____
4. kg _____
5. non rep _____
6. noct _____
7. postop _____
8. sol _____
9. top _____
10. ATC _____
11. s _____
12. syr _____

Part 3

1. ad _____
2. caps _____
3. g _____
4. ID _____
5. mEq _____
6. NR _____
7. pr _____
8. susp _____
9. tid _____
10. amp _____
11. bid _____
12. qd _____

Part 4

1. ad lib _____
2. n/v _____
3. ft _____
4. IM _____
5. mg _____
6. prn _____
7. qs _____
8. prn p _____
9. WH/SOB _____

10. gtt _____
11. mL _____
12. disp _____

Part 5

1. AM _____
2. BSA _____
3. hs _____
4. IV _____
5. mg/kg _____
6. pulv _____
7. q _____
8. qs ad _____
9. tsp _____
10. aq _____
11. stat _____
12. ung _____

Part 6

1. Ca _____
2. EtOH _____
3. KCl _____
4. MVI _____
5. NS _____
6. DW _____
7. O_2 _____
8. H_2O _____
9. LR _____
10. ½ NS _____
11. D_5W _____
12. $D_{10}W$ _____

Lab Activity #14.2: Write the organization for each of the following acronyms.

Equipment needed:
■ Pencil/pen

Time needed to complete this activity: 15 minutes

1. AAPT _____
2. ACPE _____

3. ASHP	_____	10. ISMP	_____
4. CDC	_____	11. NABP	_____
5. CMS	_____	12. NHA	_____
6. CPhT	_____	13. P&T	_____
7. DEA	_____	14. PTCB	_____
8. ExCPT	_____	15. PTEC	_____
9. FDA	_____	16. TJC	_____

Medication Safety

Objective: To make the pharmacy technician aware that the names of many medications are similar to the names of other medications and to implement best practices to help prevent medication errors.

Lab Activity #14.3: Using the ISMP List of Confused Drug Names located at http://www.ismp.org/, identify those medications that are commonly mistaken for the following drugs listed in the table.

Equipment needed:
- Computer with Internet access
- Pencil/pen

Time needed to complete this activity: 30 minutes

Medication	Mistaken for
Aciphex	
Actos	
Alkeran	
Amaryl	
aMILoride	
Anacin	
Antivert	
Aricept	
Asacol	
Avandia	
Benicar	
CeleBREX	
Celexa	
Cerebyx	
Clonazepam	
Coumadin	
Cozaar	
DAUNOrubicin	

Medication	Mistaken for
Diovan	
Effexor	
FLUoxetine	
HumaLOG	
HumuLIN	
Jantoven	
Janumet	
Januvia	
Lasix	
Leukeran	
Levothyroxine	
Lipitor	
Lodine	
LORazepam	
Methadone	
Neumega	
Neurontin	
NovoLIN	
Ortho Tri-Cyclen	
Paxil	
Plendil	
Prednisone	
Procanbid	
Tobrex	
Topamax	
Wellbutrin SR	
Yasmin	
Zantac	
Zestril	
Zetia	
Zovirax	
ZyPREXA	

Lab Activity #14.4: Medication errors in the hospital have increased because specific drug classifications and medications are now used. You have been asked to highlight the labels of those medications with a fluorescent pink marker. Indicate whether the following medications should be highlighted using the ISMP List of High-Alert Medications located at http://www.ismp.org/.

Equipment needed:
- Computer with Internet access
- Drug reference book of choice
- Pencil/pen

Time needed to complete this activity: 15 minutes

Medication	Yes	No
Actoplus Met		
Actos		
Alteplase		
Amoxicillin		
Avalide		
Avandia		
Cephalexin		
Ciprofloxacin		
Digoxin		
Humalog		
Lipitor		
Lovenox		
Magnesium sulfate injection		
Metformin		
Novolog Mix 70/30		
Oxytocin (IV)		
Plavix		
Promethazine (IV)		
Sodium chloride for injection (hypertonic)		
Total parenteral solutions		
Tricor		
Truvada		
Vytorin		
Warfarin		
Zetia		

Lab Activity #14.5: You are working in a hospital and you have been asked to serve on the Pharmacy and Therapeutics (P&T) Committee. Recently, medication errors caused by misinterpretation of pharmacy abbreviations have increased. The P&T committee has been asked to develop a list of approved abbreviations to be used in the hospital. Using the ISMP List of Error-Prone Abbreviations, Symbols, and Dose Designations located at http://www.ismp.org/, indicate whether or not the following abbreviation can be used. If it should not be used, indicate why.

Equipment needed:
- Computer with Internet access
- Pencil/pen

Time needed to complete this activity: 15 minutes

Abbreviation	Yes, It May Be Used	No, It Should Not Be Used	If No, Why?
AD			
Bid			
BT			
Cap			
D/C			
IN			
IU			
OD			
OS			
OU			
qd			
qod			
qhs			
ss			
Stat			
Susp			
Tab			
Tid			
TIW			
U			

Chapter **14 Medication Safety and Error Prevention**

Lab Activity #14.6: A patient comes to the pharmacy and states that they had difficulty taking the medication and would like to know if they can crush her medication and place it in some applesauce. Using the ISMP List of Oral Dosage Forms that Should Not Be Crushed located at http://www.ismp.org/, indicate if the following medications can be crushed.

Equipment needed:
- Computer with Internet access
- Pencil/pen

Time needed to complete this activity: 20 minutes

Medication	Can It Be Crushed?	If No, Explain
Aciphex		
Actonel		
Amoxicillin tablets		
Bactrim DS		
Boniva		
Cymbalta		
Depakote		
Dyazide		
Erythromycin stearate		
Fosamax		
Hydrea		
Imdur		
Inderal		
Keppra		
Motrin		
Naprosyn		
Nexium		
Oracea		
Paxil		
Ritalin		
Tegretol XR		
Topamax		
Toprol XL		
Xanax		
Zyban		

Lab Activity #14.7: Read and discuss each scenario with partner. Using information learned about medication errors, list the potential errors and a plan of action to implement to help prevent errors occurring for each scenario.

Equipment needed:
■ Pencil/pen

Time needed to complete this activity: 30 minutes

1. An elderly patient has been diagnosed with rheumatoid arthritis. When admitted to the hospital, they tell the nurse they take OTC NSAIDs but cannot remember the names of the medications. Because polypharmacy is a problem with many elderly adults, what steps should be taken by the hospital pharmacy?

2. An IV specialist working in a home infusion pharmacy receives an order to prepare a TPN for a 7-year-old child. When preparing the order, the IV specialist accidentally draws up the strength of the ingredients listed instead of the calculated volumes needed. What will be the consequences if this error is not caught?

3. A pharmacy technician working in a large hospital pharmacy receives a call from the critical care nurse asking for the evening dose of daptomycin for a patient who is supposed to receive the drug q8h. How should the pharmacy technician handle this situation?

4. A pharmacy IV technician in a local hospital receives a medication order for dopamine for a seriously ill baby on the pediatric floor. The nurse states that it is needed stat. What are the most important factors the pharmacy IV technician should keep in mind as they prepare the order?

Medication Reconciliation

Objective: Understand the steps required to complete a medication reconciliation form. The goal is to ensure the patient is given the correct medication at all points as they move through the health care system.

Lab Activity #14.8: With a partner, role-play the patient interview process using the patient profiles provided by your instructor. Interview your partner to complete the medication reconciliation form.

Equipment needed:
■ Medication reconciliation form
■ Pen

Time needed to complete this activity: 20 minutes

MEDICATION RECONCILIATION FORM

ADMISSION / POINT OF ENTRY RECONCILIATION

- The first nurse to interview the patient should initiate completion of this form. Additional nurses and clinicians may continue to use the same form for the same patient.
- Circle all sources of information: Patient   Caregiver   Rx bottle   EMS   Primary provider Other:_____

ALLERGIES AND ADVERSE DRUG REACTIONS : _____

ACTIVE MEDICATION LIST			Date of Admission / Point of Entry:				RECONCILIATION
List below all medications patient was taking at time of admission. *(Dosing information REQUIRED, if available.)*							Continue on Admission?
Medication Name	Dose	Route	Frequency	Last Dose (Date/Time)	Date	Initials	Circle **Y** (yes) or **N** (no)*
1.							Y N
2.							Y N
3.							Y N
4.							Y N
5.							Y N
6.							Y N
7.							Y N
8.							Y N
9.							Y N
10.							Y N
11.							Y N
12.							Y N
13.							Y N
14.							Y N
15.							Y N
OTC Medications, Herbals, etc.							
							Y N
							Y N
							Y N
							Y N

*If order to be discontinued, see Admitting Note for comments.

Medication list recorded by RN/MD/PA/NP/LPN/RPh

Initials	Print Name/Stamp	Signature	Date	Initials	Print Name/Stamp	Signature	Date

Reconciling Prescriber (MD/PA/NP/CNM)

Print Name/Stamp	Signature	Title	Date

TRANSFER RECONCILIATION	DISCHARGE RECONCILIATION
• See Physician Orders for active medication orders upon transfer. • See Medication Administration Record for last dose given.	• See Patient Discharge Plan for list of medications patient should continue after discharge. • Discharge plan should include stopped medications.
Reconciling Prescriber (Provide name, date, signature.)	**Reconciling Prescriber** (Provide name, date, signature.)

☐ Check here if multiple pages needed. Please indicate: Page ____ of ____

Pilot Number 2/06

228

Procedure

1. Verification: Obtain the patient's medication history and other medical information. This includes all medications, over-the-counter (OTC) drugs, and herbal remedies.
2. Clarification: Make sure the medications and dosages are appropriate for the patient. *The current physician's orders are compared with the patient's medication list.
3. Reconciliation: *Clinical decisions are made based on the comparison between the two drug lists. Resolving any observed discrepancies or errors through documentation and direct communication is the final step.

Procedure	Yes/No
Obtained the patient's medication history and other medical information. This includes all medications, OTC drugs, and herbal remedies.	
Ensured medication and dosages are appropriate for the patient. *The current physician's orders were compared with the patient's medication list.	
*Clinical decisions were made based on the comparison between the two drug lists. Resolved any observed discrepancies or errors through documentation and direct communication as the final step.	

*These steps are usually completed by a nurse and may be viewed by the physician, nurse, pharmacist, or trained pharmacy technician.

15 Pharmacy Operations Management

ASHP ACCREDITATION STANDARDS FOR PHARMACY TECHNICIAN EDUCATION AND TRAINING PROGRAMS

Standard 1.2: Present an image appropriate for the profession of pharmacy in appearance and behavior.

Standard 1.4: Communicate clearly and effectively, both verbally and in writing.

Standard 1.5: Demonstrate a respectful and professional attitude when interacting with diverse patient populations, colleagues, and professionals.

Standard 1.7: Apply interpersonal skills, including negotiation skills, conflict resolution, customer service, and teamwork.

Standard 1.10: Apply critical thinking skills, creativity, and innovation.

Standard 1.12: Demonstrate the ability to effectively and professionally communicate with other health care professionals, payors and other individuals necessary to serve the needs of patients and practice.

Standard 2.3: Describe the pharmacy technician's role, pharmacist's role, and other occupations in the health care environment.

Standard 3.1: Assist pharmacists in collecting, organizing, and recording demographic and clinical information for the Pharmacists; Patient Care Process.

Standard 3.2: Receive, process, and prepare prescriptions/medication orders for completeness, accuracy, and authenticity to ensure safety.

Standard 3.3: Assist pharmacist in the identification of patients who desire/require counseling to optimize the use of medication, equipment, and devices.

Standard 3.4: Prepare patient-specific medications for distribution.

Standard 3.5: Prepare non–patient-specific medications for distribution.

Standard 3.6: Assist pharmacist in preparing, storing, and distributing medication products including those requiring special handling and documentation.

Standard 3.13: Use current technology to ensure the safety and accuracy of medication dispensing.

Standard 3.31: Manage drug product inventory stored in equipment or devices used to ensure the safety and accuracy of medication dispensing.

Standard 4.2: Apply patient- and medication-safety practices in aspects of the pharmacy technician's roles.

Standard 4.4: Explain basic safety and emergency preparedness procedures applicable to the pharmacy.

Standard 4.8: Describe best practices regarding quality assurance measures according to leading quality organizations.

Standard 4.9: Verify measurements, preparation, and/or packaging of medications produced by other health care professionals.

Standard 5.1: Describe and apply state and federal laws pertaining to processing, handling, and dispensing of medications including controlled substances.

Standard 5.9: Participate in pharmacy compliance with professional standards and relevant legal, regulatory, formulary, contractual, and safety requirements.

REINFORCE KEY CONCEPTS

Terms and Definitions

Select the correct term from the following list and write the corresponding letter in the blank next to the statement.

A. American Society of Health-System Pharmacists (ASHP)
B. Automated dispensing system (ADS)
C. Medication error
D. Pharmacy Technician Certification Board (PTCB)
E. Quality assurance
F. Quality control

_____ 1. Any preventable event that may cause or lead to inappropriate medication use or patient harm

_____ 2. An association of pharmacists, pharmacy students, and technicians practicing in hospitals and health care systems, including home health care

_____ 3. Establishing systems for ensuring quality of a product

_____ 4. Electronic system used to dispense medications

_____ 5. The use of established systems to ensure quality of a product

_____ 6. An organization that offers national certification for pharmacy technicians in the United States

True or False

Write T or F next to each statement.

_____ 1. The layout, equipment placement, arrangement, responsibilities of team members, and SOPs do not factor into the way a pharmacy operates.

_____ 2. The knowledge requirements for technicians are increasing and with that comes additional leadership and advanced opportunities, as well as legal responsibilities.

_____ 3. Technician education, regulation, and basic knowledge levels are important to providing safe patient care.

_____ 4. The more knowledgeable and professional technicians become, the worse patient care will become.

_____ 5. The state boards of pharmacy require physical standards such as a sink with hot and cold running water, appropriate lighting, and minimum amounts of space in the community pharmacy.

_____ 6. Blister packing cards are used for assisted-living or long-term care facilities.

_____ 7. Each medication kept in the ADC does not have to be individually packaged.

_____ 8. Guidelines established by ASHP and USP <795> publish the layout, equipment, maintenance, training, and all procedures related to preparing IV medications.

_____ 9. Computerized systems with barcoding, NDC tracking, and other automated technology decreases productivity.

_____ 10. When proper workflow and management is put into place, a pharmacy can provide quality and safe patient care while minimizing time and expenses.

Multiple Choice

Complete each question by circling the best answer.

1. Which organization has a significant focus of "advancing the health and well-being of patients" and maintains that optimizing the role of technicians is critical to this goal?
   A. BOP
   B. NABP
   C. ASHP
   D. FDA

2. Which of the following is *not* a physical standard required by state boards of pharmacy?
   A. Carpet in the pharmacy
   B. Hot and cold running water
   C. Appropriate lighting
   D. Amount of space

3. All the following duties are typically performed by technician assigned to the front counter area in a community pharmacy *except*:
   A. Drive-thru window
   B. Answer overflow of phone calls
   C. Process prescription orders
   D. Offer OTC advice to patients

4. The last opportunity to check for accuracy of prescriptions and verify patient information is performed at this area of a community pharmacy:
   A. Drop-off window
   B. Pick-up area
   C. Filling station
   D. Compounding area

5. To help verify a patient at the pick-up area, what type of question is best to ask?
   A. Rhetorical question
   B. Final question
   C. Closed-ended question
   D. Open-ended question

6. This area of an institutional pharmacy is where pharmacists perform data entry and answer questions from other health care workers:
   A. Narcotic area
   B. CPOE area
   C. IV room
   D. Repackaging area

7. Which of the following is an advantage of using barcoding and NDC technology?
   A. Medication can be tracked
   B. Medication errors can be avoided
   C. Diversion can be avoided
   D. All the above

8. Which of the following hospital departments would *not* be stocked with pharmacy inventory?
   A. Medical/Surgical Floors (MED/SURG)
   B. Operating Room (OR)
   C. Cafeteria
   D. Emergency Department (ED)

9. The inventory pharmacy technician in a hospital pharmacy is typically responsible for the following tasks *except*:
   A. Daily inventory control
   B. Medication order entry
   C. Pricing and negotiation
   D. Formulary control

10. What would be the result if workflow in a pharmacy is interrupted constantly or there is a lack of attention to processes?
    A. Inventory would not be ordered
    B. Errors would occur
    C. Pharmacist would miss counseling opportunities
    D. All the above

Fill in the Blanks

Answer each question by completing the statement in the space provided.

1. It takes a _____ working together to keep a pharmacy and health care organization running smoothly and efficiently.

2. Changes in roles of both pharmacist and technicians are changing the way a pharmacy manages _____ tasks and patient care.

3. To meet the demands of a patient's overall wellness, today's pharmacy techs must understand not just their place in the pharmacy, but in the overall _____ system as well.

4. The pharmacy layout should incorporate a design that provides the most _____ use of workspace and allows workflow to run smoothly.

5. Satellite pharmacies will usually have their own technician and pharmacist who work in that area _____ with that health care team.

6. Barcoding and NDC technology are key to ensuring _____ and accuracy.

7. Code drugs are _____ with ready to inject syringes and bags of IV fluids and are items normally kept in EMS and code carts.

8. Often a hospital may house a special section for the _____ in case of disaster.

9. All the areas in a pharmacy must coordinate items that are required for ordering with the _____ technician or department.

10. Layout of facilities, utilization of educated and trained technicians, and standards of practice established provide a solid foundation for _____.

Matching

Match the following pharmacy technician roles with the area of a community pharmacy where each is typically performed.

_____ 1. Familiar with DME and bill for DME supplies

_____ 2. Identify patients who require counseling from the pharmacist

_____ 3. New prescription entry

_____ 4. Focus on the customer

_____ 5. Preparation of compounds

_____ 6. Package 30-day supply in a blister card

A. Data entry area
B. Store front or OTC area
C. Reconstitution or compounding area
D. Counseling and pick-up area
E. Long-term care packaging area
F. Durable and nondurable medical equipment area

Match the following pharmacy technician roles with the area of an institutional pharmacy where each is typically performed.

_____ 7. Order inventory and stock supply room

_____ 8. Fill orders manually and deliver to requesting department

_____ 9. Stock supplies for central supply and EMS

_____ 10. Store antibiotics, maintenance medication, and batteries for public emergency

_____ 11. Maintain a formulary of stocked items in the ADS

_____ 12. Specially trained personnel prepare aseptic products

_____ 13. Help maintain storage and inventory for controlled substances

_____ 14. Stock and replace OR trays and crash cart trays

_____ 15. Repackage bulk medications to unit dose

A. Narcotics area
B. Filling area with pick-up window and pneumatic tube
C. Repackaging area
D. Automated dispensing systems area
E. IV room area
F. OR tray and crash cart restocking
G. Stocking area for nonclinical area for other departments such as central supply or EMS
H. Inventory area and storeroom
I. Emergency or disaster medication supply room

Short Answer

Write a short response to each question in the space provided.

1. List five common areas located in a community pharmacy.

_____

_____

_____

2. List five common areas located in an institutional pharmacy.

_____

_____

_____

3. Explain the importance to consider workflow for efficiency and patient safety.

_____

_____

_____

4. Describe two best practices to minimize errors in the community and institutional pharmacy. List benefits with being knowledgeable and incorporating best practices.

_____

_____

_____

_____

_____

5. Explain the difference between quality control and quality assurance.

_____

_____

_____

Research Activities

Follow the instructions given in each exercise and provide a response.

1. Take a field trip to a local community pharmacy and answer the following questions:

   A. Did you notice the data entry area or "in-window" of the pharmacy? Was someone there entering prescriptions and answering phone calls?

B. Did you notice the pick-up area? Was the same person at the pick-up area also helping patients at the drive-thru area?

2. Call or take a field trip to a local closed-door pharmacy and ask the following questions:

   A. How many different areas of the pharmacy are there? Does each area have its own pharmacy technician to perform daily tasks, or are the tasks shared by all pharmacy technicians on duty?

   B. Do you cross-train pharmacy technicians for different areas in the pharmacy?

   C. What is the pharmacy workflow for your pharmacy?

   D. What advanced technology does your pharmacy use to help reduce medication errors?

   E. Does your pharmacy require pharmacy technicians to have advanced training to work in your pharmacy?

REFLECT CRITICALLY

Critical Thinking

Reply to each question based on what you have learned in the chapter.

1. It is important to always adhere to HIPAA regulations when working at the front counter. Repeating a patient's name or stating the situation with a patient where others can overhear would be in violation and result in monetary fines. What are some ways you can help maintain confidentiality while working the front counter?

2. Of the many areas in a community and institutional pharmacy, which area do you think you would enjoy the most? Why? Which do you think you would enjoy the least? Why? If you had to work in an area that you did not enjoy, what could you do to help make your role more enjoyable?

RELATE TO PRACTICE

Lab Scenarios
Pharmacy Operations Management

Objective: To review processes necessary to maintain inventory to keep disruption to the pharmacy workflow at a minimum

When putting away medication stock in the pharmacy, it should be placed in the correct location according to pharmacy protocol. It is standard practice to rotate stock while putting away new stock. To rotate stock, bring current stock forward and place new stock behind the existing stock. This allows for the most current expiration dates to be in the front and therefore dispensed first. This also helps prevent an accumulation of expired medications on the pharmacy shelfs.

While rotating stock, you may also want to take notice of any medications that will expire soon or that are expired. All pharmacies must check their inventory periodically to ensure that all medications are in date. Most often a pharmacy's standard operating procedure dictates when this task must be performed. If a medication has expired, the medication must be removed from the shelf and quarantined so that it cannot be dispensed or sold. The expired medications stay quarantined until they can be properly discarded or possibly returned to the manufacturer for a credit or refund.

Lab Activity #15.1: In your pharmacy lab, put away new inventory and rotate medication stock on the pharmacy shelves.

Equipment needed:
- Manufacturer or warehouse invoice
- Medication to be checked in
- Pen

Time needed to complete this activity: 30 minutes

Procedure:
1. Retrieve the manufacturer or warehouse invoice.
2. Account for all boxes.
3. Inspect all boxes for storage requirements.
4. Check all information against the invoice, which includes the drug name, strength, dosage form, and quantity. Also check that the expiration date is not too soon.
5. Compare the invoice with the order form to ensure that only the items requested were received.
6. Sign and date the invoice and forward it for processing per pharmacy protocol or file according to pharmacy protocol.
7. Label high-alert medications according to pharmacy protocol.
8. Place the stock in the correct location per pharmacy protocol, placing new stock behind existing stock, with the most current expiration dates in the front.
9. Return inventory cards to the medication box for future use.

Lab Activity #15.2: In your pharmacy lab, pull expired medications off the pharmacy shelves.

Equipment needed:
- Designated area for expired stock

Time needed to complete this activity: 30 minutes

Procedure:
1. Pull medications off the pharmacy shelves that will expire within the next 3 months.
2. Pull slow-moving medications off the pharmacy shelves that will expire in the next 9 months.
3. Pull medications off the pharmacy shelves that have expired.
4. Place medications in designated area for expired or return-to-manufacture bins.
5. Process paperwork per pharmacy protocol to remove these items from the pharmacy inventory.

Working in a Pharmacy

Objective: To review processes and workflow in pharmacy

Lab Activity #15.3: In your pharmacy lab, simulate working in a real pharmacy.

Equipment needed:
- Medication orders
- Prescription orders
- Pharmacy simulation lab

Time needed to complete this activity: 120 minutes

Procedure:
1. Perform duties and tasks necessary for each area you are assigned to.
2. Rotate through each area to cross-train.
3. Train a peer to perform duties and tasks for an area in the pharmacy.
4. Verify a peer's work for accuracy of dispensing medications.

Preparing an Emergency and/or Disaster Stock

Objective: To review standard operating procedures for an emergency and/or disaster in your area.

Lab Activity #15.4: In your pharmacy lab, review standard operating procedure for an emergency and/or disaster in your area and prepare supplies and medication needed for such an event.

Equipment needed:
- Standard Operating Procedure for Emergency and/or Disaster
- Pharmacy simulation lab

Time needed to complete this activity: 60 minutes

1. With a partner, review the emergency and/or disaster standard operating procedure for your pharmacy.
2. Gather or make a list of necessary supplies that would be required to be kept in the pharmacy for such an event.
3. Present and explain the protocol, the supplies/medications required, and proper storage of these items for an emergency and/or disaster for your pharmacy to your class.

16 Drug Classifications

ASHP ACCREDITATION STANDARDS FOR PHARMACY TECHNICIAN EDUCATION AND TRAINING PROGRAMS

Standard 2.5: Demonstrate basic knowledge of anatomy, physiology and pharmacology, and medical terminology relevant to the pharmacy technician's role.

Standard 5.1: Describe and apply state and federal laws pertaining to processing, handling, and dispensing of medications including controlled substances.

REINFORCE KEY CONCEPTS

Terms and Definitions

Select the correct term from the following list and write the corresponding letter in the blank next to the statement.

A. Adrenal
B. Arthritis
C. Hypercholesterolemia
D. Hypertension
E. Nephropathy
F. Osteoarthritis
G. Osteoporosis
H. Polyneuropathy
I. Schizophrenia

_____ 1. Excess cholesterol in the blood

_____ 2. Bone and joint inflammation

_____ 3. A mental condition that breaks between thoughts

_____ 4. Gland above the kidney

_____ 5. Disease of the kidneys

_____ 6. Inflammation/stiffness of the joints

_____ 7. Peripheral nerve degeneration

_____ 8. Thinning of bones

_____ 9. High blood pressure

Select the correct term from the following list and write the corresponding letter in the blank next to the statement.

A. Anemic
B. Cardiovascular
C. Esophagitis
D. Gastroesophageal
E. Hyperplasia
F. Musculoskeletal
G. Pneumonia
H. Renal
I. Rhinitis

_____ 10. Inflammation of the esophagus

_____ 11. Red blood cell deficiency

_____ 12. Inflamed lung from bacteria or viruses

_____ 13. Organ enlargement

_____ 14. Relating to the heart and blood vessels

_____ 15. Inflammation of the nasal mucous membranes

_____ 16. Relating to the stomach and esophagus

_____ 17. Relating to the kidneys

_____ 18. Relating to muscles and skeleton

Select the correct term from the following list and write the corresponding letter in the blank next to the statement.

A. Infix
B. Prefix
C. Stem
D. Suffix

_____ 19. A meaningful stem in a generic name at the beginning of the word (eg, *cef*dinir)

_____ 20. A meaningful group of letters in a generic name that allows one to classify the medication by those letters

_____ 21. A meaningful stem in a generic name in the middle of the word (eg, methyl*pred*nisolone)

_____ 22. A meaningful stem in a generic name at the end of the word (eg, peni*cillin*)

Select the correct term from the following list and write the corresponding letter in the blank next to the statement.

A. International Nonproprietary Name (INN)
B. NSAID
C. Pharmacodynamics
D. Pharmacokinetics
E. Renin-angiotensin-aldosterone-system (RAAS)
F. TALL MAN lettering
G. United States Adopted Names Council (USANC)

_____ 23. How the drug affects the body

_____ 24. Parts of generic and brand name medications that are in ALL CAPS; meant to distinguish the drug from a look-alike or sound-alike medication

_____ 25. Nonsteroidal anti-inflammatory drug, such as ibuprofen

_____ 26. The body that makes decisions on drug names

_____ 27. Helps regulate blood pressure

_____ 28. How the body affects the drug

_____ 29. A generic name

Select the correct term from the following list and write the corresponding letter in the blank next to the statement.

A. Carcinogenic effect
B. Controls
C. Double-blinded
D. Iatrogenic effect
E. Placebo effect
F. Randomization
G. Side effect
H. Tachyphylaxis
I. Teratogenic effect

_____ 30. A type of drug in which both the researchers and the subjects do not know who is receiving the active drug or a placebo.

_____ 31. An effect of the drug we do not want at the standard dose.

_____ 32. When a patient has an effect from what they think is a drug, yet there is no active ingredient.

_____ 33. Medication effect that causes birth defects.

_____ 34. Effects that produce or cause cancer.

_____ 35. The act of choosing people for the group with active medication or inactive medication in a drug trial.

_____ 36. Volunteers selected to use no medication or another medication because they are "controlling" for error in a drug trial.

_____ 37. A rapid build of the body's defenses to a drug.

_____ 38. Effects that are caused by a medical treatment.

True or False

Write T or F next to each statement.

_____ 1. The easiest way to learn the different types of classifications is to see examples.

_____ 2. A generic name is also known as a proprietary name.

_____ 3. Health professionals use the chemical name of drugs because they are easier to memorize.

_____ 4. The ISMP publishes a list titled "List of Confused Drug Names" with Tall Man lettering to help distinguish one medication from another.

_____ 5. Pharmacokinetics is how the drug affects the body.

_____ 6. A drug is often trying to get to a certain target called a receptor or a chemical binding site where the drug acts.

_____ 7. An agonist binds to a receptor but has no intrinsic activity.

_____ 8. An important way to know if a medication is safe and effective is to look at the therapeutic index.

_____ 9. Vaccines provide protection against fungus and viruses.

_____ 10. Drugs can also be classified by the drug schedules under the Controlled Substance Act (CSA).

Multiple Choice

Complete each question by circling the best answer.

1. A prefix provides a hint at the drug classification at the _____ of the drug name.
   A. end
   B. beginning
   C. middle
   D. root

2. In a double-blinded drug trial,
   A. only the researchers know who is receiving the active drug and who is receiving a placebo
   B. both the researchers and the subjects know who is receiving the active drug or a placebo
   C. both the researchers and the subjects do not know who is receiving the active drug or a placebo
   D. the subject does not know if they are receiving active drug or the placebo

3. The stem –coxib indicates the medication will specifically inhibit _____ receptors.
   A. COX-2
   B. COX-1
   C. opioid
   D. histamine

4. The stem –terol indicates a _____ receptor agonist that opens up bronchioles.
   A. histamine
   B. alpha-1
   C. beta-2
   D. cholinesterase

5. Which of the following stems relates to the structure of the drug indicating that it has a three-ring backbone?
   A. Gaba-
   B. –pine
   C. –dopa
   D. –triptan

6. The drug class benzodiazepines have the common stem:
   A. –sartan
   B. –triptan
   C. –traline
   D. –azepam

7. Angiotensin converting enzyme inhibitors (ACEI) have the common stem:
   A. –pril
   B. –sartan
   C. –statin
   D. –olol

8. Angiotensin II receptor blockers (ARBs) have the common stem:
   A. –pril
   B. –sartan
   C. –statin
   D. –olol

9. Beta-blockers used for hypertension have the common stem:
   A. –pril
   B. –sartan
   C. –statin
   D. –olol

10. Oral contraceptives with the hormone progesterone have the common stem:
   A. –mab
   B. –estr
   C. –gest
   D. gly-

Fill in the Blanks

Answer each question by completing the statement in the space provided.

1. PPIs mainly treat GERD and peptic ulcers and are generally dosed _____ daily.

2. The non-narcotic analgesic _____ can be used for musculoskeletal pain, osteoarthritis, headache, and fever.

3. Many of the opioid analgesics share similar spellings and are _____ derivatives.

4. Asthma is a condition of _____ and inflammation.

5. Medications for _____ will often indicate that it is a certain class of medication working on specific neurotransmitters like serotonin or norepinephrine.

6. In addition to hypertension, angiotensin II receptor blockers (ARBs) can be used for _____ or _____ _____ prevention.

7. We often use _____ medications like fludrocortisone and hydrocortisone (Cortef) for conditions like Addison's disease.

8. Oral contraceptives either come in _____-_____ or some form of _____-_____ combination.

9. One of the most important classes of drugs for issues with the renal system includes the _____ medications.

10. An OTC medication that can be used for anemic patients who do not have enough iron in their bodies is _____ _____.

Matching

Match each of the following drugs with the correct drug schedule in which it is classified under the Controlled Substance Act (CSA).

A. Schedule I
B. Schedule II
C. Schedule III
D. Schedule IV
E. Schedule V

_____ 1. Valium (diazepam)

_____ 2. heroin

_____ 3. Cheratussin AC (guaifenesin/codeine)

_____ 4. Vicodin (hydrocodone/acetaminophen)

_____ 5. Tylenol with codeine (acetaminophen with codeine)

Match the following suffixes with the drug class they generally belong to.

A. Penicillins
B. Antiviral
C. NSAIDs
D. Tetracyclines
E. HMG-CoA reductase inhibitors

_____ 6. -statin

_____ 7. -profen

_____ 8. -cillin

_____ 9. -cycline

_____ 10. -cyclovir

Match the following suffixes with the medical condition they generally treat.

A. Osteoporosis
B. Inflammation
C. Rheumatoid arthritis
D. Edema
E. Benign prostatic hyperplasia

_____ 11. -mab

_____ 12. -semide

_____ 13. -dronate

_____ 14. -sone

_____ 15. -steride

Short Answer

Write a short response to each question in the space provided.

1. List and describe three medication characteristics.

_____

_____

_____

2. List and describe the four phases of drug testing.

_____

_____

_____

3. List and describe the four stages an oral medication will go through, helping explain the framework of pharmacokinetics.

_____

_____

_____

_____

4. List the common stem for H_2-antagonists, what they are used to treat, and two examples.

_____

_____

5. List the common stem for proton pump inhibitors (PPIs), what they are used to treat, and two examples.

_____

_____

6. List the common stem for first-generation antihistamines, their main side effect, and two examples.

_____

_____

7. List the common stem for the medications used to treat diabetes.

_____

Research Activities

Follow the instructions given in each exercise and provide a response.

1. Access the website *https://www.ahrq.gov/research/data/meps/index.html* to answer the following questions:

   A. What does MEPS stand for?

   B. What is MEPS?

   C. How do you think these data will be useful in the pharmacy?

2. Access the website *http://www.pharmacytimes.com/contributor/tony-guerra-pharmd/2017/03/the-top-200-drugs-of-2017* to answer the following questions:

   A. What are the seven main drug groupings of drugs prescribed and what mnemonic device is listed to help remember these seven main groupings?

   B. What stems do you recognize from the chapter? Were you able place the drugs listed into a therapeutic class or list the intended treatment based on their stem?

REFLECT CRITICALLY

Critical Thinking

Reply to each question based on what you have learned in the chapter.

1. How can learning medical terminology, root words, and stems help you learn drug names and their drug classification?

2. Do you think grouping drugs by therapeutic class and by mechanism of action is helpful to learning names of drugs and what their therapeutic effect is? Why or why not? How do you plan to learn the most common drugs prescribed?

RELATE TO PRACTICE

Lab Scenarios
Drug Classifications

Objective: To review with the pharmacy technician the mechanism of action for therapeutic agents, pregnancy categories, and common stems within generic drug names and their associated drug classification or the medical condition they are generally used to treat. Additionally, to review additional aspects of the drug approval process.

DID YOU KNOW?

- In 2017, central nervous system agents were the top therapeutic class to be purchased with a total of 83,909,000.
- In 2017, 1,307,000 alternative medicines were purchased.
- In 2017, atorvastatin had the highest total number of purchases with 104,677,000.
- In 2017, lisinopril had the second highest total number of purchases with 104,221,000.

References:

Agency for Healthcare Research and Quality. Number of people with purchase in thousands by therapeutic class, United States, 1996–2017. Medical Expenditure Panel Survey. Generated interactively: September 5, 2020.

Agency for Healthcare Research and Quality. Number of people with purchase in thousands by prescribed drug, United States, 1996–2017. Medical Expenditure Panel Survey. Generated interactively: September 5, 2020.

Lab Activity #16.1: Using a drug reference book, identify common stem, the mechanism of action, and the pregnancy category of the drug classifications listed.

Equipment needed:
- *Drug Facts and Comparisons, USP DI Volume I, or Physician's Desk Reference*
- Computer with Internet access
- Pencil/Pen

Time needed to complete this activity: 60 minutes

Drug Classification	Common Stem	Mechanism of Action	Pregnancy Category
5-alpha reductase inhibitor			
ACE inhibitors			
ARBs			
Benzodiazepines			
Beta-blockers			
Bisphosphonates			
Bronchodilators			
Cholinesterase inhibitors			
DPP-4 inhibitors			
Dopamine receptor agonists			

Continued

Drug Classification	Common Stem	Mechanism of Action	Pregnancy Category
Fluoroquinolone antibiotics			
Histamine-2 antagonist			
HMG-COA reductase inhibitors (statins)			
Loop diuretics			
Macrolide antibiotics			
Meglitinides			
Mineralocorticoids			
Monoclonal antibodies			
NSAIDs			
Proton pump inhibitors			
SNRIs			
SSRIs			
Serotonin receptor agonists			
Sulfonylureas			
Tetracyclines			
Thiazide diuretics			
Thiazolidinediones			
Tricyclic antidepressants			

Lab Activity #16.2: Access the ClinCal website at *http://clincalc.com/PronounceTop200Drugs/*. With a partner, practice pronouncing the most common drugs dispensed in an outpatient setting.

Equipment needed:
- Computer with Internet access
- Pencil/pen

Time needed to complete this activity: 30 minutes

1. Which medications were difficult for you to pronounce? Which were not difficult for you?

2. After learning about drug classifications and common stems to help distinguish a drug classification, were you better able to recognize which drug belonged to each classification?

Lab Activity #16.3: Access the Medical Expenditure Panel Survey Website at *https://meps.ahrq.gov/mepsweb/*. *Prescription Drugs* and *Household Component Summary Tables* to search the Household Component tables for the *Top Prescribed Drugs*.

Equipment needed:
- Computer with Internet access
- Pencil/pen

Time needed to complete this activity: 30 minutes

1. What is the most current year for which data are available?

2. What are the 10 top prescribed drugs for that year?

3. Do you recognize a common stem for the top 10 prescribed drugs listed? List the common stems and the therapeutic class they belong to.

4. After completing this chapter, do you feel more comfortable with drug names and drug classifications? Why or why not?

Lab Activity #16.4: Access the FDA Development and Approval Process for Drugs website at *http://www.fda.gov/drugs/development-approval-process-drugs*.

Equipment needed:
■ Computer with Internet access
■ Pencil/pen

Time needed to complete this activity: 30 minutes

1. What are some of the strategies put into place for managing the risks that may be associated with some drugs?

2. Explain the accelerated drug approval process and when the FDA may apply this process.

3. Explain three approaches the FDA may utilize to encourage the development of certain drugs.

17 Therapeutic Agents for the Nervous System

REINFORCE KEY CONCEPTS

Terms and Definitions

Select the correct term from the following list and write the corresponding letter in the blank next to the statement.

A. Alzheimer disease (AD)
B. Attention-deficit/hyperactivity disorder (ADHD)
C. Epilepsy
D. Hemorrhagic stroke
E. Ischemic stroke
F. Multiple sclerosis (MS)
G. Myasthenia gravis
H. Parkinson disease (PD)
I. Polyneuropathy
J. Psychosis
K. Schizophrenia

_____ 1. A stroke caused by a brain blood vessel rupture

_____ 2. A movement disorder with the classic symptoms of tremor, rigidity, bradykinesia, and postural instability

_____ 3. A disorder characterized by inappropriate emotions and unrealistic thinking

_____ 4. A progressive form of dementia that affects memory, thinking, and behavior

_____ 5. An autoimmune disorder that affects CNS nerves; it leads to hindered motor function

_____ 6. A mental illness characterized by loss of contact with reality

_____ 7. A physiological brain disorder that affects the ability to engage in quiet, passive activities or to focus one's attention

_____ 8. A neurological disorder that occurs when many nerves malfunction; it may include painful neuropathy

_____ 9. A stroke caused by a brain blood vessel blockage

_____ 10. A neuromuscular disorder leading to skeletal muscle weakness

_____ 11. A brain disorder marked by repeated seizures over time

Select the correct term from the following list and write the corresponding letter in the blank next to the statement.

A. Blood-brain barrier (BBB)
B. Bradykinesia
C. Brainstem
D. Cerebellum
E. Cerebrospinal fluid (CSF)
F. Extrapyramidal symptoms (EPS)
G. Homeostasis
H. Insomnia
I. Neuron
J. Tardive dyskinesia (TD)

_____ 12. Hindbrain, a structure posterior to the pons and medulla oblongata responsible for posture, balance, and voluntary muscle movement

_____ 13. Unwanted, involuntary rhythmic movements recognized as a potential side effect of dopamine antagonists

_____ 14. Difficulty falling or staying asleep

_____ 15. A brain barrier that results from unique permeability characteristics of capillaries that supply brain cells

_____ 16. Often result from taking antipsychotic medications and include parkinsonism, dystonia, and tremors

_____ 17. Slowed movement

_____ 18. Continually produced and absorbed clear, watery fluid that flows in the brain ventricles around the brain surface and spinal cord

_____ 19. A section of the brain consisting of the medulla oblongata, pons, and midbrain, which connect the forebrain and cerebrum to the spinal cord

_____ 20. The body's tendency to maintain stability, as with body temperature

_____ 21. The nervous system's basic building block and cell

Select the correct term from the following list and write the corresponding letter in the blank next to the statement.

A. Autonomic nervous system (ANS)
B. Central nervous system (CNS)
C. Parasympathetic nervous system (PSNS)
D. Peripheral nervous system (PNS)
E. Somatic nervous system
F. Sympathetic nervous system (SNS)

_____ 22. An autonomic nervous system division that functions during rest

_____ 23. An autonomic nervous system division that activates during stress; the "fight or flight" response

_____ 24. The nervous system division outside the brain and spinal cord

_____ 25. The nervous system branch that carries out "automatic" body functions. It includes the sympathetic and parasympathetic systems

_____ 26. The motor neurons of the peripheral nervous system that control voluntary actions of the skeletal muscles and provide sensory input (touch, hearing, sight)

_____ 27. Consists of the brain and spinal cord; it coordinates sensory and motor body function control

True or False

Write T or F next to each statement.

_____ 1. The nervous system is a complex structure responsible for controlling and coordinating body functions.

_____ 2. The nervous system coordinates the body's actions.

_____ 3. The nervous system includes the central nervous system (CNS) and peripheral nervous system (PNS).

_____ 4. The CNS is the brain, dendrites, and spinal cord.

_____ 5. The neuron is the largest unit of the nervous system.

_____ 6. Neurotransmitters are chemicals located in and released by neurons.

_____ 7. Twelve pairs of cranial nerves originate from the brain.

_____ 8. The PNS is divided into the sympathetic and somatic systems.

_____ 9. The sympathetic nervous system responds to stressful situations.

_____ 10. The main parasympathetic nervous system neurotransmitter is dopamine.

245

System Identifier

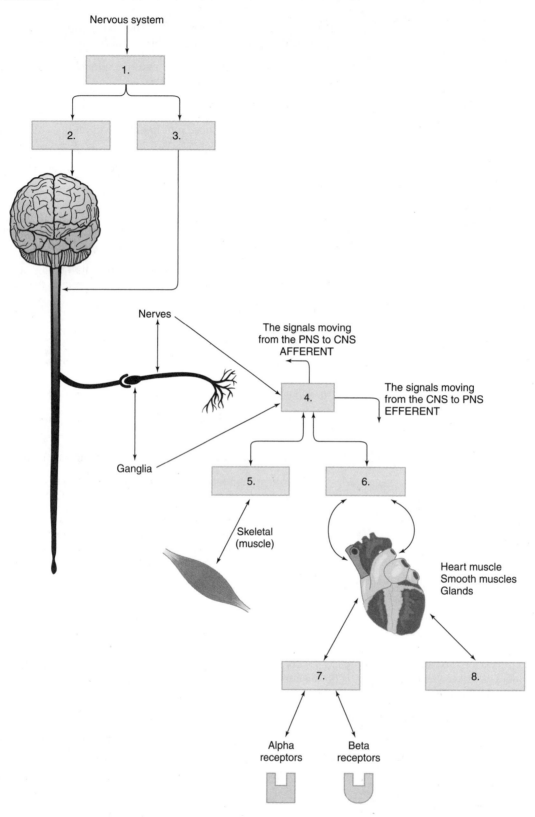

Nervous system

1.

2.

3.

Nerves

Ganglia

The signals moving
from the PNS to CNS
AFFERENT

4.

The signals moving
from the CNS to PNS
EFFERENT

5.

6.

Skeletal
(muscle)

Heart muscle
Smooth muscles
Glands

7.

8.

Alpha
receptors

Beta
receptors

Identify each component in this system and enter the term next to the corresponding number.

1. _____

2. _____

3. _____

4. _____

5. _____

6. _____

7. _____

8. _____

Multiple Choice
Complete each question by circling the best answer.

1. Drug treatments for _____ include agents that increase acetylcholine at the neuromuscular junction and suppress the immune system.
   A. depression
   B. migraines
   C. stroke
   D. myasthenia gravis

2. A medication for painful diabetic polyneuropathy would include _____.
   A. pregabalin
   B. azathioprine
   C. carbamazepine
   D. ziprasidone

3. The anticonvulsant drug _____ can be prescribed to reduce seizure frequency.
   A. rivastigmine
   B. lamotrigine
   C. benztropine
   D. sertraline

4. The gold standard treatment for Parkinson's disease is _____.
   A. amphetamine/dextroamphetamine
   B. methylphenidate
   C. levodopa/carbidopa
   D. clozapine

5. The drug _____ can improve walking in people with multiple sclerosis (MS).
   A. pramipexole
   B. eletriptan
   C. dalfampridine
   D. zolpidem

6. Antidepressants that may increase the risk of falling in patients older than 65 includes all the following *except* _____.
   A. SSRIs
   B. SNRIs
   C. TCAs
   D. MAOIs

7. Primary medications used to treat anxiety include _____ and SSRIs.
   A. acetylcholinesterase inhibitors
   B. anticholinergics
   C. dopamine agonists
   D. benzodiazepines

8. The medication _____ may alter behavior by enhancing the serotonin and norepinephrine uptake in nerve cells to help treat bipolar disorder.
   A. carbamazepine
   B. lithium
   C. sertraline
   D. divalproex

9. In addition to taking medication, individuals with insomnia may be able to help themselves by doing the following *except* _____.
   A. avoid alcohol
   B. exercise regularly
   C. increase caffeine intake
   D. learn relaxation techniques

10. Schedule II medications can be used to treat which of the following conditions?
    A. Alzheimer's disease
    B. Parkinson's disease
    C. Multiple sclerosis
    D. Attention deficit hyperactivity disorder

Fill in the Blanks
Answer each question by completing the statement in the space provided.

1. The parasympathetic system releases _____ when we are at rest.

2. The main neurotransmitters of the sympathetic nervous system (SNS) are _____ and _____.

3. Peripheral blood vessels, the heart, and eyes have _____ receptors, while _____ receptors are primarily found on smooth muscle.

4. _____ receptors are primarily found on heart muscle and _____ receptors are in the respiratory system, blood vessels, and elsewhere in the body.

5. Drugs that mimic natural sympathetic nervous system (SNS) neurotransmitters are sympathomimetics or _____.

6. _____ block drug actions and are named after the specific receptor they inhibit.

7. Parasympathomimetics are _____ drugs that mimic the parasympathetic nervous system (PSNS).

8. _____ inhibit the cholinergic reactions or block receptors.

9. Parasympathetic receptors are on _____ and _____ muscle cells and in other body areas.

10. The somatic system regulates motor nerves that control _____ skeletal muscle actions and _____ receptor impulses.

Matching

Match the following disease states with their drug treatment classes.

A. Interferons
B. Dopamine agonists
C. Acetylcholinesterase inhibitors
D. CNS stimulants
E. Anticonvulsants

_____ 1. Epilepsy

_____ 2. Alzheimer's disease

_____ 3. Multiple sclerosis

_____ 4. Parkinson's disease

_____ 5. Attention deficit/hyperactivity disorder (ADHD)

Match the following disease states with their drug treatment classes.

A. Anticonvulsants
B. Triptans
C. SSRIs
D. Antipsychotics
E. Antihistamines

_____ 6. Schizophrenia

_____ 7. Diabetic neuropathy

_____ 8. Insomnia

_____ 9. Depression

_____ 10. Migraines

Match the following drugs with the diseases they treat.

A. Parkinson's disease
B. Bipolar disorder
C. Alzheimer's disease
D. Epilepsy
E. Multiple sclerosis

_____ 11. phenytoin

_____ 12. Aricept

_____ 13. Avonex

_____ 14. Sinemet

_____ 15. Vraylar

Match the drugs with their classifications.

A. SNRI antidepressant
B. Antianxiety agent
C. Antipsychotic
D. Non-benzodiazepine hypnotic
E. SSRI antidepressant

_____ 16. Haldol

_____ 17. Celexa

_____ 18. Effexor

_____ 19. Xanax

_____ 20. Ambien

Match the following trade and generic drug names.

A. sertraline
B. olanzapine
C. temazepam
D. risperidone
E. amitriptyline

_____ 21. Restoril

_____ 22. Zoloft

_____ 23. Elavil

_____ 24. Risperdal

_____ 25. Zyprexa

Match the following trade and generic drug names.

A. escitalopram
B. sumatriptan
C. carbamazepine
D. gabapentin
E. methylphenidate

_____ 26. Imitrex

_____ 27. Ritalin

_____ 28. Lexapro

_____ 29. Neurontin

_____ 30. Tegretol

Short Answer

Write a short response to each question in the space provided.

1. For anticholinesterase medications, list the mechanism of action, an example of this type of medication, common treatments they are used for, and common side effects.

   _____

   _____

   _____

2. List four prescription drug classifications commonly used to treat painful diabetic polyneuropathy.

   _____

   _____

3. List the mechanism of action for anticonvulsants.

   _____

   _____

4. List nondrug treatment for Alzheimer's disease. Why is education for Alzheimer's disease important?

   _____

   _____

   _____

5. List non-drug treatment for Parkinson's disease.

   _____

   _____

   _____

6. List two medications used to treat Parkinson's disease that are on the American Geriatrics Society Beers Criteria.

   _____

   _____

7. List non-drug treatments for multiple sclerosis.

   _____

   _____

8. List nondrug treatments for migraines. How can these treatments be beneficial to those who suffer from migraine headaches?

   _____

   _____

   _____

   _____

Chapter **17 Therapeutic Agents for the Nervous System**

9. Name five drug therapies used in the treatment of insomnia. List an example from each type of drug therapy.

_____

_____

_____

_____

_____

10. List two medications used for smoking cessation and common medications that may alter the pharmacokinetic properties of these medications.

_____

_____

_____

Research Activities

Follow the instructions given in each exercise and provide a response.

1. Access the website *https://medlineplus.gov/caffeine.html* and answer the following questions:

A. Where is caffeine found in nature?

B. How does it affect the nervous system?

C. Who should limit or avoid caffeine?

D. Is caffeine safe to consume while pregnant? What limitations are recommended?

2. Access *http://www.alz.org/alzheimers_disease_alternative_treatments.asp*. What alternative treatments may be available to those with Alzheimer's disease?

REFLECT CRITICALLY

Critical Thinking

Reply to each question based on what you have learned in the chapter.

1. It is said that geniuses use approximately 10% of their brain capacity.

A. About what percentage does the average person use?

B. What activities can one do to create neuronal connections in the brain?

C. What role does sleep play in the ability of your brain to function at full capacity?

D. What is the meaning of the saying, "If you don't use it, you'll lose it?"

2. Many people experience a "rush of adrenaline" or a "natural high" from participating in dangerous sports. What does this mean, and what part of the nervous system is affected?

3. What is contributing to the rise in attention deficit disorder (ADD/ADHD/OCD) in children? Does it have anything to do with preservatives or hormones in food?

RELATE TO PRACTICE

Lab Scenarios
Therapeutic Agents for the Nervous System

Objective: To review with the pharmacy technician terms associated with the nervous system and review the brand and generic names, indications, dosage forms, routes of administration, and recommended daily dosage of medications used to treat disorders of the nervous system

---

DID YOU KNOW?

- 1 in 9 people aged 45 years and older experience subjective cognitive decline.
- Alzheimer's disease is the sixth leading cause of death.
- Epilepsy affects 3 million adults and 470,000 children.
- 0.6% of children aged 0 to 17 have had a diagnosis of epilepsy or seizure disorder.
- Approximately 1 in 100 people have obsessive compulsive personality disorder, with twice as many men diagnosed than women.
- 1 in 25 Americans aged 18 or older have a serious mental illness.
- 10.8% of children 5 to 17 years of age were diagnosed with ADHD between 2015 and 2017.

References:
https://www.cdc.gov/aging/data/infographic/2018/aggregated-cognitive-decline.html
https://iocdf.org/wp-content/uploads/2014/09/OCPD-1.pdf
https://www.cdc.gov/nchs/fastats/alzheimers.htm
https://www.cdc.gov/nchs/fastats/adhd.htm
https://www.cdc.gov/epilepsy/about/fast-facts.htm
https://www.cdc.gov/mentalhealth/learn/

Lab Activity #17.1: Define the following terms associated with the nervous system.

Equipment needed:
- Medical dictionary
- Pencil/pen

Time needed to complete this activity: 30 minutes

1. Absence seizures _____

2. Afferent _____

3. Akinetic seizures _____

4. Anxiety disorder _____

5. Axon _____

6. Bipolar disorder _____

7. Cell body _____

8. Convulsion _____

9. Dementia _____

10. Dendrites _____

11. Depression _____

12. Dyskinesia _____

13. Efferent _____

14. Generalized anxiety disorder _____

15. Mania _____

16. Migraine _____

17. Myoclonic seizures _____

18. Neurotransmitter _____

19. Nerve terminal _____

20. OCD _____

21. Panic disorder _____

22. Partial seizures _____

23. Petit mal seizures _____

24. Phobia _____

25. Post-traumatic stress disorder (PTSD) _____

26. Social anxiety disorder _____

27. Status epilepticus _____

28. Tonic-clonic seizures _____

Lab Activity #17.2: Using a drug reference book, identify the brand name, drug classification, indications, dosage forms, routes of administration, and recommended daily dosage for the *most common* medications used to treat conditions affecting the nervous system.

Equipment needed:
- *Drug* Facts and Comparisons or *Physicians' Desk Reference*
- Pencil/pen

Time needed to complete this activity: 60 minutes

Generic Name	Brand Name	Classification	Indication(s)	Dose Form(s)	Route(s)	Recommended Daily Dosage	Auxiliary Labeling
Alprazolam							
Amitriptyline							
Amphetamine/ dextroamphetamine							
Aripiprazole							
Bupropion							
Citalopram							
Clonazepam							
Dexmethylphenidate HCl							
Diazepam							
Divalproex sodium							
Donepezil HCl							
Duloxetine							
Escitalopram oxalate							
Fluoxetine HCl							
Gabapentin							

Generic Name	Brand Name	Classification	Indication(s)	Dose Form(s)	Route(s)	Recommended Daily Dosage	Auxiliary Labeling
Lamotrigine							
Levetiracetam							
Lisdexamfetamine dimesylate							
Lorazepam							
Memantine HCl							
Methylphenidate							
Oxcarbazepine							
Paroxetine							
Phenytoin							
Pregabalin							
Quetiapine fumarate							
Risperidone							
Ropinirole HCl							
Sertraline HCl							
Sumatriptan							
Topiramate							
Trazodone HCl							
Venlafaxine HCl							
Zolpidem tartrate							

Chapter **17** Therapeutic Agents for the Nervous System

Lab Activity #17.3: Using a drug reference book, identify MAOIs, food interactions with MAOIs, and auxiliary labels for MAOIs.

Equipment needed:
- *Drug Facts and Comparisons, Physicians' Desk Reference,* or Internet access
- Pencil/pen

Time needed to complete this activity: 30 minutes

1. List the brand and generic names of MAOIs that are used therapeutically.

   _____

   _____

   _____

2. What conditions are MAOIs used to treat?

   _____

   _____

   _____

3. What amino acid should be avoided while taking MAOIs?

   _____

4. Therefore, what foods contain the amino acid and should be avoided?

   _____

   _____

   _____

5. What auxiliary labels should be placed on MAOI prescriptions?

   _____

   _____

   _____

6. What can happen if the amino acid is not avoided while taking an MAOI? List signs and symptoms that may indicate a high level of the amino acid.

   _____

   _____

   _____

Record-Keeping and Pharmacy Law for Therapeutic Agents for the Nervous System

Objective: To review with the pharmacy technician record-keeping and the legal requirements of ordering and receiving Schedule II medications pertaining to drugs used to treat the nervous system

Lab Activity #17.4: Using DEA Form 222, fill out the form and properly file in the pharmacy.

Equipment needed:
- Sample DEA Form 222
- *Red Book Online* or the online *FDA National Drug Code Directory*
- Blue or black pen

Time needed to complete this activity: 30 minutes

Procedure

1. Your pharmacist has asked you to create an order for C-II medications. Using a blue or black pen, enter the name of the supplier; the supplier's street address, city, and state; and the date the DEA Form 222 is being filled out.

2. Enter the number of packages, the bottle size, and the name of the medication on the DEA Form 222.

   - 1 bottle of 100 capsules of Adderall XR 10 mg
   - 2 bottles of 100 tablets of amphetamine salt combo 20 mg
   - 2 bottles of 100 tablets of dexmethylphenidate HCl 5 mg
   - 1 bottle of 100 tablets of methylphenidate HCl 20 mg
   - 2 bottles of 100 capsules of Vyvanse 20 mg
   - 2 bottles of 100 capsules of Vyvanse 40 mg

3. Using the *Red Book Online* or the online *FDA National Drug Code Directory,* find the NDC for the drugs being ordered and properly fill in the NDC number on the DEA Form 222.

4. Sign the document.

No order form may be issued for Schedule I and II substances unless a completed application form has been received, (21 CFR 1305.04).

OMB APPROVAL
No. 1117-0010

TO: (Name of Supplier)

STREET ADDRESS

CITY and STATE

DATE

TO BE FILLED IN BY SUPPLIER
SUPPLIERS DEA REGISTRATION No.

TO BE FILLED IN BY PURCHASER

LINE No.	No. of Packages	Size of Package	Name of Item	National Drug Code	Packages Shipped	Date Shipped
1						
2						
3						
4						
5						
6						
7						
8						
9						
10						

◄ LAST LINE COMPLETED *(MUST BE 10 OR LESS)*

SIGNATURE OF PURCHASER OR ATTORNEY OR AGENT

Date Issued	DEA Registration No.	Name and Address of Registrant
20010101	DEAREGNO	VOID VOID VOID

Schedules
XXXXXXXXXXXXX

VOID VOID VOID
VOID VOID VOID

Registered as a	No. of this Order Form
XXXXXXXXXXXX	000000005

VOID VOID VOID
VOID VOID VOID

DEA Form -222
(Oct. 2004)

U.S. OFFICIAL ORDER FORMS - SCHEDULES I & II
DRUG ENFORCEMENT ADMINISTRATION
SUPPLIER'S Copy 1

107051797

The pharmacist approved and then sent the C-II order. After the order arrived, the pharmacist verified the contents and quantities received and then asked you to properly file the paperwork.

A. What two pieces of paperwork should be filed?

_____

B. How long must these files be retained in your pharmacy?

_____

Lab Activity #17.5: Identify what is missing from the following prescriptions and the measures needed to correct the errors.

Equipment needed:
■ Pen

Time needed to complete this activity: 30 minutes

Rx 1:

Dr. Andre Sheen
1100 Brentwood Blvd, Suite M780
St. Louis, MO 63144
314-527-0000
DEA FS1234563

Michael Smith   January 18, 202X
2624 Main Blvd,
St. Louis, MO 63144
DOB 08/14/64

Rx: Abilify
         i qd po   Disp #30

Ref x 3   *Andre Sheen, MD*

Identify the missing information and how it can be corrected.

_____

_____

_____

Rx 2:

Dr. David Douglas
2101 Woodward Drive, Suite 205
St. Louis, MO 63144
314-527-2536

Jane Jones
4401 West Avenue,
St. Louis, MO 63144
DOB:

Rx: Imitrex 50mg
         i po, may repeat once 2 hours after first dose   Disp #9

Ref x 3   _____

Identify the missing information and how it can be corrected.

_____

_____

_____

256

Rx 3:

Dr. Pamela Parsons
5874 North Ave, Suite 126
St. Louis, MO 63144
314-527-8547
DEA FP1234563

9654 Any Street,
St. Louis, MO 63144
DOB 05/23/57

Rx: Risperidone 2mg
         i qd   Disp #30

Ref x 3   *Pamela Parsons, MD*

Identify the missing information and how it can be corrected.

_____

_____

_____

Rx 4:

Dr. Andre Sheen
1100 Brentwood Blvd, Suite M780
St. Louis, MO 63144
314-527-0000

Jane Smith   March 9, 202X
2624 Main Blvd,
St. Louis, MO 63144
DOB:

Rx: Ambien
         i 1° a hs x 10d   Disp #10

Ref x 0   *Andre Sheen, MD*

Identify the missing information and how it can be corrected.

_____

_____

_____

Rx 5:

Dr. Anna Johnson
1100 Brentwood Blvd, Suite M780
St. Louis, MO 63144

Jane Jones
852 East Ave,
St. Louis, MO 63144
DOB 02/20/72

Rx: Wellbutrin XL
        i qam
                                                          Disp #30

Ref x 3   *Anna Johnson, MD*

Identify the missing information and how it can be corrected.

_____

_____

_____

Lab Activity #17.6: Fill out the perpetual inventory log for each of the prescriptions.

Equipment needed:
- Blue or black pen

Time needed to complete this activity: 30 minutes

Prescription label 1:

Your Friendly Pharmacy
1234 Park Avenue
St. Louis, MO 63144
314-555-1000

Rx 1001

Michael Smith   Date 01/15/2X
2624 Main Blvd,
St. Louis, MO 63144   Dr. A. Sheen

DOB 08/14/62

Concerta ER 36mg Tablets
Take one tablet by mouth daily.   30 Tablets

Refills: 0   Manufacturer: McNeil

Fill out the perpetual inventory log for this prescription.

Drug: Concerta ER 36 mg	Manufacturer: McNeil
Dosage Form: Tablets	NDC: 50458-586-01

Date	Rx #	Patient Name	Quantity Dispensed	Balance on Hand	Initials	Verified
				200		

Prescription label 2:

Your Friendly Pharmacy
1234 Park Avenue
St. Louis, MO 63144
314-555-1000

Rx 1002

Michael Smith
2624 Main Blvd,
St. Louis, MO 63144

Date 01/20/2X

Dr. A. Sheen

DOB 08/14/62

Dextroamphetamine, Amphetamine (mixed salts) 10mg Tablets

Take one tablet by mouth twice daily.

60 Tablets

Refills: 0

Manufacturer: CorePharma

Fill out the perpetual inventory log for this prescription.

Drug: Dextroamphetamine, amphetamine (mixed salts) 10 mg	Manufacturer: CorePharma
Dosage Form: Tablets	NDC: 64720-132-10

Date	Rx #	Patient Name	Quantity Dispensed	Balance on Hand	Initials	Verified
				420		

Prescription label 3:

```
                         Your Friendly Pharmacy
                            1234 Park Avenue
                           St. Louis, MO 63144
                              314-555-1000
Rx 1003

Michael Smith                                    Date 02/10/2X
2624 Main Blvd,
St. Louis, MO 63144                              Dr. A. Sheen

DOB 08/14/62

Methylphenidate ER 20mg Tablets
Take one tablet by mouth twice daily.                60 Tablets

Refills: 0                          Manufacturer: MD Pharmaceuticals
```

Fill out the perpetual inventory log for this prescription.

Drug: Methylphenidate ER 20 mg	Manufacturer: MD Pharmaceuticals
Dosage Form: Tablets	NDC: 43567-562-07

Date	Rx #	Patient Name	Quantity Dispensed	Quantity Remaining	Initials	Verified
				440		

Prescription label 4:

```
                         Your Friendly Pharmacy
                            1234 Park Avenue
                           St. Louis, MO 63144
                              314-555-1000
Rx 1004

Michael Smith                                    Date 02/20/2X
2624 Main Blvd,
St. Louis, MO 63144                              Dr. A. Sheen

DOB 08/14/62

Adderall XR 30mg Capsules
Take one capsule by mouth daily.                     30 Capsules

Refills: 0                               Manufacturer: Shire
```

Fill out the perpetual inventory log for this prescription.

Drug: Adderall XR 30 mg	Manufacturer: Shire
Dosage Form: Capsules	NDC: 54092-391-01

Date	Rx #	Patient Name	Quantity Dispensed	Quantity Remaining	Initials	Verified
				170		

Prescription label 5:

> **Your Friendly Pharmacy**
> 1234 Park Avenue
> St. Louis, MO 63144
> 314-555-1000
>
> Rx 1005
>
> Michael Smith   Date 03/15/2X
> 2624 Main Blvd,
> St. Louis, MO 63144   Dr. A. Sheen
>
> DOB 08/14/62
>
> Vyvanse 30mg Capsules
> Take one capsule by mouth every morning.   30 Capsules
>
> Refills: 0   Manufacturer: Shire

Fill out the perpetual inventory log for this prescription.

Drug: Vyvanse 30 mg	Manufacturer: Shire
Dosage Form: Capsule	NDC: 59417-0103-10

Date	Rx #	Patient Name	Quantity Dispensed	Quantity Remaining	Initials	Verified
				310		

18 Therapeutic Agents for the Endocrine System

REINFORCE KEY CONCEPTS

Terms and Definitions

Select the correct term from the following list and write the corresponding letter in the blank next to the statement.

A. Aldosterone
B. Calcitonin
C. Catecholamines
D. Homeostasis
E. Hormones
F. Thyroxine (T_4)
G. Triiodothyronine (T_3)
H. Vasopressin

_____ 1. A thyroid hormone derived from tyrosine (amino acid) that influences the metabolic rate

_____ 2. A thyroid hormone that helps to regulate blood concentrations of calcium and phosphate and promotes the formation of bone

_____ 3. Another term used for antidiuretic hormone (ADH)

_____ 4. The equilibrium pertaining to the balance of fluid levels, pH level, osmotic pressures, and concentrations of various substances

_____ 5. Chemical substances produced and secreted by an endocrine duct into the bloodstream that result in a physiological response at a specific target tissue

_____ 6. The principal mineralocorticoid in the body that maintains sodium and potassium homeostasis by stimulating the kidneys to conserve sodium and excrete potassium

_____ 7. A thyroid hormone that helps regulate growth and development and controls metabolism and body temperature; it is mainly produced through the metabolism of thyroxine

_____ 8. Hormones produced in the brainstem, nervous system, and adrenal glands that help the body respond to stress and prepare the body for the "fight-or-flight" response; they are important in regulating heart rate, blood pressure, and nervous system functions

Select the correct term from the following list and write the corresponding letter in the blank next to the statement.

A. Adrenal cortex
B. Adrenal medulla
C. Body mass index (BMI)
D. Comorbidity
E. Endocrine glands
F. Endocrinologist
G. Exocrine glands
H. Glucometer
I. Pancreas
J. Parenteral

_____ 9. Glands that produce hormones sent to the target organ or tissue via a tube or duct outside the body

_____ 10. A measure of body fat based on height and weight of a patient.

_____ 11. An endocrine gland that produces both insulin and glucagon

_____ 12. A portion of the adrenal gland that secretes steroids, including mineralocorticoids, glucocorticoids, and sex steroids

_____ 13. Glands that produce hormones that enter the bloodstream to reach their target or act at target sites near the area of hormone release

_____ 14. A device used to test blood sugar levels in patients with diabetes mellitus (DM)

_____ 15. A concomitant, but not necessarily related, medical condition existing simultaneously with another condition

_____ 16. A term indicating administration of a substance by a route other than by mouth

_____ 17. An inner part of the adrenal gland that synthesizes and secretes the catecholamines norepinephrine and epinephrine

_____ 18. A physician who specializes in the treatment of conditions of the endocrine system

Select the correct term from the following list and write the corresponding letter in the blank next to the statement.

A. Hyperglycemia
B. Hypertension
C. Hypocalcemia
D. Hypoglycemia
E. Hypokalemia
F. Oogenesis
G. Orthostatic hypotension
H. Ovulation

_____ 19. Production or development of an egg

_____ 20. Excessively low concentration of glucose in the blood

_____ 21. The release of an egg from the ovary

_____ 22. Elevated concentration of glucose in the blood

_____ 23. Low concentration of potassium in the blood

_____ 24. Low concentration of calcium in the blood

_____ 25. Low blood pressure that occurs upon standing up

_____ 26. Elevated blood pressure

Select the correct term from the following list and write the corresponding letter in the blank next to the statement.

A. Acromegaly
B. Addison disease
C. Cretinism
D. Dwarfism
E. Exophthalmos
F. Gastroparesis
G. Gigantism
H. Goiter
I. Graves' disease
J. Hyperthyroidism
K. Hypopituitary dwarfism
L. Insulin resistance
M. Myxedema
N. Peripheral neuropathy
O. Type 1 diabetes mellitus (T1DM)
P. Type 2 diabetes mellitus (T2DM)

_____ 27. A condition caused by excessive growth hormone production during adulthood

_____ 28. A condition caused by thyroid hormone hypersecretion; symptoms include diffuse goiter, exophthalmos, and skin changes

_____ 29. A condition in which the development of the brain and body is inhibited by a congenital lack of thyroid hormone secretion

_____ 30. A condition associated with a decrease in overall adult thyroid function; also known as hypothyroidism

_____ 31. An eyeball prominence (protrusion) from the orbit; increased thyroid hormone is a common cause of bilateral presentation

_____ 32. Damage to nerves of the peripheral nervous system

_____ 33. A condition of excessive growth hormone production during childhood or adolescence that results in excessive height and body tissue growth

_____ 34. Short stature due to a deficiency in growth hormone during childhood

_____ 35. A form of diabetes mellitus associated with insulin resistance and a relative deficiency of insulin; people with T2DM can be treated with oral therapies, noninsulin injectable medications, and insulin

_____ 36. A condition in which the thyroid gland is enlarged because of a lack of iodine

_____ 37. Excessive secretion of thyroid hormone

_____ 38. Delayed gastric emptying

_____ 39. A form of diabetes mellitus associated with an absolute deficiency of insulin production by the pancreas; people with T1DM require insulin therapy

_____ 40. A condition characterized by a growth hormone deficiency during adolescence, resulting in short stature and decreased organ size

_____ 41. The resistance of body tissues (skeletal muscle and fat) to insulin effects; insulin resistance is associated with the development of type 2 diabetes mellitus

_____ 42. A condition resulting in decreased levels of adrenocortical hormones (eg, mineralocorticoids and glucocorticoids), which causes symptoms such as muscle weakness and weight loss

True or False

Write T or F next to each statement.

_____ 1. The Greek word for hormone means "that which sets in motion."

_____ 2. The parathyroid gland secretes a hormone called parathyroid hormone (PTH), which helps maintain adequate potassium levels.

_____ 3. The adrenal glands secrete calcitonin and thyroxine, which responds to stress of the body.

_____ 4. The largest endocrine gland is the pancreas.

_____ 5. The "islets of Langerhans" in the pancreas contain alpha cells that produce glucose and alpha cells that produce insulin.

_____ 6. A feedback system maintains hormone levels in a normal range.

_____ 7. The hypothalamus stimulates the pituitary gland by neuronal impulses and regulates most endocrine activity.

_____ 8. The major mineral potassium is important for the proper functioning of muscle contractions, nerve impulses, and blood clotting.

_____ 9. The parathyroid glands are essential in helping the body cope with stress.

_____ 10. Many endocrine system conditions are due to too much or too little production of a hormone by a gland of the endocrine system.

System Identifier

Identify each organ in this system and enter the term next to the corresponding number.

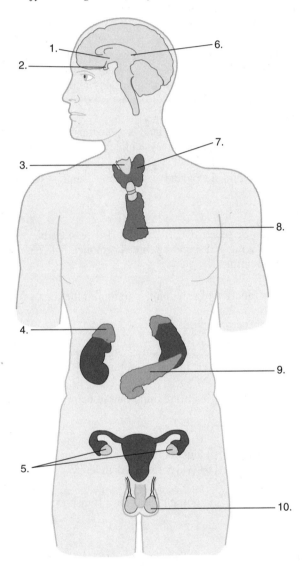

1. _____

2. _____

3. _____

4. _____

5. _____

6. _____

7. _____

8. _____

9. _____

10. _____

Multiple Choice

Complete each question by circling the best answer.

1. PTU and methimazole are used for the treatment of:
   A. Diabetes
   B. Osteoporosis
   C. Hyperthyroidism
   D. Hypothyroidism

2. The drugs _____ and _____ are synthetic forms of ADH and are typically prescribed to treat diabetes insipidus.
   A. corticotropin and prolactin
   B. vasopressin and desmopressin acetate
   C. levothyroxine and liothyronine
   D. doxercalciferol and calcitriol

3. The most common treatment for Graves' disease in the United States is _____.
   A. Glucophage (metformin)
   B. radioactive iodine
   C. exercise
   D. Declomycin (demeclocycline)

4. Hypothyroidism can be treated with the drug _____.
   A. Tapazole (methimazole)
   B. Humatrope (somatropin)
   C. Sandostatin (octreotide)
   D. Synthroid (levothyroxine)

5. Hectorol (doxercalciferol) and Rocaltrol (calcitriol) are used for the treatment of:
   A. Diabetes
   B. Hyperparathyroidism
   C. Hyperthyroidism
   D. Estrogen replacement

6. The mineralocorticoid drug fludrocortisone acetate can be used for the treatment of:
   A. Graves' disease
   B. Cushing's disease
   C. diabetes mellitus
   D. Addison's disease

7. The long-acting insulin _____ is three times as concentrated as Lantus (insulin glargine) and has shown to be more effective at controlling blood sugar.
   A. Toujeo
   B. Apidra
   C. Levemir
   D. Afrezza

8. The insulin _____ is the same as that in Humulin but is inhaled rather than injected subcutaneously.
   A. Apidra
   B. Toujeo
   C. Levemir
   D. Afrezza

9. The following brand name medications are combination oral drugs for T2DM *except*:
   A. Janumet
   B. Glucovance
   C. Glucophage
   D. Duetact

10. The medication _____ is approved for patients with obesity who are exercising and eating a reduced-calorie diet.
    A. ActoPlus Met (pioglitazone–metformin)
    B. Oseni (alogliptin–pioglitazone)
    C. Xenical (orlistat)
    D. Sensipar (cinacalcet)

Fill in the Blanks

Answer each question by completing the statement in the space provided.

1. The _____ plays a key role in the regulation of several functions, such as water balance, metabolism of fat and carbohydrates, body temperature, appetite, and emotions.

2. The _____ gland is analogous to the control tower of the endocrine system.

3. The pineal gland produces and secretes _____.

4. The _____ gland is responsible for producing and secreting three hormones: T4, T3, and calcitonin.

5. The function of calcitonin is to inhibit the removal of _____ from bone.

6. The _____ glands are the primary regulators of calcium levels in the blood through PTH release.

7. The adrenal glands are important in helping the body cope with _____.

8. Diabetes insipidus is a _____ disorder caused by ADH (vasopressin) deficiency.

9. Insulin is important in the transportation of _____ into the cell.

10. Gestational diabetes mellitus (GDM) occurs in women during _____.

Matching

Match the drugs with their indications.

_____ 1. Synthroid
(levothyroxine
sodium (T₄))

_____ 2. Glucophage
(metformin)

_____ 3. Cortef
(hydrocortisone)

_____ 4. Tapazole
(methimazole)

_____ 5. Sensipar
(cinacalcet)

A. Addison's disease
B. Hyperthyroidism
C. Hypothyroidism
D. Hypercalcemia
E. Type 2 diabetes
  mellitus

Match the trade and generic drug names.

_____ 6. Glucotrol

_____ 7. Rocaltrol

_____ 8. Medrol

_____ 9. Sandostatin

_____ 10. Actos

A. calcitriol
B. octreotide
C. pioglitazone
D. glipizide
E. methylprednisolone

Match the type of insulin with its main category.

_____ 11. Humulin 70/30

_____ 12. Humulin R

_____ 13. Lantus

_____ 14. NovoLog

_____ 15. Humulin N

A. Rapid-acting
B. Short-acting
C. Intermediate-acting
D. Long-acting
E. Premixed

Match the trade and generic drug names.

_____ 16. Amaryl

_____ 17. Tradjenta

_____ 18. Onglyza

_____ 19. Invokana

_____ 20. Farxiga

A. saxagliptin
B. glimepiride
C. linagliptin
D. dapagliflozin
E. canagliflozin

Short Answer

Reply to each question based on what you have learned in the chapter.

1. List the three hormones the thyroid gland produces that affect metabolism.

   _____

   _____

2. List the differences between the endocrine and exocrine glands.

   _____

   _____

3. List three functions hormones perform throughout the body and how they do it.

   _____

   _____

   _____

   _____

4. List the three signaling pathways that influence the endocrine system and the production of hormones.

   _____

   _____

5. List two hormones stored in the posterior portion of the pituitary gland and how they affect the body.

   _____

   _____

6. List the classic hyperglycemia symptoms that can lead to a T1DM diagnosis.

   _____

   _____

7. List the first-line treatment for patients with diabetes mellitus (DM).

_____

_____

Research Activities

Follow the instructions given in each exercise and provide a response.

1. To help manage additional risks the American Heart Association lists guidelines for Living Heathy with Diabetes. Access the website *https://www.heart.org/en/health-topics/diabetes/prevention--treatment-of-diabetes/living-healthy-with-diabetes* and answer the following:

   A. List two ways to manage weight to help reduce the risk of obesity and cardiovascular disease.

   B. How much physical activity is recommended to help lower the risk of developing diabetes?

   C. What other lifestyle changes are recommend to help maintain your health and reduce the risk of developing and/or managing diabetes?

2. Access the website *http://www.ncbi.nlm.nih.gov/pmc/articles/PMC2769828/*. Read the article about type 3 diabetes mellitus that would enable you to answer the following questions:

   A. What is Alzheimer's disease (AD)?

   B. What scientific findings lead researchers to link Alzheimer's disease to diabetes mellitus?

   C. How could medications currently used for diabetes mellitus be used to help prevent Alzheimer's disease in the future?

REFLECT CRITICALLY

Critical Thinking

Reply to each question based on what you have learned in the chapter.

1. Diabetes mellitus (type 2) has been prevalent in your family for the past few years. What lifestyle choices have you made that could contribute to being diagnosed with this disease? What lifestyle changes can you make to help avoid being diagnosed with this disease?

2. Why is it important for pharmacy technicians to be familiar with the various glucometers available to those with diabetes mellitus? How can pharmacy technicians help those with diabetes mellitus and the supplies they would need to help them check blood glucose levels?

RELATE TO PRACTICE

Lab Scenarios
Therapeutic Agents for the Endocrine System

Objective: To review with the pharmacy technician the organs of the endocrine system; in addition, to review the brand and generic names, indications, dosage forms, routes of administration, and daily dosing of medications used to treat disorders of the endocrine system

---

DID YOU KNOW?

- 34 million American have diabetes, but 1 in 5 do not know they have it.
- Approximately 88 million people 20 years of age and older have prediabetes.
- 1.4 million Americans are diagnosed yearly with diabetes.
- The total cost of diagnosed diabetes was $327 billion yearly.
- Diabetes is the seventh leading cause of death.

Reference:
https://www.cdc.gov/diabetes/library/socialmedia/infographics.html

Lab Activity #18.1: Define the following terms associated with the endocrine system.

Equipment needed:
- Medical dictionary
- Pencil/pen

Time needed to complete this activity: 30 minutes

1. Cushing's disease

   _____

2. Diabetes insipidus

   _____

3. Diabetes mellitus

   _____

4. Gestational diabetes

   _____

5. Glucose

   _____

6. Graves' disease

   _____

7. Hashimoto's thyroiditis

   _____

8. Hypercalcemia

   _____

9. Insulin-dependent diabetes mellitus (IDDM)

   _____

10. Non–insulin-dependent diabetes mellitus (NIDDM)

    _____

11. Pheochromocytoma

    _____

12. Thyroid dysgenesis

    _____

13. Thyroiditis

    _____

14. Thyrotoxicosis

    _____

Lab Activity #18.2: Using a drug reference book, identify the brand name, drug classification, indications, dosage forms, routes of administration, and recommended daily dosage of the *most common* medications used to treat conditions affecting the endocrine system.

Equipment needed:
- *Drug Facts and Comparisons* or *Physicians' Desk Reference*
- Pencil/pen

Time needed to complete this activity: 60 minutes

Generic Name	Brand Name	Classification	Indication(s)	Dose Form(s)	Route(s)	Recommended Daily Dosage	Auxiliary Label(s)
Canagliflozin							
Exenatide							
Glimerpiride							

Continued

Generic Name	Brand Name	Classification	Indication(s)	Dose Form(s)	Route(s)	Recommended Daily Dosage	Auxiliary Label(s)
Glipizide							
Glyburide							
Insulin Aspart							
Insulin Detemir							
Insulin Glargine							
Insulin Lispro							
Levothyroxine							
Liraglutide							
Metformin HCl							
Metformin HCl/ Sitagliptin Phosphate							
Phentermine/ topiramate							
Pioglitazone HCl							
Sitagliptin Phosphate							
Thyroid							

Lab Activity #18.3: Using a drug reference, identify the generic name, manufacturer, product size availability, NDC, and AWP.

Equipment needed:
- Computer with Internet access
- *Red Book Online*
- Pencil/pen

Time needed to complete this activity: 60 minutes

Brand (Trade) Name	Generic Name	Manufacturer	Product Size Availability	NDC	AWP
Humalog					
Humalog KwikPen					
NovoLog					
NovoLog FlexPen					
Apidra					
Apidra SoloStar					
Humulin R					
Novolin R					
Humulin N					
Novolin N					
Lantus					
Lantus SoloStar					

Continued

Brand (Trade) Name	Generic Name	Manufacturer	Product Size Availability	NDC	AWP
Levemir					
Levemir FlexPen					
Toujeo SoloStar					

You are to recommend one insulin product from each insulin category for the inpatient pharmacy. Using the information you gathered for the table on the previous page and information learned from previous chapters, answer the following questions to help you determine which product to recommend:

A. For each of the insulin categories, which product (vial or pen) would be most cost effective?

B. List advantages and disadvantages of using a community insulin vial for the inpatient floor.

C. List advantages and disadvantages of using a community insulin pen for the inpatient floor.

D. List advantages and disadvantages of using an insulin vial for each patient.

E. List advantages and disadvantages of using an insulin pen for each patient.

F. Considering the advantages and disadvantages listed, which would be safer to use (vial or pen) for the inpatient setting?

G. For each of the insulin categories, which product would you recommend the inpatient pharmacy to dispense?

Using Therapeutic Agents for the Endocrine System

Objective: To review with the pharmacy technician prescription orders, dosage calculations, and sterile product preparation.

Lab Activity #18.4: Answer the questions based on the prescription orders for each question.

Equipment needed:
- *Drug Facts and Comparisons* or *Physician's Desk Reference*
- Pencil/pen
- Calculator

Time needed to complete this activity: 30 minutes

The following are approved DAW codes:

DAW 0: no product selection indicated
DAW 1: substitution not allowed by provider
DAW 2: substitution allowed: patient-requested product dispensed
DAW 3: substitution allowed: pharmacist-selected product dispensed
DAW 4: substitution allowed: generic drug not in stock
DAW 5: substitution allowed: brand drug dispensed as generic
DAW 6: override
DAW 7: substitution not allowed: brand drug mandated by law
DAW 8: substitution allowed: generic drug not available in marketplace
DAW 9: other

1. Rx 1:
   Humulin-R U-100 insulin, 2 vials
   40 units SC qam and 30 units ac evening meal
   Ref × 3

   A. How much will be dispensed (use metric quantities)?

   _____

   B. How many days will the medication last?

   _____

   C. How many refills are permitted on the prescription?

   _____

   D. What DAW code will be used?

   _____

   E. Write directions as they would appear on the medication label.

   _____

   F. What auxiliary label(s) should be affixed to the medication label?

   _____

   _____

   _____

2. Rx 2:
   Lantus insulin, 1 vial
   12 units SC before dinner
   Ref × 1

   A. How much will be dispensed (use metric quantities)?

   _____

   B. How many days will the medication last?

   _____

   C. How many refills are permitted on the prescription?

   _____

   D. What DAW code will be used?

   _____

   E. Write directions as they would appear on the medication label.

   _____

   F. What auxiliary label(s) should be affixed to the medication label?

   _____

   _____

   _____

3. Rx 3:
   Glucophage 500-mg tab, 30-day supply
   1 g qam and qpm ac
   Ref × 6
   Patient has requested brand name

   A. How much will be dispensed?

   _____

   B. How many days will the medication last?

   _____

   C. How many refills are permitted on the prescription?

   _____

273

D. What DAW code will be used?

_____

E. Write directions as they would appear on the medication label.

_____

_____

F. What auxiliary label(s) should be affixed to the medication label?

_____

_____

_____

4. Rx 4:
   Synthroid 0.1 mg, #30
   100 mcg qam, no later than 10 am
   Ref × 3
   Brand name medically necessary

   A. How much will be dispensed?

   _____

   B. How many days will the medication last?

   _____

   C. How many refills are permitted on the prescription?

   _____

   D. What DAW code will be used?

   _____

   E. Write directions as they would appear on the medication label.

   _____

   _____

   F. What auxiliary label(s) should be affixed to the medication label?

   _____

   _____

   _____

5. Rx 5:
   Prednisone 10-mg tablets
   i qid × 2d; i tid × 2d; i bid × 2d; i qd × 2d; ss qd × 2d
   Ref: 0

   A. How much will be dispensed?

   _____

   B. How many days will the medication last?

   _____

   C. How many refills are permitted on the prescription?

   _____

   D. What DAW code will be used?

   _____

   E. Write directions as they would appear on the medication label.

   _____

   _____

   F. What auxiliary label(s) should be affixed to the medication label?

   _____

   _____

   _____

Lab Activity #18.5: Calculate the quantity of the ingredients needed to prepare the following dilutions.

Equipment needed:
■ Calculator
■ Pencil/pen
■ Paper
■ *Handbook on Injectable Drugs*

Time needed to complete this activity: 30 minutes

1. Dilution #1
   A. The pharmacy has in stock a 10-mL vial of Humulin R insulin with a concentration of 100 units/mL. How much of the 100 units/mL Humulin R insulin and how much diluent are needed to prepare 10 mL of a dilution with a concentration of 10 units/mL?

   What diluents can be used?

   _____

Humulin R Insulin 100 units/mL amount:

_____

Diluent amount: _____

B. Using the dilution made in part A, how much Humulin R insulin 10 units/mL and how much diluent are needed to prepare 30 mL of a second dilution with a concentration of 1 unit/mL?

What diluents can be used?

_____

Humulin R Insulin 10 units/mL amount:

_____

Diluent amount: _____

2. Dilution #2

The pharmacy has in stock hydrocortisone 100 mg/2 mL. How much of the hydrocortisone 100 mg/2 mL and how much diluent are needed to prepare 8 mL of a 5 mg/mL hydrocortisone solution?

What diluents can be used?

_____

Hydrocortisone 100 mg/2 mL amount:

_____

Diluent amount: _____

Lab Activity #18.6: Using the calculations from Lab Activity 18.5, question 1, prepare a dilution of insulin using sterile compounding procedures.

Equipment needed:
- Alcohol swabs (sterile)
- Diluent
- Laminar airflow hood
- Empty sterile 10-mL vial
- Empty sterile 30-mL vial
- Personal protection equipment (PPE)
- Non-shedding disposable towels
- 70% isopropyl alcohol
- Sterile water
- Waterless alcohol-based hand rub
- Aseptic cleaning wipes
- Sharps container
- Humulin R insulin 10-mL vial
- Sink with running hot and cold water
- Syringes with needles
- Vented needles
- Labels

Procedure

1. Gather all materials needed for activity.
2. All items must be wiped down with aseptic cleaning wipes before entering the IV room.
3. Wash hands properly using aseptic technique.
4. Don PPEs in the proper sequence.
5. Clean laminar flow workbench in the proper manner, using the correct supplies and techniques.
6. Collect the medication to be compounded.
7. Check expiration dates on both the vial and sterile vials.
8. Place ingredients in the laminar flow hood.
9. Swab the rubber top of the diluent and empty sterile vial with alcohol. Allow the alcohol to dry.
10. Make sure the needle is firmly attached to the syringe.
11. Prepare the syringe by adding the amount of air that will be equal to the amount of diluent to be withdrawn into the syringe.
12. Hold the syringe with the thumb and the index and middle fingers.
13. Remove cap from needle.
14. Insert the needle at a 45-degree angle into the rubber stopper of the vial with beveled part of the needle facing upward.
15. Hold the vial with the hand opposite the hand that is holding the syringe.
16. Invert the vial.
17. Push the plunger, forcing the air in the syringe into the vial, and release gently, allowing the fluid to be drawn into the syringe.
18. Tap the syringe to force air bubbles out of it.
19. Draw up the correct amount of diluent needed to dilute the insulin to correct concentration.
20. Pull back on the plunger to clear the neck of the syringe. Remove the needle and replace with a vented needle.
21. Remove all excess air from syringe.
22. Insert vented needle of the syringe at a 45-degree angle into the rubber top of the empty sterile vial and transfer the diluent.
23. Swab the rubber top of the insulin vial and sterile vial (with diluent in it) with alcohol. Allow the alcohol to dry.
24. Make sure the needle is firmly attached to the syringe.
25. Prepare the syringe by adding the amount of air that will be equal to the amount of insulin to be withdrawn into the syringe.
26. Hold the syringe with the thumb and the index and middle fingers.
27. Remove cap from needle.
28. Insert the needle at a 45-degree angle into the rubber stopper of the vial with beveled part of the needle facing upward.
29. Hold the vial with the hand opposite the hand that is holding the syringe.
30. Invert the vial.
31. Push the plunger, forcing the air in the syringe into the vial, and release gently, allowing the fluid to be drawn into the syringe.
32. Tap the syringe to force air bubbles out of it.

275

33. Draw up the correct amount of insulin needed to dilute the insulin to correct concentration.
34. Pull back on the plunger to clear the neck of the syringe. Remove the needle and replace with a vented needle.
35. Remove all excess air from syringe.
36. Insert vented needle of the syringe at a 45-degree angle into the rubber top of the sterile vial and transfer the insulin.
37. Gently swirl to mix.
38. Discard syringes into sharps container.
39. Properly label vial with correct concentration and expiration date.
40. Repeat steps 6 through 39 to perform the second dilution to 1 unit/mL.
41. Remove PPEs in the proper sequence and discard.
42. Record initials, date, and time on the cleaning log.

Time needed to complete this activity: 45 minutes

1. What information would to be on the label for the dilution you just made?

   _____

   _____

2. What BUD would be assigned to this dilution?

   _____

Glucose Testing

Objective: To introduce glucometers and related supplies to the pharmacy technician and the procedure for testing blood glucose levels; to review and apply information learned about diabetes mellitus

Lab Activity #18.7: Answer the following questions to predict a normal, high, or low blood glucose level.

   Equipment needed:
   ■ Pencil/pen
   ■ Paper

   Time needed to complete this activity: 15 minutes

1. At what time did you eat your last meal/snack? _____

   _____

2. Do you smoke? _____

   _____

3. Have you had coffee or other caffeine today? If so, at

   what time? _____

4. Do you have any medical conditions? _____

   _____

A. If you have diabetes, what medications are you currently on and have you taken them today?

B. If you have high blood pressure, what medications are you currently on and have you taken them today?

5. Are you currently taking any OTC or herbal products or prescription medications? If so, which ones?

   _____

   _____

   _____

6. Based on your answers from the previous questions and your knowledge of foods, medications, and health conditions that affect blood glucose, do you think your blood glucose level will be normal, high, or low if you checked it right now? Why?

   _____

   _____

   _____

Lab Activity #18.8: Using a glucose monitor, test your blood glucose level. Answer the questions based on the information given in Lab Activity #18.7 and your glucose reading.

   Equipment needed:
   ■ Glucose monitor
   ■ Glucose strips
   ■ Lancet device
   ■ Lancets
   ■ Alcohol swabs
   ■ Gauze/cotton balls
   ■ Bandage
   ■ Sharps container
   ■ Pencil/pen

Procedure

1. Clean workspace in proper manner, using correct supplies and techniques.
2. Gather all materials needed for activity.
3. Wash hands properly.
4. Assemble equipment.

5. Select puncture site.
6. Gently rub finger to promote circulation.
7. Clean site with alcohol swab and allow to dry.
8. Firmly grasp finger.
9. Hold lancet device at a 90-degree angle (perpendicular) to patient's finger and make a rapid, deep puncture on the fingertip.
10. Wipe away first drop of blood with a clean gauze/cotton ball.
11. Apply gentle pressure to cause blood to flow freely.
12. Collect sample.
13. Clean site with clean gauze/cotton ball.
14. Apply pressure with clean gauze/cotton ball.
15. Record reading.
16. Check for bleeding, then apply bandage.
17. Dispose of material in proper containers.
18. Clean work area.
19. Properly wash hands using correct procedures and techniques

Time needed to complete this activity: 30 minutes

Optimal Blood Glucose Level	Category
Less than 100 mg/dL	Fasting
Less than 140 mg/dL	2 hours after a meal

1. Glucose reading: _____ mg/dL

2. Is your blood glucose level within the optimal blood glucose guidelines?

_____

3. What factors may have contributed to your blood glucose level?

_____

_____

4. Was your prediction from Lab Activity #18.7, question 6 correct? Why or why not?

_____

_____

_____

5. As a pharmacy technician, how could you help those with diabetes mellitus while working in a pharmacy?

_____

_____

_____

Insulin Syringes

Objective: To introduce insulin syringes to the pharmacy technician

Lab Activity #18.9: Fill in the table below about insulin syringes.

Equipment needed:
- Pencil/pen
- 1-cc, ½-cc, ⅓-cc insulin syringes

Time needed to complete this activity: 15 minutes

Insulin syringes look very much like the syringes you learned about in Chapter 12 except the points of measurement are not in milliliters. The points of measurement for an insulin syringe are marked as units since insulin is measured in units. An insulin syringe has three parts: the needle, barrel, and plunger. They come in three main sizes, 1 cc, ½ cc, and ⅓ cc. The smallest size syringe should be used for the dose needed. Several needle lengths and gauges are also available for insulin syringes. Be sure to check with the patient what their dose of insulin is and their preference for the needle length and gauge so that they receive the correct insulin syringe. Using the insulin syringes available to you, fill in the table below.

Syringe size	Number of Units Syringe Holds	Needle Length	Gauge of Needle
⅓ cc			
½ cc			
1 cc			

19 Therapeutic Agents for the Musculoskeletal System

ASHP ACCREDITATION STANDARDS FOR PHARMACY TECHNICIAN EDUCATION AND TRAINING PROGRAMS

Standard 1.2: Present an image appropriate for the profession of pharmacy in appearance and behavior.

Standard 1.3: Demonstrate active and engaged listening skills.

Standard 1.4: Communicate clearly and effectively, both verbally and in writing.

Standard 1.5: Demonstrate a respectful and professional attitude when interacting with diverse patient populations, colleagues, and professionals.

Standard 1.7: Apply interpersonal skills, including negotiation skills, conflict resolution, customer service, and teamwork.

Standard 1.10: Apply critical thinking skills, creativity, and innovation.

Standard 2.5: Demonstrate basic knowledge of anatomy, physiology and pharmacology, and medical terminology relevant to the pharmacy technician's role.

Standard 3.1: Assist pharmacists in collecting, organizing, and recording demographic and clinical information for the Pharmacists; Patient Care Process.

Standard 3.2: Receive, process, and prepare prescriptions/medication orders for completeness, accuracy, and authenticity to ensure safety.

Standard 3.3: Assist pharmacists in the identification of patients who desire/require counseling to optimize the use of medications, equipment, and devices.

Standard 5.1: Describe and apply state and federal laws pertaining to processing, handling, and dispensing of medications including controlled substances.

REINFORCE KEY CONCEPTS

Terms and Definitions

Select the correct term from the following list and write the corresponding letter in the blank next to the statement.

A. Analgesic
B. Antipyretic
C. Arthroplasty
D. Cyclooxygenase (COX)
E. Euphoria
F. Gout
G. Miosis
H. Opioid analgesic
I. Osteoarthritis (OA)
J. Osteoporosis
K. Prostaglandin
L. (Bone) resorption
M. Reye syndrome
N. Uric acid

_____ 1. Either of two related enzymes that control prostaglandin production

_____ 2. A mediator responsible for the features of inflammation, such as swelling, pain, stiffness, redness, and warmth

_____ 3. The water-insoluble end product of purine metabolism; deposition of uric acid as crystals in the joints and kidneys causes gout

_____ 4. Feeling or state of intense excitement and happiness

_____ 5. An analgesic medication that activates opioid receptors

_____ 6. A drug that relieves pain

_____ 7. Degeneration of joint cartilage and the underlying bone

_____ 8. A medical condition in which the bones become brittle and fragile from loss of bone density and poor microarchitecture

_____ 9. A life-threatening metabolic disorder in young children of uncertain cause. Aspirin use may precipitate the syndrome.

_____ 10. A painful form of arthritis characterized by defective metabolism of uric acid

_____ 11. A drug that prevents or reduces fever

_____ 12. Removal of osseous tissue by osteoclasts

_____ 13. Constriction of the pupil of the eye

_____ 14. Surgical reconstruction or replacement of a joint

Select the correct term from the following list and write the corresponding letter in the blank next to the statement.

A. Bone fracture
B. Bone marrow
C. Cancellous bone
D. Compact bone
E. Fascicles
F. Ligament
G. Motor nerve
H. Muscle fiber
I. Neuromuscular junction
J. Skeletal muscle
K. Skeletal system
L. Spongy bone
M. Subchondral bone
N. Synovium
O. Tendon

_____ 15. A bundle such as muscle fibers

_____ 16. Muscle that is connected to the skeleton to form part of the mechanical system that moves the limbs and other parts of the body

_____ 17. Rigid bone, which makes up most of the skeleton; also known as cortical bone

_____ 18. A flexible but inelastic cord of strong fibrous collagen tissue that attaches a muscle to a bone

_____ 19. The hard structure (bones and cartilages) that provides a frame for the body

_____ 20. Bone located below the cartilage, particularly within a joint

_____ 21. A meshwork of spongy bone typically found at the core of vertebral bones in the spine and the ends of long bones; also called spongy bone

_____ 22. The junction between a nerve fiber and the muscle it supplies

_____ 23. A fibrous connective tissue that connects to bones

_____ 24. Muscle cell

_____ 25. A thin membrane in synovial (freely moving) joints that lines the joint capsule and secretes synovial fluid

_____ 26. Meshwork of spongy bone typically found at the core of vertebral bones in the spine and the ends of long bones, also known as cancellous bone

_____ 27. A break or rupture of a bone

_____ 28. A nerve carrying impulses from the brain or spinal cord to a muscle or gland

_____ 29. A fatty network of connective tissue that fills the cavities of bones

True or False

Write T or F next to each statement.

_____ 1. Skeletal muscles attach to bones to enable movement, such as walking, talking, and chewing food.

_____ 2. Osteoporosis is the most common form of joint disease.

_____ 3. Treatment of patients with osteoarthritis should focus on controlling pain and other symptoms to minimize disability and preserve quality of life.

_____ 4. Acetaminophen is abbreviated APAP in the United States.

_____ 5. The first company to market aspirin was St. Joseph.

_____ 6. Prescribers and patients use NSAIDs for mild to moderate pain and inflammation.

_____ 7. Opioid medications are not controlled substances.

_____ 8. The prognosis of osteoporosis can be good when treated with dietary changes, exercise, and medication.

_____ 9. Weight loss, abstaining from alcohol, and adopting a low-purine diet can be beneficial for those with gout.

_____ 10. Individuals with liver disease may take 4000 mg of acetaminophen daily.

System Identifier I

Label the following parts of the structure of a typical bone and the internal structure of a long bone.

1. _____

2. _____

3. _____

4. _____

5. _____

6. _____

279

7. _____   10. _____

8. _____   11. _____

9. _____   12. _____

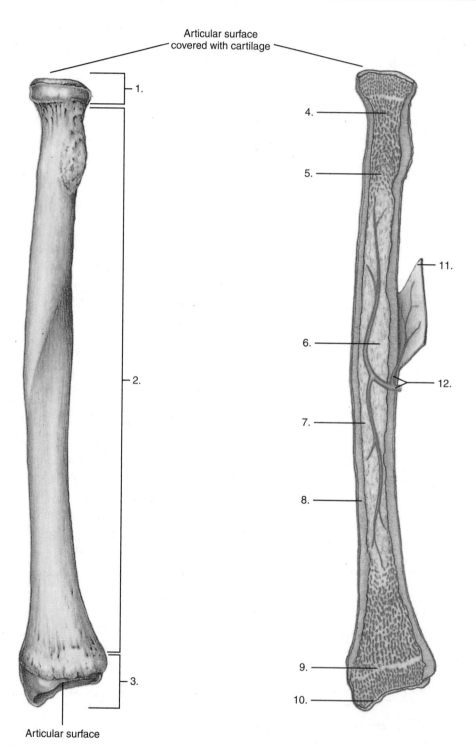

Articular surface
covered with cartilage

1.

2.

3.

Articular surface

4.

5.

11.

6.

12.

7.

8.

9.

10.

(A) The structure of a typical long bone.

(B) Internal structure of a long bone.

From Solomon EP: *Introduction to human anatomy and physiology,* ed 3, St Louis, 2009, Saunders.

System Identifier II

Label the following parts of the muscle.

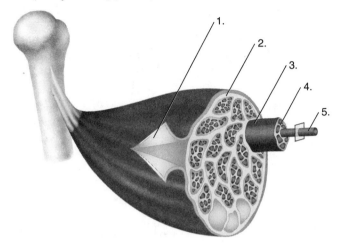

1. _____
2. _____
3. _____
4. _____
5. _____

From Solomon EP: *Introduction to human anatomy and physiology*, ed 3, St Louis, 2009, Saunders.

Multiple Choice

Complete each question by circling the best answer.

1. _____ is the analgesic of choice for osteoarthritis pain.
   A. Ibuprofen
   B. Hydrocodone
   C. Aspirin
   D. Acetaminophen

2. Aspirin should not be given to children because its use in that age group has been linked to:
   A. Toxic shock syndrome
   B. Reye's syndrome
   C. Chickenpox
   D. Sudden infant death syndrome (SIDS)

3. Which of the following is true about nonsteroidal anti-inflammatories (NSAIDs)?
   A. All NSAIDs are available in lesser strengths over the counter (OTC).
   B. They are highly addictive.
   C. They reduce fever.
   D. They increase inflammation.

4. Relafen (nabumetone) and Indocin (indomethacin) are both:
   A. NSAIDs
   B. Opioid analgesics
   C. COX-2 selective inhibitors
   D. Bisphosphonates

5. Which of the following is *not* a potential side effect of corticosteroids?
   A. Inflammation
   B. Increased blood sugar
   C. High blood pressure
   D. Fluid retention

6. The following auxiliary label should be placed on an NSAID prescription:
   A. Take on an empty stomach.
   B. Caution: Federal law prohibits the transfer of this drug to any person other than the patient.
   C. Rotate injection site.
   D. Take with food or milk.

7. Which of the following can be used topically to help treat muscle strains and osteoarthritis?
   A. Benadryl (diphenhydramine)
   B. Duragesic (fentanyl)
   C. Tiger Balm (camphor and menthol)
   D. Motrin (ibuprofen)

8. For combination opioid medications with acetaminophen, it is the acetaminophen that limits the maximum amount to _____ daily.
   A. 4 g
   B. 3 g
   C. 2 g
   D. 1 g

9. The drug _____ is an oral treatment of osteoporosis.
   A. Miacalcin (calcitonin)
   B. Evista (raloxifene)
   C. Forteo (teriparatide)
   D. Prolia (denosumab)

10. Oral bisphosphonate medications should be taken:
   A. With milk
   B. With a meal
   C. On an empty stomach
   D. With orange juice

Fill in the Blanks

Answer each question by completing the statement in the space provided.

1. Advanced _____ is one of the strongest risk factors associated with osteoarthritis.

2. Acetaminophen _____ is the most common cause of acute liver failure in the United States.

3. Aspirin can increase _____ risk, and prescribers should consider this danger.

4. Naturally occurring and exogenous steroids reduce _____ by binding to steroid receptors.

5. Most consider _____ the prototypical opioid pain medication.

6. An acceptable intake of vitamin D and calcium are critical co-therapies for _____.

7. Drug therapies for _____ include colchicine, NSAIDs, and corticosteroids.

8. Prescribers can use skeletal muscle relaxants for _____ injuries.

9. _____ capsules and tablets vary enough to cause differences in efficacy and side effects if changing between dosage forms.

10. Surgeons will use neuromuscular blocking agents with _____ for surgery to relax skeletal muscles to induce _____.

Short Answer

Write a short response to each question in the space provided.

1. Explain how the enzyme cyclooxygenase affects the body. What is the difference between a cyclooxygenase (COX)-1 inhibitor and a COX-2 inhibitor?

_____

_____

_____

_____

_____

_____

2. What medication can cause Reye's syndrome? When may this condition develop? What symptoms or reactions may develop with this condition?

_____

_____

3. What three properties do aspirin and NSAIDs have?

A. _____

B. _____

C. _____

4. What three problems can be caused by the overuse of NSAIDs?

A. _____

B. _____

C. _____

5. List two drugs that can be used to reverse the opioid agonist effects.

A. _____

B. _____

Matching

Match the following trade and generic drug names.

_____ 1. Motrin

_____ 2. Dilaudid

_____ 3. Anectine

_____ 4. Naprosyn

_____ 5. Boniva

_____ 6. Uloric

_____ 7. Lioresal

_____ 8. Soma

_____ 9. Lodine

_____ 10. Robaxin

A. febuxostat
B. etodolac
C. ibuprofen
D. naproxen
E. hydromorphone
F. ibandronate
G. methocarbamol
H. baclofen
I. succinylcholine
J. carisoprodol

Match the drugs with their classifications.

_____ 11. Colcrys
(colchicine)

_____ 12. Mobic
(meloxicam)

_____ 13. Celebrex
(celecoxib)

_____ 14. Duragesic
(fentanyl)

_____ 15. Evista (raloxifene)

_____ 16. Flexeril
(cyclobenzaprine)

_____ 17. Foxamax
(alendronate)

_____ 18. Zemuron
(rocuronium)

_____ 19. Miacalcin
(calcitonin
salmon)

_____ 20. Benuryl
(probencid)

_____ 21 Zyloprim
(allopurinol)

_____ 22. Prolia
(denosumab)

_____ 23. Forteo
(teriparatide)

A. Skeletal muscle
relaxant
B. Calcitonin hormone
analogue
C. Monoclonal
antibody
D. NSAID
E. Opioid analgesic
F. Bisphosphonate
G. Antigout agent
H. Uricosuric agent
I. COX-2 inhibitor
J. Parathyroid
hormone analogue
K. Neuromuscular
blocker
L. Xanthine oxidase
inhibitor
M. Selective estrogen
receptor modulator

Research Activities

Follow the instructions given in each exercise and provide a response.

1. Access the website *https://www.knowyourdose.org/common-medicines/*.

   A. Approximately how many over-the-counter and prescription products are available with the ingredient acetaminophen?

   B. List 5 examples of over-the-counter products that contain acetaminophen.

C. List five examples of prescription products that contain acetaminophen.

D. Why would it be important for the pharmacy to ensure patients know about additional products containing acetaminophen?

2. Access the website *http://pubs.niaaa.nih.gov/publications/Medicine/medicine.htm*.

   A. List the medications used for the musculoskeletal system that interact with alcohol.

   B. For each of the medications listed, what is the possible reaction when taken with alcohol?

REFLECT CRITICALLY

Critical Thinking

Reply to each question based on what you have learned in the chapter.

1. TV advertisements sometimes can be deceiving. Picture this: A person is rowing a boat across a lake, and their arms become sore. They reach the dock where their friend is waiting for them. The rower complains about their arms, and the friend recommends Tylenol for their sore muscles. What is wrong with this picture?

2. Osteoporosis occurs most commonly in postmenopausal women. What change occurred to help cause this? What can women do to help prevent this?

283

Lab Scenarios

Therapeutic Agents for the Skeletal System

Objective: To review with the pharmacy technician terms associated with the musculoskeletal system and review the brand and generic names, indications, dosage forms, routes of administration, and recommended daily dosage of medications used to treat disorders of the musculoskeletal system

---

DID YOU KNOW?

■ 54.4 million adults and almost 300,000 children in the United States have been diagnosed with some form of arthritis, rheumatoid arthritis, gout, lupus, or fibromyalgia.

■ 5.1% of men and 24.5% of women age 65 and over have osteoporosis of the femur, neck, or lumbar spine.

References:

https://www.rheumatology.org/Learning-Center/Statistics

https://www.cdc.gov/nchs/fastats/osteoporosis.htm

https://www.arthritis.org/getmedia/e1256607-fa87-4593-aa8a-8db4f291072a/2019-abtn-final-march-2019.pdf

Lab Activity #19.1: Define the following terms associated with the musculoskeletal system.

Equipment needed:
■ Medical dictionary
■ Pencil/pen

Time needed to complete this activity: 30 minutes

1. Amyotrophic lateral sclerosis (ALS) _____

2. Cerebral palsy _____

3. Hyperuricemia _____

4. Multiple sclerosis _____

5. Muscle strain _____

6. Myoglobin _____

7. Myositis _____

8. Osteoblasts _____

9. Osteoclasts _____

10. Osteopenia _____

11. Paget's disease _____

12. Paralysis _____

13. Rhabdomyolysis _____

14. Rheumatoid arthritis _____

15. Spasticity _____

16. Systemic lupus erythematosus _____

17. Trigeminal neuralgia _____

Lab Activity #19.2: Using a drug reference book, identify the brand name, drug classification, indications, dosage forms, routes of administration, and recommended daily dosage of the *most common* medications used to treat conditions affecting the musculoskeletal system.

Equipment needed:
■ *Drug Facts & Comparisons* or *Physicians' Desk Reference*
■ Pencil/pen

Time needed to complete this activity: 60 minutes

Generic Name	Brand Name	Classification	Indication(s)	Dose Form(s)	Route(s)	Recommended Daily Dosage	Auxiliary Label(s)
Acetaminophen							
Alendronate sodium							
Allopurinol							
Aspirin							
Baclofen							
Carisoprodol							
Celecoxib							
Cyclobenzaprine HCl							
Diclofenac Sodium							
Hydrocodone/APAP							
Ibuprofen							
Meloxicam							
Methocarbamol							
Morphine sulfate							
Naproxen							
Oxycodone							
Tizanidine							
Tramadol							

Chapter **19** **Therapeutic Agents for the Musculoskeletal System**

Lab Activity #19.3: Using a drug reference book, identify the generic name, storage requirements, and expiration date (at room temperature) for neuromuscular blocking agents.

Equipment needed:
- *Handbook on Injectable Drugs*
- Pencil/pen

Time needed to complete this activity: 30 minutes

Brand Name	Generic Name	Storage Requirements	Expiration Date
Anectine			
Nimbex			
Norcuron			
Zemuron			
Tracrium			
Pavulon			

Using Therapeutic Agents for the Musculoskeletal System

Objective: To review with the pharmacy technician prescription orders, dosage calculations, customer service, laws and regulations, and code of ethics

Lab Activity #19.4: Answer the questions based on the prescription orders for each question.

Equipment needed:
- *Drug Facts and Comparisons* or *Physicians' Desk Reference*
- Pencil/pen
- Calculator

Time needed to complete this activity: 30 minutes

The following are approved DAW codes:

DAW 0: no product selection indicated
DAW 1: substitution not allowed by provider
DAW 2: substitution allowed: patient requested product dispensed
DAW 3: substitution allowed: pharmacist selected product dispensed
DAW 4: substitution allowed: generic drug not in stock
DAW 5: substitution allowed: brand drug dispensed as generic
DAW 6: override
DAW 7: substitution not allowed: brand drug mandated by law
DAW 8: substitution allowed: generic drug not available in marketplace
DAW 9: other

1. Rx 1:
Mobic 7.5 mg #30
i tab po qd
Ref: 0

A. How much will be dispensed?

_____

B. How many days will the medication last?

_____

C. How many refills are permitted on the prescription?

_____

D. What DAW code will be used?

_____

E. Write directions as they would appear on the medication label.

_____

_____

F. What auxiliary label(s) should be affixed to the medication label?

_____

_____

_____

2. Rx 2:
   Zanaflex 4 mg #21
   i tab po q8h
   Ref: 0

   A. How much will be dispensed?

   _____

   B. How many days will the medication last?

   _____

   C. How many refills are permitted on the prescription?

   _____

   D. What DAW code will be used?

   _____

   E. Write directions as they would appear on the medication label.

   _____

   _____

   F. What auxiliary label(s) should be affixed to the medication label?

   _____

   _____

   _____

3. Rx 3:
   Actonel 35 mg #4
   i tab po weekly
   Ref: 2

   A. How much will be dispensed?

   _____

   B. How many days will the medication last?

   _____

   C. How many refills are permitted on the prescription?

   _____

   D. What DAW code will be used?

   _____

   E. Write directions as they would appear on the medication label.

   _____

   _____

   F. What auxiliary label(s) should be affixed to the medication label?

   _____

   _____

4. Rx 4:
   Skelaxin 800 mg #42
   i tab po q8h
   Ref: 0
   Brand name medically necessary

   A. How much will be dispensed?

   _____

   B. How many days will the medication last?

   _____

   C. How many refills are permitted on the prescription?

   _____

D. What DAW code will be used?

_____

E. Write directions as they would appear on the medication label.

_____

_____

F. What auxiliary label(s) should be affixed to the medication label?

_____

_____

_____

5. Rx 5:
   Flexeril 10 mg
   i tab po tid ×2 weeks
   Ref: 0

A. How much will be dispensed?

_____

B. How many days will the medication last?

_____

C. How many refills are permitted on the prescription?

_____

D. What DAW code will be used?

_____

E. Write directions as they would appear on the medication label.

_____

_____

F. What auxiliary label(s) should be affixed to the medication label?

_____

_____

_____

6. Rx 6:
   Soma 350 mg
   i tab po tid and hs ×1 week
   Ref: 0

A. How much will be dispensed?

_____

B. How many days will the medication last?

_____

C. How many refills are permitted on the prescription?

_____

D. What DAW code will be used?

_____

E. Write directions as they would appear on the medication label.

_____

_____

F. What auxiliary label(s) should be affixed to the medication label?

_____

_____

_____

7. Rx 7:
   Robaxin 500 mg #56
   ii tab po qid
   Ref: 0

A. How much will be dispensed?

_____

B. How many days will the medication last?

_____

C. How many refills are permitted on the prescription?

_____

D. What DAW code will be used?

_____

E. Write directions as they would appear on the medication label.

_____

_____

F. What auxiliary label(s) should be affixed to the medication label?

_____

_____

_____

8. Rx 8:
Motrin 600 mg #15
i tab po tid
Ref: 0
Patient requested brand

A. How much will be dispensed?

_____

B. How many days will the medication last?

_____

C. How many refills are permitted on the prescription?

_____

D. What DAW code will be used?

_____

E. Write directions as they would appear on the medication label.

_____

_____

F. What auxiliary label(s) should be affixed to the medication label?

_____

_____

_____

9. Rx 9:
Naprosyn 500 mg #90
i tab po tid
Ref × 5

A. How much will be dispensed?

_____

B. How many days will the medication last?

_____

C. How many refills are permitted on the prescription?

_____

D. What DAW code will be used?

_____

E. Write directions as they would appear on the medication label.

_____

_____

F. What auxiliary label(s) should be affixed to the medication label?

_____

_____

_____

10. Rx 10:
Fosamax #4
i tab po weekly
Ref × 6

A. How much will be dispensed?

_____

B. How many days will the medication last?

_____

C. How many refills are permitted on the prescription?

_____

D. What DAW code will be used?

_____

E. Write directions as they would appear on the medication label.

_____

_____

F. What auxiliary label(s) should be affixed to the medication label?

_____

_____

_____

Lab Activity #19.5: Read each scenario. Role-play each scenario with a partner and/or your instructor, incorporating pharmacy laws and regulations, pharmacy protocols, and your role to help alert pharmacists to information that would help them perform their duties. Also consider the pharmacy technician code of ethics and good customer service practices when responding to and interacting with patients. When in doubt, always refer to the pharmacist.

Equipment needed:
- Knowledge of pharmacy laws and regulations and pharmacy protocols
- Pencil/pen

Time needed to complete this activity: 45 minutes

1. Scenario #1
   You are a pharmacy technician working at the local grocery store pharmacy when a patient walks up to the pharmacy counter with a 12-pack of beer and informs you they are there to pick up their prescription. When ringing up the patient, you notice that the medication they are picking up is a prescription for cyclobenzaprine.

2. Scenario #2
   You are a pharmacy technician at the local community pharmacy when a patient approaches your pharmacy counter requesting a refill for acetaminophen/codeine. When looking at the prescription in your pharmacy database, you notice that they have one refill remaining, but the prescription was filled two days earlier for a 10-day supply.

3. Scenario #3
   You are a pharmacy technician at the local community pharmacy when a patient walks up to the pharmacy counter to pick up their prescription. After pulling the prescription from the prescription pick-up bin you notice the medication is for carisoprodol. Pharmacy protocol is to verify controlled substance pick-up with a valid photo ID. When you ask for the patient's ID, they inform you they do not have their ID with them.

20 Therapeutic Agents for the Cardiovascular System

ASHP ACCREDITATION STANDARDS FOR PHARMACY TECHNICIAN EDUCATION AND TRAINING PROGRAMS

Standard 2.5: Demonstrate basic knowledge of anatomy, physiology and pharmacology, and medical terminology relevant to the pharmacy technician's role.
Standard 2.6: Perform mathematical calculations essential to the duties of pharmacy technicians in a variety of settings.
Standard 3.1: Assist pharmacists in collecting, organizing, and recording demographic and clinical information for the Pharmacists; Patient Care Process.
Standard 3.2: Receive, process, and prepare prescriptions/medication orders for completeness, accuracy, and authenticity to ensure safety.
Standard 5.1: Describe and apply state and federal laws pertaining to processing, handling, and dispensing of medications including controlled substances.

REINFORCE KEY CONCEPTS

Terms and Definitions

Select the correct term from the following list and write the corresponding letter in the blank next to the statement.

A. Aorta
B. Artery
C. Atrium
D. Capillary
E. Cardiac muscle
F. Coronary artery
G. Endocardium
H. Epicardium
I. Lumen
J. Myocardium
K. Pericardium
L. Pulmonary artery
M. Vein
N. Vena cava
O. Ventricle

_____ 1. The entry chamber on both sides of the heart

_____ 2. The outer layer of the heart wall; the inner layer of the pericardium

_____ 3. The middle muscular layer of the heart wall; it consists of cardiac muscle tissue

_____ 4. One of the two large veins that carry deoxygenated blood from the upper (superior vena cava) and lower (inferior vena cava) parts of the body to the right atrium of the heart

_____ 5. A vessel that carries oxygenated blood from the heart to the tissues of the body

_____ 6. A channel within a tube (e.g., a blood vessel)

_____ 7. An tiny vessel that connects the ends of the smallest arteries (arterioles) to the smallest veins (venules), where exchange of nutrients, waste products, oxygen (O_2), and carbon dioxide (CO_2) occurs

_____ 8. One of the two lower chambers of the heart

_____ 9. The thin membrane that lines the interior of the heart; the inner layer of the heart wall

_____ 10. A fluid-filled membrane that surrounds the heart; also called the pericardial sac

_____ 11. The great arterial trunk that carries blood from the heart to be distributed to tissues of the body

_____ 12. One of two vessels formed as terminal branches of the pulmonary trunk; conveys unaerated blood to the lungs

_____ 13. Either of two arteries that arise from the aorta (one from the left side and one from the right side) and supply the tissues of the heart itself

_____ 14. A vessel that carries deoxygenated blood to or toward the heart

_____ 15. A type of muscle tissue found only in the heart

Select the correct term from the following list and write the corresponding letter in the blank next to the statement.

A. Aldosterone
B. Angiotensin II
C. Enzyme
D. High-density lipoprotein (HDL)
E. Low-density lipoprotein (LDL)
F. Low-density lipoprotein receptor (LDLR)
G. Renin
H. Thrombin
I. Triglyceride

_____ 16. A lipid (fat) and protein combined molecule. It is associated with an increased probability of developing atherosclerosis

_____ 17. A steroid hormone secreted by the adrenal cortex that regulates the salt and water balance in the body

_____ 18. A blood coagulation enzyme from prothrombin; reacts with fibrinogen and converts it to fibrin, which is essential in the formation of blood clots; levels are tested by performing a prothrombin time or partial thromboplastin time blood test

_____ 19. A blood-plasma lipoprotein composed of a high proportion of protein with little triglyceride and cholesterol and associated with a decreased probability of developing atherosclerosis

_____ 20. A protein released by the kidney in response to low sodium levels or blood volume

_____ 21. A protein that accelerates a reaction by reducing the amount of energy required to initiate the reaction

_____ 22. The dominant form of body-stored fat consisting of three fatty acid molecules and a molecule of the alcohol glycerol

_____ 23. A peptide hormone that causes vasoconstriction and a subsequent increase in blood pressure

_____ 24. A protein found mainly on liver cells that binds to and removes blood LDL

Select the correct term from the following list and write the corresponding letter in the blank next to the statement.

A. Blood pressure
B. Cardiac output (CO)
C. Diastole
D. Dysrhythmias
E. Essential hypertension
F. Heart failure (HF)
G. Hypertension
H. Hypotension
I. Orthostatic hypotension
J. Peripheral resistance
K. Secondary hypertension
L. Systole
M. Tachycardia
N. Stent
O. Syndrome
P. Thrombosis
Q. Vasoconstriction
R. Vasodilation

_____ 25. A heart that cannot keep up with demand; failure of the heart to pump blood with normal efficiency

_____ 26. The period when the heart is contracting, specifically when the left ventricle of the heart contracts

_____ 27. The most common form of hypertension; it occurs in the absence of any evident cause

_____ 28. Hypertension that results from an underlying identifiable cause

_____ 29. A rapid heart rate, usually defined as greater than 100 beats per minute

_____ 30. The formation or presence of a blood clot in a blood vessel

_____ 31. Blood vessel widening resulting from muscular vessel wall relaxation

_____ 32. Vascular resistance to the flow of blood in peripheral arterial vessels

_____ 33. A temporary, often rapid lowering of blood pressure, usually related to standing up suddenly

_____ 34. The period when the heart is in a state of relaxation and dilation

_____ 35. A tube inserted into a vessel or passageway to keep it open

_____ 36. Low blood pressure

_____ 37. Abnormal or irregular heart rhythms

_____ 38. The amount of blood, in liters, the heart pumps through the circulatory system in a minute

292

_____ 39. Blood vessel narrowing resulting from contraction of the vessel muscular walls

_____ 40. A set of conditions that occur together

_____ 41. High blood pressure

_____ 42. The pressure of the blood within the arteries

Select the correct term from the following list and write the corresponding letter in the blank next to the statement.

A. Aneurysm
B. Angina
C. Arteriosclerosis
D. Atherosclerosis
E. Coagulation
F. Embolus
G. Heterozygous familial hypercholesterolemia (HeFH)
H. Hyperlipidemia
I. Myocardial infarction (MI)
J. Stroke
K. Transient ischemic attack (TIA)

_____ 43. Chest pain due to an inadequate supply of oxygen to the heart muscle

_____ 44. A neurological event in which the signs and symptoms of a stroke appear but resolve within a short time

_____ 45. A balloon-like bulge or dilation of an artery due to weakening of the arterial wall

_____ 46. Myocardial tissue death due to sudden deprivation of oxygenated blood flow, often a result of a blood clot plugging a coronary artery; also known as a heart attack

_____ 47. A condition characterized by thickening, loss of elasticity (hardening), and calcification of the arterial walls

_____ 48. A clump of material, often a blood clot, that travels from one part of the body to another and obstructs a blood vessel; can consist of any material, including bacteria or air

_____ 49. A condition marked by an increase in bloodstream cholesterol that can lead to atherosclerosis, or artery hardening

_____ 50. The sudden death of brain cells due to oxygen deprivation a blockage (ischemic) or rupture (hemorrhagic) of an artery to the brain impairs blood flow

_____ 51. The process of progressive thickening and hardening of the walls of medium-sized and large arteries because of fat deposits on their inner lining, a specific arteriosclerosis

_____ 52. A genetic disorder based on a gene that encodes LDLR; very high LDL levels within the blood characterize this disorder

_____ 53. Solidification or change from a fluid state to a solid state, as in the formation of a blood clot

Select the correct term from the following list and write the corresponding letter in the blank next to the statement.

A. Anticoagulant
B. Antihyperlipidemics
C. Fibrates
D. Nicotinic acid
E. Nitrates
F. PCSK9
G. Statin
H. Thrombolytic

_____ 54. A class of drugs used to treat heart conditions, such as angina

_____ 55. A diverse group of pharmaceuticals used in the treatment of hyperlipidemia or excess lipids in the blood

_____ 56. A member of the vitamin B complex; also known as niacin

_____ 57. A medication used to break up a thrombus or blood clot

_____ 58. An agent used to prevent the formation of blood clots

_____ 59. An informal term for HMG-CoA reductase inhibitors referring to the last six letters in the name of each medication name in the class used for the treatment of hyperlipidemia, primarily to lower LDL cholesterol

_____ 60. An enzyme that binds to and breaks down LDLR

_____ 61. An antihyperlipidemic drug class that primarily lowers triglycerides

293

True or False

Write T or F next to each statement.

_____ 1. A normal heart beats 160 to 200 times per minute.

_____ 2. The right atrium receives fully oxygenated blood from the lungs via the pulmonary veins.

_____ 3. The cardiac conduction system provides the electrical charge that makes the heart pump.

_____ 4. Most of the body's blood supply is cycled through the heart in 5 minutes.

_____ 5. The adrenal glands release norepinephrine and epinephrine to increase heart rate.

_____ 6. Blood pressure can rise in a dehydrated patient, or blood pressure can fall with excess body fluid.

_____ 7. High blood pressure is also known as the "silent killer" because it has no obvious signs.

_____ 8. Diet and exercise can lower lipid content.

_____ 9. Non-drug therapy for those with chronic hypotension may include medication to help decrease blood pressure.

_____ 10. Sublingual nitroglycerin tablets must be kept in a dry area and in the original light-protected glass container.

System Identifier

Identify each component in the heart system and enter the term next to the corresponding number.

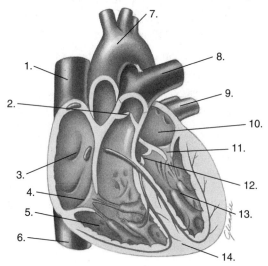

From Gerdin J: *Health careers today,* ed 5, St Louis, 2012, Mosby.

1. _____

2. _____

3. _____

4. _____

5. _____

6. _____

7. _____

8. _____

9. _____

10. _____

11. _____

12. _____

13. _____

14. _____

Multiple Choice

Complete each question by circling the best answer.

1. Tenormin, Inderal, and Lopressor are all classified as:
   A. Angiotensin-converting enzyme (ACE) inhibitors
   B. Beta-blockers
   C. Calcium channel blockers
   D. Diuretics

2. Which of the following medications may cause orthostatic hypotension as a side effect?
   A. Norvasc (amlodipine)
   B. Aldomet (methyldopa)
   C. Diovan (valsartan)
   D. Vasotec (enalapril)

3. The cardiac glycoside _____ can be used to treat chronic heart failure and arrhythmias.
   A. Lasix (furosemide)
   B. Lanoxin (digoxin)
   C. Lopressor (metoprolol)
   D. Lotensin (benazepril)

4. Which of the following diuretics will most likely not cause a loss of potassium?
   A. Zaroxolyn (metolazone)
   B. Lasix (furosemide)
   C. Bumex (bumetanide)
   D. Aldactone (spironolactone)

5. Torsemide, acetazolamide, and triamterene are classified as:
   A. Thrombolytics
   B. Diuretics
   C. Nitrates
   D. Antiplatelet agents

6. Gemfibrozil, simvastatin, and ezetimibe are classified as:
   A. Antihypertensives
   B. Antiarrhythmics
   C. Anticoagulants
   D. Antihyperlipidemics

7. A dry, hacking cough that does not resolve over time is a side effect of:
   A. Calcium channel blockers
   B. ARBs
   C. ACE inhibitors
   D. Beta-blockers

8. An antidote for an overdose of Lanoxin (digoxin) is:
   A. diuretics
   B. Digibind
   C. digitalis
   D. Digitonin

9. In addition to treating hypertension, _____ can be used for migraine prophylaxis and treatment of some tremors.
   A. Norvasc (amlodipine)
   B. ProAmatine (midodrine)
   C. Inderal (propranolol)
   D. Questran (cholestyramine)

10. Nitrostat tablets should be administered by which route?
    A. PO
    B. SL
    C. SubQ
    D. PR

Fill in the Blanks

Answer each question by completing the statement in the space provided.

1. The cardiac cycle is an event series that occurs in one complete _____ and has two sequences, systole and diastole.

2. The parasympathetic nervous system _____ the heart, while the sympathetic nervous system _____ heart rate.

3. Hormones can also _____ blood pressure.

4. Body fluid volume can change based on _____ intake.

5. When peripheral resistance increases, _____ increases.

6. The first-line therapy for most hypertensive patients includes a _____ diuretic.

7. _____ performs many vital functions, including steroid hormone and cell membrane synthesis.

8. Warfarin interferes with _____ -dependent coagulation factor synthesis (II, VII, IX, and X) in the liver.

9. TIAs are treated by improving arterial brain blood flow so that a _____ can be avoided.

10. One of the most common drug treatments for heart failure is _____.

Matching

Match the classes of drugs or drugs with their indication.

_____ 1. Antihyperlipidemics

_____ 2. Arrhythmic agents

_____ 3. Antiplatelet agents

_____ 4. Antihypertensives

_____ 5. Anticoagulants

A. quinidine, procainamide, amiodarone
B. heparin, warfarin
C. ACE inhibitors, ARBs, beta-blockers, calcium channel blockers, diuretics
D. Bile acid sequestrants, HMG-CoA reductase inhibitors, fibrates, PCSK9 inhibitors
E. clopidogrel, aspirin

Match the drug with the generic name.

_____ 6. Praluent

_____ 7. Lovaza

_____ 8. Lovenox

_____ 9. Xarelto

_____ 10. Pradaxa

_____ 11. Bumex

_____ 12. Altace

_____ 13. Minipress

_____ 14. Tricor

_____ 15. Niaspan ER

A. rivaroxaban
B. prazosin
C. alirocumab
D. niacin
E. enoxaparin
F. bumetanide
G. fenofibrate
H. omega-3 fatty acids
I. ramipril
J. dabigatran

Drug Names

Give the generic names for the following drugs.

1. Mevacor _____

2. Norpace _____

3. Lanoxin _____

4. Dyrenium _____

5. Lotensin _____

6. Hytrin _____

7. Quinidex _____

8. Zestril _____

9. Cozaar _____

10. Cardizem _____

Short Answer

Reply to each question in the space provided.

1. What are four common classifications of agents used to treat heart conditions?

_____

_____

2. How do angiotensin receptor blockers (ARBs) work? List the common suffix for ARBs.

_____

_____

_____

3. How do ACE inhibitors help reduce blood pressure? List the common suffix for ACE inhibitors.

_____

_____

_____

_____

4. How do calcium channel blockers (CCBs) help reduce blood pressure?

_____

_____

_____

5. How do beta-blockers help reduce blood pressure? List the common suffix for beta blockers.

_____

_____

_____

6. How to HMG-CoA reductase inhibitors help reduce HDL cholesterol levels? List the common suffix for HMG-CoA reductase inhibitors.

_____

_____

_____

7. Which antihyperlipidemic drug is also used to treat type 2 diabetes?

_____

8. Food containing vitamin K may counteract the effectiveness of the drug warfarin. List foods that contain vitamin K.

_____

_____

_____

Research Activities

Follow the instructions given in each exercise and provide a response.

1. Access the website *http://www.americanheart.org/*. What is tPA? How does this drug help stroke victims recover? What are the symptoms of a stroke? What acronym is used to help remember these symptoms?

2. Access the website *http://www.americanheart.org/*. What are the symptoms of a heart attack? List five ways to help reduce the risk of a heart attack.

3. Access the website *https://jamanetwork.com/journals/jama/fullarticle/1791497*. From the article, what are the recommendations for the management of hypertension? What evidence led researchers to these recommendations?

REFLECT CRITICALLY

Critical Thinking

Reply to each question based on what you have learned in the chapter.

1. "An aspirin a day keeps a heart attack away." What are some everyday activities people can do to "keep a heart attack away?"

2. You have just finished your lunch, which consisted of a double cheeseburger, extra-large fries, and a cola. Name all the body systems that will be affected by that "yummy" meal.

3. "I feel like I'm having a heart attack," someone says to you. How do you know for sure? What symptoms do you look for?

297

RELATE TO PRACTICE

Lab Scenarios
Therapeutic Agents for the Cardiovascular System

Objective: To review with the pharmacy technician terms associated with the cardiovascular system and review the brand and generic names, indications, dosage forms, routes of administration, and recommended daily dosage of medications used to treat disorders of the cardiovascular system

---

DID YOU KNOW?

- 30.3 million (12.1%) of adults have some form of heart disease.
- Heart disease is the leading cause of death for both men and women.
- Approximately 108 million adults have hypertension.
- Stroke is the fifth leading cause of death.
- 7.8 million adults have suffered from a stroke.
- 11.8% of adults age 20 years and older suffer from high serum cholesterol ($\geq$240 mg/dL)

References:

https://www.cdc.gov/nchs/fastats/heart-disease.htm
https://www.cdc.gov/bloodpressure/facts.htm#:~:text=Rates%20of%20High%20Blood%20Pressure%20Control%20Vary%20by%20Sex%20and%20Race&text=A%20greater%20percent%20of%20men,pressure%20than%20women%20(43%25).&text=High%20blood%20pressure%20is%20more,or%20Hispanic%20adults%20(36%25).
https://www.cdc.gov/nchs/fastats/stroke.htm
https://www.cdc.gov/nchs/fastats/cholesterol.htm

Lab Activity #20.1: Define the following terms associated with the cardiovascular system.

Equipment needed:
- Medical dictionary
- Pencil/pen

Time needed to complete this activity: 45 minutes

1. Aneurysm _____

2. Anoxia _____

3. Aorta _____

4. Atrial fibrillation _____

5. Atrial flutter _____

6. Bradycardia _____

7. Cardiomyopathy _____

8. Deep vein thrombosis (DVT) _____

9. Embolic stroke _____

10. Endocarditis _____

11. Hemorrhagic stroke _____

12. Hyperkalemia _____

13. Hypernatremia _____

14. Hypokalemia _____

15. Hyponatremia _____

16. Hypoxia _____

17. Infarction _____

18. Ischemia _____

19. Mitral valve prolapse _____

20. Mitral valve stenosis _____

21. Peripheral vascular disease _____

22. Phlebitis _____

23. Plaque _____

24. Prehypertension _____

25. Raynaud's disease _____

26. Rheumatic heart disease _____

27. Stable angina _____

28. Supraventricular tachycardia _____

29. Thrombophlebitis _____

30. Thrombotic stroke _____

31. Thrombus _____

32. Unstable angina _____

33. Variant _____

34. Ventricular fibrillation _____

35. Ventricular tachycardia _____

298

Lab Activity #20.2: Using a drug reference book, identify the brand name, drug classification, indications, dosage forms, routes of administration, and recommended daily dosage of the *most common* medications used to treat conditions affecting the cardiovascular system.

Equipment needed:
- *Drug Facts & Comparisons* or *Physicians' Desk Reference*
- Pencil/pen

Time needed to complete the exercise: 60 minutes

Generic Name	Brand Name	Classification	Indication(s)	Dosage Form(s)	Route(s)	Daily Recommended Dosage	Auxiliary Label(s)
Amiodarone HCl							
Amlodipine besylate							
Aspirin							
Atenolol							
Atorvastatin							
Benazepril HCl							
Carvedilol							
Clonidine							
Clopidogrel bisulfate							

Continued

Generic Name	Brand Name	Classification	Indication(s)	Dosage Form(s)	Route(s)	Daily Recommended Dosage	Auxiliary Label(s)
Dabigatran etexilate Mesylate							
Digoxin							
Diltiazem HCl							
Doxazosin mesylate							
Enalapril maleate							
Ezetimibe							
Fenofibrate							
Furosemide							
Gemfibrozil							
Hydralazine HCl							
Isosorbide							

Generic Name	Brand Name	Classification	Indication(s)	Dosage Form(s)	Route(s)	Daily Recommended Dosage	Auxiliary Label(s)
Lisinopril							
Losartan potassium							
Lovastatin							
Metoprolol							
Nebivolol HCl							
Nifedipine							
Nitroglycerin							
Olmesartan medoxomil							
Omega-3-acid ethyl esters							
Pravastatin sodium							

Continued

Generic Name	Brand Name	Classification	Indication(s)	Dosage Form(s)	Route(s)	Daily Recommended Dosage	Auxiliary Label(s)
Propranolol HCl							
Quinapril							
Ramipril							
Rivaroxaban							
Rosuvastatin calcium							
Simvastatin							
Terazosin							
Valsartan							
Valsartan/HCTZ							
Verapamil HCl							
Warfarin							

Using Therapeutic Agents for the Cardiovascular System

Objective: To review with the pharmacy technician contra-indications, prescription/medication orders, and dosage calculations

Lab Activity #20.3: Using information learned and resources available, identify over-the-counter (OTC) products that can affect blood pressure and products available for those with hypertension.

Equipment needed:
- *Drug Facts & Comparisons* or *Pocket Guide for Nonprescription Product Therapeutics*
- Pencil/pen

Time needed to complete the exercise: 45 minutes

1. Which OTC products can affect blood pressure?

2. As a pharmacy technician, how can you help those with hypertension ensure they do not take OTC products that can affect blood pressure?

3. List available decongestant OTC products available specifically for those with hypertension.

Lab Activity #20.4: Answer the questions based on the prescription orders for each question.

Equipment needed:
- Calculator
- *Drug Facts and Comparisons* or *Physicians' Desk Reference*
- Pencil/pen

Time needed to complete this activity: 30 minutes

The following are approved DAW codes:

DAW 0: no product selection indicated
DAW 1: substitution not allowed by provider
DAW 2: substitution allowed: patient requested product dispensed
DAW 3: substitution allowed: pharmacist selected product dispensed
DAW 4: substitution allowed: generic drug not in stock
DAW 5: substitution allowed: brand drug dispensed as generic

DAW 6: override
DAW 7: substitution not allowed: brand drug mandated by law
DAW 8: substitution allowed: generic drug not available in marketplace
DAW 9: other

1. Rx 1:
Crestor 20 mg #30
i tab po qd
Ref ×5

A. How much will be dispensed?

_____

B. How many days will the medication last?

_____

C. How many refills are permitted on the prescription?

_____

D. What DAW code will be used?

_____

E. Write directions as they would appear on the medication label.

_____

_____

F. What auxiliary label(s) should be affixed to the medication label?

_____

_____

_____

2. Rx 2:
Mevacor 40 mg #30
i tab po qpm
Ref ×3

A. How much will be dispensed?

_____

B. How many days will the medication last?

_____

303

C. How many refills are permitted on the prescription?

_____

D. What DAW code will be used?

_____

E. Write directions as they would appear on the medication label.

_____

_____

F. What auxiliary label(s) should be affixed to the medication label?

_____

_____

_____

3. Rx 3:
   Coreg 25 mg #60
   i tab po bid
   Ref ×2

A. How much will be dispensed?

_____

B. How many days will the medication last?

_____

C. How many refills are permitted on the prescription?

_____

D. What DAW code will be used?

_____

E. Write directions as they would appear on the medication label.

_____

_____

F. What auxiliary label(s) should be affixed to the medication label?

_____

_____

_____

4. Rx 4:
   Zocor 40 mg #31
   i tab po qpm
   Ref ×5
   Brand Name Medically Necessary

A. How much will be dispensed?

_____

B. How many days will the medication last?

_____

C. How many refills are permitted on the prescription?

_____

D. What DAW code will be used?

_____

E. Write directions as they would appear on the medication label.

_____

_____

F. What auxiliary label(s) should be affixed to the medication label?

_____

_____

_____

5. Rx 5:
Tricor 145 mg #30
i tab po qd
Ref ×5
Patient is allergic to soy, which is an inactive ingredient in Tricor.

A. How much will be dispensed?

_____

B. How many days will the medication last?

_____

C. How many refills are permitted on the prescription?

_____

D. What DAW code will be used?

_____

E. Write directions as they would appear on the medication label.

_____

_____

F. What auxiliary label(s) should be affixed to the medication label?

_____

_____

_____

6. Rx 6:
Lopressor 100 mg #30
i tab po qd
Ref ×5
Patient has requested brand name only.

A. How much will be dispensed?

_____

B. How many days will the medication last?

_____

C. How many refills are permitted on the prescription?

_____

D. What DAW code will be used?

_____

E. Write directions as they would appear on the medication label.

_____

_____

F. What auxiliary label(s) should be affixed to the medication label?

_____

_____

_____

7. Rx 7:
Diovan 80 mg #31
i tab po daily
Ref ×3
Patient is on vacation and forgot his medicine at home.

A. How much will be dispensed?

_____

B. How many days will the medication last?

_____

C. How many refills are permitted on the prescription?

_____

D. What DAW code will be used?

_____

E. Write directions as they would appear on the medication label.

_____

_____

F. What auxiliary label(s) should be affixed to the medication label?

_____

_____

8. Rx 8:
   Zestril 2.5 mg #32
   i tab po qd
   Ref ×5

   A. How much will be dispensed?

   _____

   B. How many days will the medication last?

   _____

   C. How many refills are permitted on the prescription?

   _____

   D. What DAW code will be used?

   _____

   E. Write directions as they would appear on the medication label.

   _____

   F. What auxiliary label(s) should be affixed to the medication label?

   _____

   _____

9. Rx 9:
   Benicar HCT 20/12.5, #31
   i tab po daily
   Ref ×2

   A. How much will be dispensed?

   _____

   B. How many days will the medication last?

   _____

   C. How many refills are permitted on the prescription?

   _____

   D. What DAW code will be used?

   _____

E. Write directions as they would appear on the medication label.

   _____

   _____

F. What auxiliary label(s) should be affixed to the medication label?

   _____

   _____

   _____

10. Rx 10:
    Toprol XL 50 mg #31
    i tab po qd
    Ref ×2

    A. How much will be dispensed?

    _____

    B. How many days will the medication last?

    _____

    C. How many refills are permitted on the prescription?

    _____

    D. What DAW code will be used?

    _____

    E. Write directions as they would appear on the medication label.

    _____

    _____

    F. What auxiliary label(s) should be affixed to the medication label?

    _____

    _____

    _____

Lab Activity #20.5: Answer each question using the IV medication order provided.

Equipment needed:
■ Calculator
■ *Trissel's Handbook of Injectable Drugs*
■ Pencil/pen

Time needed to complete this activity: 30 minutes

Answer the questions based on the following medication order:

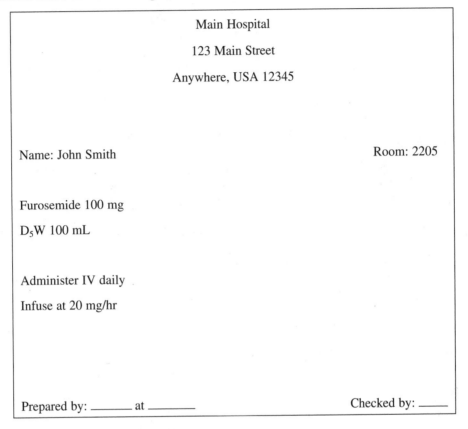

Main Hospital

123 Main Street

Anywhere, USA 12345

Name: John Smith   Room: 2205

Furosemide 100 mg

D_5W 100 mL

Administer IV daily

Infuse at 20 mg/hr

Prepared by: _____ at _____   Checked by: _____

1. You have the following in stock in your pharmacy. Which one will you use to make the IV bag? _____

NDC 70121-**1163**-1

**Furosemide
Injection, USP**

20 mg / 2 mL

(10 mg/mL)

FOR IV OR IM USE

2 mL SINGLE DOSE VIAL
        Rx only

WARNING: USE ONLY IF SOLUTION IS CLEAR AND COLORLESS. PROTECT FROM LIGHT. Store at 20° to 25°C (68° to 77°F); excursions permitted between 15° to 30°C (59° to 86°F) [see USP Controlled Room Temperature]. Directions for Use: See Package Insert. Mfg. Lic. No. G/28/1539
Manufactured by:
Amneal Pharmaceuticals Pvt. Ltd.,
Parenteral Unit Ahmedabad, India
Rev. 10-2016-00

Unvarnished Area for, Lot. & Exp.
(18 mm x 6.2 mm)

From NIH: US National Library of Medicine, *Daily Med,* https://dailymed.nlm.nih.gov/dailymed/index.cfm

Chapter **20** **Therapeutic Agents for the Cardiovascular System**

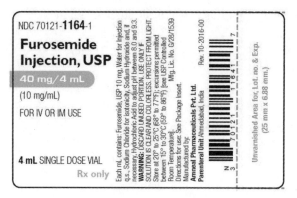

From NIH: US National Library of Medicine, *Daily Med,* https://dailymed.nlm.nih.gov/dailymed/index.cfm

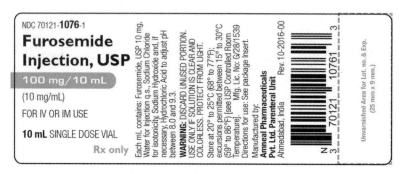

From NIH: US National Library of Medicine, *Daily Med,* https://dailymed.nlm.nih.gov/dailymed/index.cfm

2. How many milliliters of furosemide will you draw up to make the IV bag?

_____

3. How should this IV be stored after preparation?

_____

4. How long is this IV stable after preparing?

_____

5. Over how many hours will this IV bag be infused?

_____

21 Therapeutic Agents for the Respiratory System

REINFORCE KEY CONCEPTS

Terms and Definitions

Select the correct term from the following list and write the corresponding letter in the blank next to the statement.

A. Alveoli
B. Bronchi
C. Bronchioles
D. Cilia
E. Diaphragm

_____ 1. Small branches that divide from the bronchus in the lungs

_____ 2. Tiny air sacs in the lungs where oxygen and carbon dioxide exchange takes place

_____ 3. A dome-shaped, muscular partition separating the thorax from the abdomen that plays a major role in breathing

_____ 4. The major lung air passages that diverge from the windpipe

_____ 5. Short, microscopic, hairlike structures

Select the correct term from the following list and write the corresponding letter in the blank next to the statement.

A. Allergen
B. Aspiration
C. Dyspnea
D. Expiration
E. Influenza
F. Inspiration
G. Sputum

_____ 6. The act of breathing out; exhalation

_____ 7. Fluid (mucus) expectorated from the lungs and bronchial tissues

_____ 8. A substance that causes an allergic reaction

_____ 9. A respiratory tract infection caused by an influenza virus

_____ 10. To draw a foreign substance into the respiratory tract during inhalation

_____ 11. The act of breathing in; inhalation

_____ 12. Difficult or labored breathing

Select the correct term from the following list and write the corresponding letter in the blank next to the statement.

A. Anticholinergic
B. Antihistamine
C. Antitussive
D. Decongestant
E. Expectorant
F. Prophylactic

_____ 13. A drug that shrinks the swollen membranes in the nasal cavity, making it easier to breathe

_____ 14. A drug or other compound that inhibits the effects of histamine; often used to treat allergies

_____ 15. Treatment given before an event or exposure to prevent the condition or symptom

_____ 16. A drug that helps remove mucous secretions from the respiratory system; it loosens and thins sputum and bronchial secretions for ease of expectoration

309

_____ 17. An agent that inhibits the physiological action of acetylcholine

_____ 18. A drug that can decrease the central nervous system coughing reflex

True or False

Write T or F next to each statement.

_____ 1. Opioids can suppress the respiratory rate.

_____ 2. The lungs fill the entire space in the chest cavity.

_____ 3. The diaphragm separates the chest cavity from the abdominal area.

_____ 4. Breathing is a voluntary mechanism.

_____ 5. The respiratory rate of a child and an adult are the same.

_____ 6. The most common bacterial organism causing community-acquired pneumonia is *Mycobacterium tuberculosis.*

_____ 7. Older adults are at a high risk for pneumonia, especially after an injury.

_____ 8. Tuberculosis is a leading cause of morbidity and mortality worldwide.

_____ 9. With reduced smoking rates, death rates from lung cancer have increased in recent years.

_____ 10. Individuals who have high blood pressure should not take Sudafed regularly.

System Identifier

Identify each anatomical part in this system and enter the term next to the corresponding number.

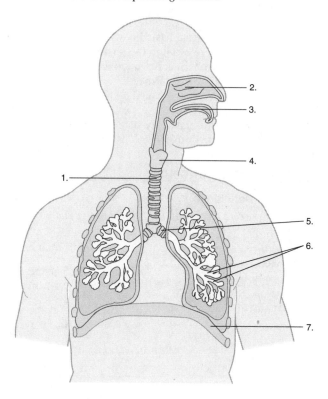

1. _____

2. _____

3. _____

4. _____

5. _____

6. _____

7. _____

Multiple Choice

Complete each question by circling the best answer.

1. The body's pH level must remain close to:
   A. 1.7
   B. 5.6
   C. 6.5
   D. 7.4

2. To loosen mucus so that it can be expelled through coughing, a patient can take a (an):
   A. Antitussive
   B. Expectorant
   C. Antihistamine
   D. Decongestant

3. The most frequent acute illness in the United States is:
   A. Pneumonia
   B. Influenza
   C. Common cold
   D. Tuberculosis

4. *Rhinorrhea* is the medical name for a (an):
   A. Allergy
   B. Cold
   C. Sore throat
   D. Runny nose

5. In life-threatening cases, injectable _____ can open the airways.
   A. fexofenadine
   B. acetylcysteine
   C. streptomycin
   D. epinephrine

6. For severe influenza, a prescriber may give _____ at early onset (usually within 48 hours) to help shorten the course or lessen illness severity.
   A. antibiotics
   B. antivirals
   C. decongestants
   D. methylxanthines

7. The short-acting beta-agonist _____ routinely work as a "rescue" inhaler.
   A. Qvar Redihaler (beclomethasone)
   B. Pulmicort Flexhaler (budesonide)
   C. Flovent HFA (fluticasone)
   D. Xopenex HFA (levalbuterol)

8. Emphysema can be caused by:
   A. Exposure to environmental hazards
   B. Smoking
   C. Genetic disposition
   D. All of the above

9. Which of the following decongestants can cause rebound congestion?
   A. Afrin (oxymetazoline)
   B. Xyzal (levocetirizine)
   C. Xolair (omalizumab)
   D. Beclovent (beclomethasone)

10. Which of the following is a prophylactic agent for asthma and a nasal preparation for seasonal rhinitis and congestion?
    A. fluticasone
    B. budesonide
    C. cromolyn sodium
    D. montelukast

Fill in the Blanks

Answer each question by completing the statement in the space provided.

1. Drinking plenty of _____ and getting enough _____ are important parts of nondrug treatment of the common cold.

2. Gargling with _____ _____ can help relieve a sore throat.

3. Many decongestants can worsen nasal congestion with _____ congestion if patients use them for more than three consecutive days.

4. An _____ is an abnormal response of the immune system to an unrecognized, typically harmless substance.

5. Postnasal drip comes from _____ accumulating in the back of the nose and throat.

6. Patients might use _____ with certain inhalers to allow patients to inhale, not exhale, into the device.

7. Metered dose inhalers (MDIs) move medication into the lungs with the _____ hydrofluoroalkane (HFA).

8. The three general _____ types include chronic bronchitis, emphysema, and asthma.

9. Immunocompromised patients also are at a higher risk of _____ development.

10. Chemotherapy is a _____ treatment modality for many types and stages of lung cancer.

Matching

Matching I

Match the following classes of drugs with their mechanisms of action.

_____ 1. Antitussives

_____ 2. Mucolytics

_____ 3. Decongestants

_____ 4. Corticosteroids

_____ 5. Anticholinergics

A. Help clear respiratory passages
B. Act as anti-inflammatory agents
C. Break up mucus in patients with COPD
D. Inhibit the action of acetylcholine
E. Suppress coughing

Match the disease states with their drug treatments.

_____ 6. Tuberculosis (TB)

_____ 7. Asthma prophylaxis

_____ 8. Common cold

_____ 9. COPD

_____ 10. Cough

A. Sudafed (pseudoephedrine)
B. Mucinex (guaifenesin)
C. isoniazid
D. Flovent HFA (fluticasone propionate)
E. Atrovent HFA (ipratropium bromide)

Match the brand name with the generic name.

_____ 11. Nasonex

_____ 12. Singulair

_____ 13. Flovent HFA

_____ 14. Theo-24

_____ 15. Ventolin HFA

_____ 16. Beconase AQ

_____ 17. Patanase

_____ 18. Tamiflu

_____ 19. Serevent Diskus

_____ 20. Spiriva

_____ 21. Advair Diskus

_____ 22. Symbicort

_____ 23. Myambutol

_____ 24. NasalCrom

_____ 25. Flumadine

A. theophylline
B. beclomethasone
C. mometasone
D. salmeterol xinafoate powder
E. formoterol/budesonide
F. albuterol
G. olopatadine
H. fluticasone/salmeterol
I. rimantadine
J. montelukast
K. ethambutol
L. tiotropium
M. oseltamivir
N. cromolyn sodium
O. fluticasone propionate

Short Answer

Reply to each question based on what you have learned in the chapter.

1. List the primary functions of the upper respiratory tract.

   _____

   _____

2. List the common symptoms of a cold and two preventative efforts to help ward off a cold.

   _____

   _____

3. List symptoms and reactions of an allergy.

   _____

   _____

4. List the classic signs of asthma.

   _____

   _____

5. List two drugs used for the treatment of non–small cell lung cancer.

   _____

   _____

Research Activities

Follow the instructions given in each exercise and provide a response.

1. Visit the website *http://www.lung.org/stop-smoking/about-smoking/health-effects/secondhand-smoke.html*. What are the effects of secondhand smoke in children? In lung cancer patients?

2. Access the website *http://www.cdc.gov/flu/about/viruses/change.htm*. What is "antigenic drift"? Why does this allow for reoccurrence of the flu? How can an "antigenic shift" cause a flu pandemic?

REFLECT CRITICALLY

Critical Thinking

Reply to each question based on what you have learned in the chapter.

1. Electronic cigarettes (e-cigarettes) have become very popular among smokers. What are potential benefits and hazards of e-cigarettes? Do you think this is a better option than cigarettes?

2. What are the health benefits of having plants in your home and office?

3. While having dinner in a restaurant, you see a person who may be choking. You quickly go over to help. What is the first question you should ask the person? Why?

4. Pseudoephedrine now must be sold by a pharmacist and is kept behind the pharmacy counter. Why is the sale of pseudoephedrine now controlled?

5. Why do some people become ill with the flu even if they have received the flu vaccine?

RELATE TO PRACTICE

Lab Scenarios

Therapeutic Agents for the Respiratory System

Objective: To review with the pharmacy technician terms associated with the respiratory system and review the brand and generic names, indications, dosage forms, routes of administration, and recommended daily dosage of medications used to treat disorders of the respiratory system

313

References:
https://www.cdc.gov/nchs/fastats/copd.htm
https://www.cdc.gov/nchs/fastats/asthma.htm

Lab Activity #21.1: Define the following terms associated with the respiratory system.

Equipment needed:
- Medical dictionary
- Pencil/pen

Time needed to complete this activity: 30 minutes

1. Acute bronchitis _____

2. Allergic asthma _____

3. Allergic rhinitis _____

4. Anaphylaxis _____

5. Asthma _____

6. Bronchiolitis _____

7. COPD _____

8. Emphysema _____

9. Hypersensitivity pneumonitis _____

10. Mesothelioma _____

11. Metered dose inhaler _____

12. Nebulizer _____

13. Non–small cell lung cancer _____

14. Pneumonia _____

15. PPD skin test _____

16. Severe acute respiratory syndrome (SARS) _____

17. Small cell lung cancer _____

18. Tuberculosis _____

19. Wheezing _____

Lab Activity #21.2: Using a drug reference book, identify the brand name, drug classification, indications, dosage forms, routes of administration, and recommended daily dosage of the *most common* medications used to treat conditions affecting the respiratory system.

Equipment needed:
- *Drug Facts & Comparisons* or *Physicians' Desk Reference*
- Pencil/pen

Time needed to complete this activity: 60 minutes

Generic Name	Brand Name	Classification	Indication(s)	Dosage Form(s)	Route(s)	Recommended Daily Dosage	Auxiliary Label(s)
Albuterol							
Albuterol sulfate/ Ipratropium bromide							
Beclomethasone							
Budesonide							

Generic Name	Brand Name	Classification	Indication(s)	Dosage Form(s)	Route(s)	Recommended Daily Dosage	Auxiliary Label(s)
Budesonide/Formoterol							
Cetirizine HCl							
Diphenhydramine HCl							
Fluticasone							
Fluticasone propionate/ Salmeterol xinafoate							
Guaifenesin							
Ipratropium bromide							
Levocetirizine Dihydrochloride							
Loratadine							
Mometasone							
Montelukast							
Tiotropium							
Triamcinolone							

Using Therapeutic Agents for the Respiratory System

Objective: To review with the pharmacy technician prescription orders and dosage calculations

Lab Activity #21.3: Answer the questions based on the prescription orders for each question.

Equipment needed:
- *Drug Facts and Comparisons* or *Physician's Desk Reference*
- Pencil/pen
- Calculator

Time needed to complete this activity: 30 minutes

The following are approved DAW codes:

DAW 0: no product selection indicated
DAW 1: substitution not allowed by provider
DAW 2: substitution allowed: patient requested product dispensed
DAW 3: substitution allowed: pharmacist selected product dispensed
DAW 4: substitution allowed: generic drug not in stock
DAW 5: substitution allowed: brand drug dispensed as generic
DAW 6: override
DAW 7: substitution not allowed: brand drug mandated by law
DAW 8: substitution allowed: generic drug not available in marketplace
DAW 9: other

1. Rx 1:
Spiriva HandiHaler (1 HandiHaler, 30 capsules)
i qd
Ref ×5

A. How much will be dispensed?

_____

B. How many days will the medication last?

_____

C. How many refills are permitted on the prescription?

_____

D. What DAW code will be used?

_____

E. Write directions as they would appear on the medication label.

_____

F. What auxiliary label(s) should be affixed to the medication label?

_____

_____

_____

2. Rx 2:
Singulair 5mg, #30
i tab qpm
Ref ×6

A. How much will be dispensed?

_____

B. How many days will the medication last?

_____

C. How many refills are permitted on the prescription?

_____

D. What DAW code will be used?

_____

E. Write directions as they would appear on the medication label.

_____

_____

F. What auxiliary label(s) should be affixed to the medication label?

_____

_____

3. Rx 3:
Xopenex 0.63 mg/3mL, 1 box (24 vials/box)
i vial in neb q8h
Ref ×2

A. How much will be dispensed?

_____

B. How many days will the medication last?

_____

C. How many refills are permitted on the prescription?

_____

D. What DAW code will be used?

_____

316

E. Write directions as they would appear on the medication label.

_____

_____

F. What auxiliary label(s) should be affixed to the medication label?

_____

_____

_____

4. Rx 4:
   ProAir HFA (200 metered doses)
   i to ii inhalations q 4 to 6 h prn SOB and 15 min before
       exercise
   Ref ×3

   A. How much will be dispensed?

   _____

   B. How many days will the medication last?

   _____

   C. How many refills are permitted on the prescription?

   _____

   D. What DAW code will be used?

   _____

   E. Write directions as they would appear on the medication label.

   _____

   _____

   F. What auxiliary label(s) should be affixed to the medication label?

   _____

   _____

5. Rx 5:
   Combivent Respimat (120 metered doses)
   i inhalation qid
   Ref ×6

   A. How much will be dispensed?

   _____

   B. How many days will the medication last?

   _____

   C. How many refills are permitted on the prescription?

   _____

   D. What DAW code will be used?

   _____

   E. Write directions as they would appear on the medication label.

   _____

   _____

   F. What auxiliary label(s) should be affixed to the medication label?

   _____

   _____

6. Rx 6:
   Flovent HFA (120 metered doses)
   ii inhalations bid
   Ref ×3

   A. How much will be dispensed?

   _____

   B. How many days will the medication last?

   _____

   C. How many refills are permitted on the prescription?

   _____

   D. What DAW code will be used?

   _____

Chapter **21** **Therapeutic Agents for the Respiratory System**

E. Write directions as they would appear on the medication label.

_____

_____

F. What auxiliary label(s) should be affixed to the medication label?

_____

_____

_____

7. Rx 7:
Azmacort (240 metered doses)
ii inhalations qid
Ref ×2

A. How much will be dispensed?

_____

B. How many days will the medication last?

_____

C. How many refills are permitted on the prescription?

_____

D. What DAW code will be used?

_____

E. Write directions as they would appear on the medication label.

_____

_____

F. What auxiliary label(s) should be affixed to the medication label?

_____

_____

_____

8. Rx 8:
Beconase AQ (180 metered sprays)
ii spr in each nost bid
Ref ×3

A. How much will be dispensed?

_____

B. How many days will the medication last?

_____

C. How many refills are permitted on the prescription?

_____

D. What DAW code will be used?

_____

E. Write directions as they would appear on the medication label.

_____

_____

F. What auxiliary label(s) should be affixed to the medication label?

_____

_____

9. Rx 9:
Advair Diskus 250/50 (60 blisters)
i inhalation qam and qpm
Ref ×5

A. How much will be dispensed?

_____

B. How many days will the medication last?

_____

C. How many refills are permitted on the prescription?

_____

D. What DAW code will be used?

_____

E. Write directions as they would appear on the medication label.

_____

_____

F. What auxiliary label(s) should be affixed to the medication label?

_____

_____

_____

10. Rx 10:
 Pulmicort Respules 0.25 mg, 2 cartons (30 respules/ carton)
 i respule in neb bid
 Ref ×3

A. How much will be dispensed?

_____

B. How many days will the medication last?

_____

C. How many refills are permitted on the prescription?

_____

D. What DAW code will be used?

_____

E. Write directions as they would appear on the medication label.

_____

_____

F. What auxiliary label(s) should be affixed to the medication label?

_____

_____

_____

319

22 Therapeutic Agents for the Gastrointestinal System

ASHP ACCREDITATION STANDARDS FOR PHARMACY TECHNICIAN EDUCATION AND TRAINING PROGRAMS

Standard 2.5: Demonstrate basic knowledge of anatomy, physiology and pharmacology, and medical terminology relevant to the pharmacy technician's role.

Standard 2.6: Perform mathematical calculations essential to the duties of pharmacy technicians in a variety of settings.

REINFORCE KEY CONCEPTS

Terms and Definitions

Select the correct term from the following list and write the corresponding letter in the blank next to the statement.

A. Absorption
B. Amino acids
C. Antiemetics
D. Carbohydrates
E. Chyme
F. Digestion
G. Emesis
H. Excretion
I. Fistulae
J. Ingestion
K. Peristalsis
L. Surface area

_____ 1. The resulting soupy mixture (semifluid) after food mixes with stomach acids and digestive enzymes

_____ 2. Permanent abnormal passageways between two organs or between an organ and the outside

_____ 3. A drug that prevents or treats nausea and vomiting

_____ 4. Extent of an object's surface in contact with its surroundings

_____ 5. Movement of nutrients, fluids, and medications from the gastrointestinal tract into the bloodstream

_____ 6. A medical term for vomiting

_____ 7. The mechanical, chemical, and enzymatic action of breaking food into molecules for metabolism

_____ 8. Chemical compounds that contain carbon, hydrogen, and oxygen; examples include sugars, glycogen, starches, and cellulose

_____ 9. Taking in food, liquid, or other substances (eg, medications)

_____ 10. Molecules that are the building blocks of proteins

_____ 11. Tubular muscle contraction and relaxation of the esophagus, stomach, and intestines to move substances through the gastrointestinal tract

_____ 12. Elimination of waste products mainly through stools and urine

True or False

Write T or F next to each statement.

_____ 1. The gastrointestinal system is controlled by the sympathetic system.

_____ 2. The stomach's acidity can impact drug and mineral absorption.

_____ 3. Some medications need to be administered parenterally to bypass the stomach and its acidic environment.

_____ 4. The small intestine is about 6 feet in length and is responsible for the final digestion steps.

_____ 5. Antacids like calcium carbonate and magnesium hydroxide work within a few hours to increase gastric pH and relieve occasional dyspepsia or heartburn.

_____ 6. Histamine-2 antagonists like famotidine and ranitidine or proton pump inhibitors like esomeprazole and omeprazole start their work slowly but need less frequent dosing.

_____ 7. The antacid can chelate to some antibiotics and reduce its absorption.

_____ 8. H$_2$-antagonists are medications used to treat constipation.

_____ 9. The primary nondrug treatment for IBS includes avoiding specific irritants and triggers including foods or stress.

_____ 10. Most antiemetics do not require a prescription.

System Identifier

Identify each organ/anatomical part in this system and enter the term next to the corresponding number.

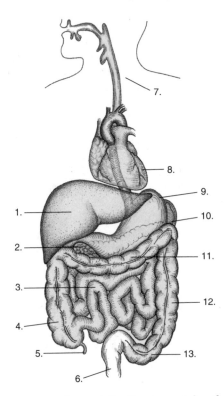

From Potter PA, Perry AG: _Fundamentals of nursing,_ ed 8, St. Louis, 2013, Mosby.

1. _____

2. _____

3. _____

4. _____

5. _____

6. _____

7. _____

8. _____

9. _____

10. _____

11. _____

12. _____

13. _____

Multiple Choice

Complete each question by circling the best answer.

1. Absorption primarily takes place in the:
   A. Stomach
   B. Large intestine
   C. Pancreas
   D. Small intestine

2. This digestive juice is produced by the liver and stored in the gallbladder to help the body absorb fats and fat-soluble vitamins:
   A. Saliva
   B. Bile
   C. Chyme
   D. Lipase

3. Which of the following is _not_ a common condition that affects the gastrointestinal system?
   A. Heartburn
   B. Appendicitis
   C. Constipation
   D. Diarrhea

4. Mylicon (simethicone) is indicated for:
   A. Flatulence
   B. Diarrhea
   C. Heartburn
   D. Constipation

5. Aluminum can cause:
   A. Flatulence
   B. Diarrhea
   C. Heartburn
   D. Constipation

6. Which of the following is a prescription drug for diarrhea?
   A. Pepto-Bismol (bismuth subsalicylate)
   B. Lomotil (diphenoxylate/atropine)
   C. Metamucil (psyllium)
   D. Imodium AD (loperamide)

7. First-line recommendations for _H. pylori_ in patients who are allergic to penicillin include:
   A. A PPI, clarithromycin, and metronidazole
   B. A PPI, clarithromycin, and amoxicillin
   C. A PPI, bismuth salicylate, tetracycline, and metronidazole
   D. Bismuth salicylate, clarithromycin, and metronidazole

321

8. The patient must read and sign a patient–physician agreement form before receiving a prescription for:
   A. Dulcolax (bisacodyl)
   B. Tigan (trimethobenzamide)
   C. Lotronex (alosetron)
   D. Reglan (metoclopramide)

9. If a patient is vomiting, the physician may prescribe:
   A. Axid (nizatidine)
   B. Colace (docusate)
   C. Compazine (prochlorperazine)
   D. Lomotil (diphenoxylate/atropine)

10. If a chemotherapy patient has chemotherapy-induced vomiting, the physician may prescribe:
    A. Zofran (ondansetron)
    B. Dramamine (meclizine)
    C. Naloxegol (movantik)
    D. Amitiza (lubiprostone)

Fill in the Blanks

Answer each question by completing the statement in the space provided.

1. The _____ intestinal pH allows for good nutrient absorption.

2. Hyperacidity _____ like antacids, histamine-2 blockers, and proton pump inhibitors help heartburn, upset stomach, and gastroesophageal reflux disease (GERD).

3. Laxatives and antidiarrheals can speed up or slow the _____ for acute or chronic constipation and diarrhea.

4. Immunosuppressants and steroid anti-inflammatories serve to treat the _____ bowel conditions like Crohn's disease and ulcerative colitis.

5. Combinations of _____ and acid reducers combine to treat the *Helicobacter pylori* often found in gastric and duodenal ulcers.

6. Proton pump Inhibitors (PPIs) mainly treat _____ and _____ ulcers.

7. Resting and drinking clear fluids such as Pedialyte until the _____ subsides are commonly suggested to prevent dehydration and electrolyte loss.

8. Narcotic pain medications, antidepressants, anticonvulsants, calcium channel blockers, and aluminum-containing antacids can cause _____.

9. Poor food _____ causes flatulence as undigested food reaches bacteria in the small intestine or colon.

10. A common side effect of chemotherapy is _____

Matching
Matching I

Match the following trade and generic drug names.

_____ 1. Pepto-Bismol

_____ 2. Prevacid

_____ 3. Aciphex

_____ 4. Imodium

_____ 5. Humira

_____ 6. Tagamet

_____ 7. Protonix

_____ 8. Lomotil

_____ 9. Pentasa

_____ 10. Senna Plus

_____ 11. Colazal

_____ 12. Asacol

A. rabeprazole
B. psyllium
C. loperamide
D. bismuth subsalicylate
E. adalimumab
F. lansoprazole
G. infliximab
H. mesalamine
I. balsalazide
J. cimetidine
K. docusate/senna
L. lubiprostone
M. atropine/diphenoxylate
N. mesalamine
O. pantoprazole

322

_____ 13. Remicade

_____ 14. Metamucil

_____ 15. Amitiza

Matching II
Match the following drug classes with the correct example.

_____ 16. Pepcid (famotidine)

_____ 17. Dexilant (dexlansoprazole)

_____ 18. Cimzia (certolizumab)

_____ 19. Reglan (metoclopramide)

_____ 20. Azulfidine (sulfasalazine)

_____ 21. Movantik (naloxegol)

_____ 22. Tysabri (natalizumab)

_____ 23. Miralax (polyethylene glycol)

_____ 24. Tums (calcium carbonate)

_____ 25. Colace (docusate)

_____ 26. Citrucel (methylcellulose)

_____ 27. Senokot (senna)

A. Tumor necrosis factor
B. Antiemetic
C. H_2-antagonist
D. 5-Aminosalicilate
E. Proton pump inhibitor
F. Opioid antagonist
G. Stimulant laxative
H. Osmotic Laxative
I. Emollient Laxative
J. Bulk-Forming laxative
K. Alpha-4 Integrin Antagonist
L. Antacid

Short Answer
Write a short response to each question in the space provided.

1. List two drugs that antacids will interact with and prevent proper absorption.

_____

_____

2. List three non-drug treatments to treat peptic ulcer disease (PUD).

_____

_____

_____

3. Explain the difference between irritable bowel syndrome (IBS) and irritable bowel disease (IBD).

_____

_____

4. List two non-drug treatments for diarrhea.

_____

_____

5. List the vitamins and minerals that can interact with the absorption of medications in the gastrointestinal tract.

_____

_____

_____

Research Activities
Follow the instructions given in each exercise and provide a response.

1. Lotronex is a medication that must be dispensed with a medication guide. Access and read the medication guide located at _https://www.fda.gov/downloads/drugs/drugsafety/ucm088624.pdf_. Why do you think it's important for patients to receive the medication guide? How can you be sure the patient receives it and receives counseling from the pharmacist?

2. Access the website *https://www.accessdata.fda.gov/scripts/cdrh/cfdocs/cfcfr/cfrsearch.cfm?fr=201.308.* What new label requirement must be in red letters on bottles of ipecac syrup? Why must this label be a part of the labeling requirements for this product?

REFLECT CRITICALLY

Critical Thinking

Reply to each question based on what you have learned in the chapter.

1. It has been stated that you must chew your food "32 times." How does not chewing your food affect digestion in the stomach?

2. A hectic and stressful lifestyle can contribute to many "stomach problems" such as indigestion and acid reflux. What lifestyle changes can be made to reduce these problems?

3. What constitutes good oral hygiene? Is flossing that important? How can flossing impact the Gastrointestinal system?

4. Chemotherapy and radiation can have many adverse effects on patients, including Gastrointestinal system effects (eating, swallowing, saliva production). What prescription and OTC products are available to help with these unwanted effects? As a pharmacy technician, how could you help support these patients?

RELATE TO PRACTICE

Lab Scenarios

Therapeutic Agents for the Gastrointestinal System

Objective: To review with the pharmacy technician terms associated with the Gastrointestinal system and review the brand and generic names, indications, dosage forms, routes of administration, and recommended daily dosage of medications used to treat disorders of the Gastrointestinal system

---

DID YOU KNOW?

- 14.8 million adults have been diagnosed with an ulcer in the digestive system.
- It is estimated that 25 to 45 million Americans are affected by IBS.
- GERD affects approximately 20% of the adult US population.

References:
https://www.cdc.gov/nchs/fastats/digestive-diseases.htm
https://www.aboutibs.org/facts-about-ibs.html
https://www.niddk.nih.gov/health-information/health-statistics/digestive-diseases

Lab Activity #22.1: Define the following terms associated with the Gastrointestinal system.

Equipment needed:
- Medical dictionary
- Pencil/pen

Time needed to complete this activity: 30 minutes

1. Appendicitis _____

2. Constipation _____

3. Diarrhea _____

4. Duodenal ulcer_____

5. Celiac disease _____

6. Crohn's disease _____

7. Gastric ulcer _____

8. Gastritis _____

9. Gastroesophageal reflux disease (GERD) _____

10. Hiatal hernia_____

11. Inflammatory bowel syndrome (IBS) _____

12. Intrinsic factor (IF) _____

13. Irritable bowel disease (IBD)_____

14. Laryngopharyngeal reflux _____

15. Lipids _____

16. Peptic ulcer _____

17. Peptic ulcer disease (PUD) _____

18. Reflux _____

19. Stomatitis _____

20. Ulcer _____

21. Ulcerative colitis _____

22. Villus _____

23. Xerostomia _____

Lab Activity #22.2: Using a drug reference book, identify the brand name, drug classification, indications, dosage forms, routes of administration, and recommended daily dosage of the *most common* medications used to treat conditions affecting the Gastrointestinal system.

Equipment Needed:
- *Drug Facts & Comparisons* or *Physicians' Desk Reference*
- Pencil/pen

Time needed to complete this activity: 60 minutes

Generic Name	Brand Name	Classification	Indication(s)	Dose Form(s)	Route(s)	Daily Recommended Dosage	Auxiliary Label(s)
Dexlansoprazole							
Docusate							
Esomeprazole							
Famotidine							
Lansoprazole							
Mesalamine							
Omeprazole							
Ondansetron							
Pantoprazole sodium							
Promethazine HCl							
Rabeprazole							

325

Lab Activity #22.3: Using resources available, complete the following table of common OTC drug products for the Gastrointestinal system.

Equipment needed:
- Computer with Internet access
- Paper
- Pencil/pen
- *Pocket Guide for Nonprescription Product Therapeutics*

Time needed to complete this activity: 60 minutes

Brand Name	Active Ingredient(s)	Dosage Forms Available	Patient Information	Recommended Dosage	Rx Strength Availability
Gastrointestinal Problems					
Alka-Seltzer					
Axid AR					
Gaviscon					
Milk of Magnesia					
Miralax					
Mylanta					
Pepcid					
Pepto-Bismol					
Prevacid					
Prilosec					
Tagamet HB					
Zantac 75					
Motion Sickness					
Bonine					
Dramamine					

Brand Name	Active Ingredient(s)	Dosage Forms Available	Patient Information	Recommended Dosage	Rx Strength Availability
Intestinal Discomfort					
Beano					
Gas-X					
Lactaid					
Mylicon					
Constipation					
Benefiber					
Castor oil					
Colace					
Dulcolax					
FiberCon					
Fleet					
Metamucil					
Senokot					
Surfak					
Diarrhea					
Imodium AD					
Pedialyte					

Using Therapeutic Agents for the Gastrointestinal System

Objective: To review with the pharmacy technician medication orders and dosage calculations

Lab Activity #22.4: Answer each question using the IV medication order provided.

Equipment needed:
- Calculator
- *Trissel's Handbook of Injectable Drugs*
- Pencil/pen

Time needed to complete this activity: 30 minutes

Answer the questions based on the following medication order:

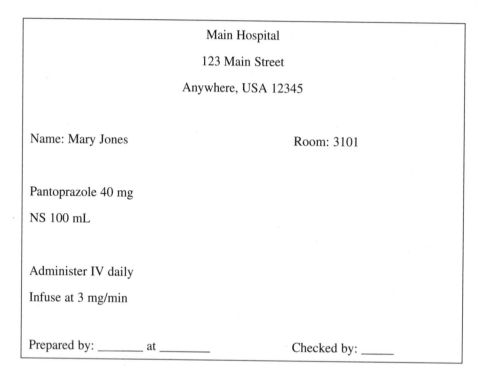

Main Hospital

123 Main Street

Anywhere, USA 12345

Name: Mary Jones   Room: 3101

Pantoprazole 40 mg

NS 100 mL

Administer IV daily

Infuse at 3 mg/min

Prepared by: _____ at _____   Checked by: _____

1. You have the following in stock in your pharmacy, which should be reconstituted with 10 mL of NS. What will the concentration be after reconstitution?

_____

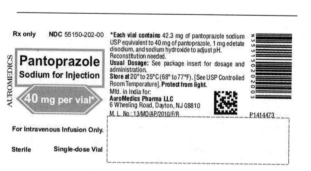

From NIH: US National Library of Medicine, *Daily Med,* https://dailymed.nlm.nih.gov/dailymed/index.cfm

2. How many mL of pantoprazole will be needed to make this IV infusion?

_____

3. How many vials will you need to make this IV infusion?

_____

4. How should this IV be stored after preparation?

_____

5. How long is this IV stable after preparing?

_____

6. How long will this IV infusion last?

_____

23 Therapeutic Agents for the Renal System

ASHP ACCREDITATION STANDARDS FOR PHARMACY TECHNICIAN EDUCATION AND TRAINING PROGRAMS

Standard 2.5: Demonstrate basic knowledge of anatomy, physiology and pharmacology, and medical terminology relevant to the pharmacy technician's role.
Standard 3.1: Assist pharmacists in collecting, organizing, and recording demographic and clinical information for the Pharmacists; Patient Care Process.
Standard 3.2: Receive, process, and prepare prescriptions/medication orders for completeness, accuracy, and authenticity to ensure safety.
Standard 5.1: Describe and apply state and federal laws pertaining to processing, handling, and dispensing of medications including controlled substances.

REINFORCE KEY CONCEPTS

Terms and Definitions

Select the correct term from the following list and write the corresponding letter in the blank next to the statement.

A. Acidosis
B. Alkalosis
C. Anions
D. Cations
E. Erythropoietin
F. Ions
G. Plasma
H. Renin
I. Urinary acidification

_____ 1. The conversion of urine to a more acidic content

_____ 2. An enzyme secreted by and stored in the kidneys that promotes the production of the protein angiotensin

_____ 3. An increase in the blood's acidity, resulting from the accumulation of acid or loss of bicarbonate; the blood's pH is lower

_____ 4. Negatively charged ions

_____ 5. An increase in the blood's alkalinity, resulting from the accumulation of alkali or reduction of acid content; the blood's pH is higher

_____ 6. A hormone that kidneys secrete that increases the rate of red blood cell production

_____ 7. The colorless fluid portion of the blood

_____ 8. Positively charged ions

_____ 9. Atoms or molecules with a net electrical charge (positive or negative)

Select the correct term from the following list and write the corresponding letter in the blank next to the statement.

A. Collecting duct
B. Interstitial space
C. Nephron
D. Renal artery
E. Renal vein
F. Tubular reabsorption
G. Tubular secretion

_____ 10. One of the pair of arteries that branch from the abdominal aorta; each kidney has one renal artery

_____ 11. A function of the nephron in which ions, toxins, and water are secreted into the collecting duct to be excreted

_____ 12. The filtering unit of the kidneys

_____ 13. The conservation of protein, glucose, bicarbonate, and water from the glomerular filtrate by the tubules

_____ 14. A series of tubules in the kidneys that connect the nephrons to the ureter

_____ 15. Small, narrow spaces between tissues

_____ 16. The vein in which filtered blood from the kidneys is sent back into the body's circulatory system; each kidney has one renal vein

329

Select the correct term from the following list and write the corresponding letter in the blank next to the statement.

A. Dialysate
B. Dialysis
C. Diuretic
D. Micturition
E. Osmosis
F. Stress incontinence
G. Urge incontinence

_____ 17. Urination

_____ 18. The fluid into which material passes by way of the membrane in dialysis

_____ 19. Urinary incontinence due to involuntary bladder contractions that result in an urgent need to urinate

_____ 20. The passage of a solute through a semipermeable membrane to remove toxic materials and to maintain fluid, electrolyte, and pH levels when the kidneys malfunction

_____ 21. Involuntary emission of urine when the pressure in the abdomen suddenly increases

_____ 22. The diffusion of water from low-solute concentrations to higher-solute concentrations across a semipermeable membrane

_____ 23. An agent that increases urine output and excretion of water

Select the correct term from the following list and write the corresponding letter in the blank next to the statement.

A. Chronic kidney disease (CKD)
B. Edema
C. Lithotripsy
D. Nosocomial infection
E. Peritonitis
F. Ureteroscopy
G. Urethritis
H. Urolithiasis

_____ 24. A treatment with ultrasound shock waves to break kidney stones into small particles

_____ 25. Solid mineral deposits that form stones in the urinary tract

_____ 26. An infection that originates in the hospital or institutional setting

_____ 27. A condition that reduces the kidneys' ability to function properly

_____ 28. An examination of the upper urinary tract, usually performed with an endoscope passed through the urethra

_____ 29. An inflammation of the peritoneum, typically caused by a bacterial infection

_____ 30. An excess of watery fluid in the cavities or tissues of the body

_____ 31. An inflammation of the urethra

True or False

Write T or F next to each statement.

_____ 1. The shape of the kidneys is similar to the shape of a kidney bean.

_____ 2. When the kidney is full, the person feels the need to urinate.

_____ 3. The body excretes approximately 1000 to 2000 mL of urine per day.

_____ 4. Each kidney contains thousands of microscopic nephrons.

_____ 5. It is possible for people to survive with one functioning kidneys.

_____ 6. As a kidney ages, it is better able to compensate for fluid imbalances.

_____ 7. Drinking plenty of water is one of the most effective ways to take care of the urinary system.

_____ 8. The nephrons actively filter blood 12 hours a day.

_____ 9. Thiazides and thiazide-like diuretics decrease urinary excretion of sodium and chloride ions by blocking ionic reabsorption in the distal convoluted tubule.

_____ 10. Incontinence tends to affect women more than men.

System Identifier

Identify each main organ/anatomical part in the urinary system and enter the term next to the corresponding number.

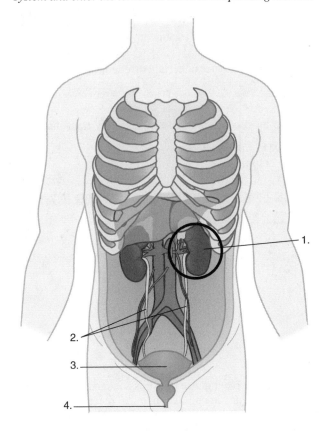

1. _____

2. _____

3. _____

4. _____

Multiple Choice

Complete each question by circling the best answer.

1. Kidney reabsorption regulates _____ content.
   A. potassium
   B. sodium
   C. phosphate
   D. magnesium

2. What volume of blood products do the kidneys filter each day?
   A. 1 gallon
   B. 5 gallons
   C. 45 gallons
   D. 100 gallons

3. Albumins and antibodies are components of:
   A. plasma
   B. blood
   C. hemoglobin
   D. All the above

4. The one-way reabsorption of sodium and chloride from the loop of Henle is called:
   A. ion exchange
   B. osmosis
   C. active transport
   D. tubular secretion

5. The kidneys are also responsible for the production of

   _____, which helps maintain water balance in the body.
   A. erythropoietin
   B. aldosterone
   C. renin
   D. hilus

6. Those who have end-stage renal disease (ESRD) may

   be prescribed _____ to help overcome anemia.
   A. Rocaltrol (calcitriol)
   B. Renagel (sevelamer)
   C. Vitamin K
   D. Epogen (epoetin alfa)

7. Which of the following is *not* used as preventative for kidney stones?
   A. Zyloprim (allopurinol)
   B. Klor-Con (potassium chloride)
   C. Thiazide diuretics
   D. Urocit-K (potassium citrate)

8. Which of the following is *not* a means of cleansing the blood of patients with ESRD?
   A. hemodialysis
   B. peritoneal dialysis
   C. nocturnal dialysis
   D. oxydialysis

9. The most common side effect of all diuretics is:
   A. frequent urination
   B. infrequent urination
   C. increased thiamine levels
   D. decreased thiamine levels

10. For symptomatic fungal UTIs, _____ can be prescribed.
    A. Keflex (cephalexin)
    B. Diflucan (fluconazole)
    C. Cipro (ciprofloxacin)
    D. Macrobid (nitrofurantoin)

Fill in the Blanks

Answer each question by completing the statement in the space provided.

1. The four important _____ functions of the body are absorption, distribution, metabolism, and excretion.

2. Acidosis occurs when too many free _____ ions are present in body fluids, and alkalosis occurs when there is either retention of _____ or excessive loss of hydrogen ions.

3. _____ are primarily responsible for the regulation of fluids, solutes, and wastes within the body.

4. The acid content in urine is between a pH of _____ and _____.

5. Kidneys maintain _____ by balancing electrolyte levels.

6. When kidney function declines, less _____ leads to decreased red blood cell production and anemia.

7. Kidney stones can pass naturally through the _____ without treatment.

8. Two general types of peripheral edema are _____ and _____.

9. The most common cause of a urinary tract infection (UTI) is the bacterium _____ _____ from the colon.

10. The most common incontinence nondrug therapy is _____ exercises.

Matching

Match the following ions with their function.

_____ 1. Calcium (Ca^{2+})

_____ 2. Potassium (K^+)

_____ 3. Magnesium (Mg^{2+})

_____ 4. Sodium (Na^+)

_____ 5. Chloride (Cl^-)

_____ 6. Bicarbonate (HCO_3^-)

_____ 7. Phosphate (PO_4^{3-})

A. Maintains water balance, nerve impulse transmission, and regulation of acid–base balance; participates in cellular chemical reactions

B. Aids as a buffer to balance acid–base regulation in cells; promotes normal neuromuscular action and participates in carbohydrate metabolism; essential for formation and strength of bones and teeth; also needed for many biochemical pathways

C. Necessary for glycogen deposits in the liver and skeletal muscles; aids in nerve impulse and cardiac conduction; helps in contraction in skeletal and smooth muscles

D. The most important chemical buffer; essential for the proper acid–base balance

E. Aids in cardiac and skeletal muscle excitability, enzyme activities, and neurochemical activities

F. Bone and teeth formation, cell membrane integrity, cardiac conduction, nerve impulse conduction, muscle contraction, hormone secretion

G. The main anion in the transport of sodium, hydrogen, and potassium; essential to acid–base balance

Match the following trade names with their generic drug names.

_____ 8. Thalitone

_____ 9. Lasix

_____ 10. Aldactone

_____ 11. Diamox

_____ 12. Levaquin

_____ 13. Demadex

_____ 14. Ditropan

_____ 15. Urispas

_____ 16. Midamor

_____ 17. Vesicare

A. spironolactone
B. acetazolamide
C. chlorthalidone
D. levofloxacin
E. furosemide
F. amiloride
G. oxybutynin
H. solifenacin
I. torsemide
J. flavoxate

Match the following drugs with their classification.

_____ 18. Bumex (bumetanide)

_____ 19. Dyrenium (triamterene)

_____ 20. Zaroxolyn (metolazone)

_____ 21. Toviaz (fesoterodine)

_____ 22. Diamox (acetazolamide)

_____ 23. Pyridium (phenazopyridine)

_____ 24. Osmitrol (mannitol)

_____ 25. Microzide (hydrochlorothiazide)

_____ 26. Renagel (sevelamer)

_____ 27. Epogen (epoetin alfa)

_____ 28. Feosol (ferrous sulfate)

_____ 29. Rocaltrol (calcitriol)

_____ 30. Detrol (tolterodine)

_____ 31. Macrobid (nitrofurantoin)

A. Potassium-sparing diuretic
B. Carbonic anhydrase inhibitor
C. Loop diuretic
D. Thiazide-like diuretic
E. Antimuscarinic
F. Osmotic diuretic
G. Thiazide diuretic
H. Urinary analgesic
I. Hematopoietic
J. Phosphorous-binding
K. Overactive bladder agent
L. Antibiotic
M. Vitamin D analog
N. Iron supplement

Short Answer

Write a short response to each question in the space provided.

1. Who is at high risk for renal failure?

_____

_____

_____

2. List two important functions of the nephron.

_____

_____

3. Name the six main classes of diuretics used to treat edema.

_____

_____

_____

_____

_____

4. List the mechanism of action for potassium-sparing diuretics.

_____

_____

_____

5. List the mechanism of action for loop diuretics.

_____

_____

_____

6. List the mechanism of action for osmotics.

_____

_____

_____

7. List the mechanism of action for thiazide and thiazide-like diuretics.

_____

_____

_____

8. List the mechanism of action for carbonic anhydrase inhibitors.

_____

_____

_____

Research Activities

Follow the instructions given in each exercise and provide a response.

1. Visit the website *https://www.mayoclinic.org/healthy-lifestyle/nutrition-and-healthy-eating/in-depth/water/art-20044256*. Investigate how much water you should drink in a day.

   A. How much water is recommended for men and women daily? How does this differ from the "eight glasses per day" recommendation?

   B. What are the health benefits of water?

   C. What factors affect daily water intake?

   D. What foods can you eat to help meet the recommended daily water intake?

   E. Is it possible to drink too much water? Why or why not?

2. Visit the website *http://www.nlm.nih.gov/medlineplus/dialysis.html*. Investigate what dialysis is and how it works.

   A. What are the two types of kidney dialysis discussed?

B. What does dialysis help the kidneys do?

C. How does each type of dialysis work?

REFLECT CRITICALLY

Critical Thinking

Reply to each question based on what you have learned in the chapter.

1. Nosocomial urinary tract infections are a very common hospital-acquired infection. Who would be more at risk for acquiring this type of infection? What are some ways to prevent the spread of this type of infection?

2. If a UTI is left untreated, how will the infection progress?

   A. What are some common symptoms of a UTI?

   B. What drug therapy (prescription, OTC, and alternative medications) could be used to help treat a UTI?

3. Diabetes can be complicated by hypertension and kidney failure. A change in the patient's diet is always recommended. Apply your knowledge of the disease and devise a list of lifestyle changes that would benefit a diabetic patient.

RELATE TO PRACTICE

Lab Scenarios
Therapeutic Agents for the Renal Systems

Objective: To review with the pharmacy technician the organs of the renal system; in addition, to review the brand and generic names, indications, dosage forms, routes of administration, and daily dosing of medications used to treat disorders of the renal system

---

DID YOU KNOW?

- It is estimated that 37 million or 15% adults have chronic kidney disease.
- 1 in 3 adults with diabetes and 1 in 5 adults with high blood pressure may also have chronic kidney disease.
- Approximately 661,000 Americans have kidney failure with 468,000 of these are on dialysis.

References:

https://www.cdc.gov/kidneydisease/basics.html

https://www.cdc.gov/diabetes/pubs/pdf/kidney_factsheet.pdf

https://www.niddk.nih.gov/health-information/health-statistics/kidney-disease

Lab Activity #23.1: Define the following terms associated with the urinary system.

Equipment needed:
- Medical dictionary
- Pencil/pen

Time needed to complete this activity: 45 minutes

1. Anuria _____

2. Blood urea nitrogen (BUN) _____

3. Cystitis _____

4. Dehydration _____

5. Electrolyte _____

6. End-stage renal disease _____

7. Excretion _____

8. Hyperchloremia _____

9. Hyperkalemia _____

10. Hypernatremia _____

11. Hyperphosphatemia _____

12. Hypocalcemia _____

13. Hypochloremia _____

14. Hypokalemia _____

15. Hyponatremia _____

16. Hypophosphatemia _____

17. Incontinence _____

18. Kidney stones _____

19. Oliguria _____

20. Polyuria _____

21. Pyelonephritis _____

22. Renal osteodystrophy _____

23. Uremia _____

24. Urethritis _____

Lab Activity #23.2: Using a drug reference book, identify the brand name, drug classification, indications, dosage forms, routes of administration, and recommended daily dosage of the *most common* medications used to treat conditions affecting the renal system.

Equipment needed:
- *Drug Facts & Comparisons* or *Physicians' Desk Reference*
- Pencil/pen

Time needed to complete this activity: 60 minutes

Generic Name	Brand Name	Classification	Indication(s)	Dosage Form(s)	Route(s)	Recommended Daily Dosage	Auxiliary Label(s)
Cephalexin							
Chlorthalidone							
Ciprofloxacin							
Darifenacin							
Fesoterodine							
Furosemide							

Generic Name	Brand Name	Classification	Indication(s)	Dosage Form(s)	Route(s)	Recommended Daily Dosage	Auxiliary Label(s)
Hydrochlorothiazide							
Hydrochlorothiazide/ Triamterene							
Levofloxacin							
Nitrofurantoin							
Oxybutynin							
Phenazopyridine							
Potassium							
Solifenacin							
Spironolactone							
Tolterodine							
Trospium							

Chapter **23 Therapeutic Agents for the Renal System**

Lab Activity #23.3: Using a drug reference, identify the brand name, manufacturer, product size availability, and storage requirements for these temperature-sensitive medications.

Equipment needed:
- Computer with Internet access
- Pencil/pen
- *Red Book Online*
- *Trissel's Handbook of Injectable Drugs*

Time needed to complete this activity: 30 minutes

Generic Name	Brand Name	Manufacturer	Product Size Availability	Storage Requirements
Darbepoetin alfa				
Epoetin alfa				
Mannitol				
Onabotulinum toxin A				

Why is it important to pay attention to the storage requirements and store them properly?

_____

_____

_____

Using Therapeutic Agents for the Renal System

Objective: To review with the pharmacy technician prescription orders, dosage calculations, and auxiliary labeling

Lab Activity #23.4: Answer the questions based on the prescription order.

Equipment needed:
- Calculator
- *Physician's Desk Reference* or *Drug Facts and Comparisons*
- Pencil/pen

Time needed to complete this activity: 30 minutes

Answer the questions based on the following prescription order:

Dr. Jack Davidson

2145 Main Street

St. Louis, MO 63144

314-987-0100

Name: _Dorra James_   Date: _July 12, 202X_

Address: _145 Anywhere St, St Louis, MO_   DOB: _Sept 10, 1994_

Rx: _Pyridium_

200 mg tid pc for two days

Macrobid

100 mg bid x7 days

Refills: _none_   _Jack Davidson, MD_

DEA no _____

---

1. How many prescriptions are written on this prescription order?

   _____

2. For the first medication written, answer the following questions:

   A. What is the name of the drug written?

   _____

   B. Is this medication available as a generic? If so, what is the generic name?

   _____

   C. What medication will be dispensed?

   _____

   D. What directions should appear on the prescription label?

   _____

E. What quantity will be dispensed?

   _____

F. How many refills are available for this prescription?

   _____

G. What auxiliary labels need to go on this prescription?

   _____

3. For the second medication written, answer the following questions:

   A. What is the name of the drug written?

   _____

   B. Is this medication available as a generic? If so, what is the generic name?

   _____

339

C. What medication will be dispensed?

_____

D. What directions should appear on the prescription label?

_____

E. What quantity will be dispensed?

_____

F. How many refills are available for this prescription?

_____

G. What auxiliary labels need to go on this prescription?

_____

24 Therapeutic Agents for the Reproductive System

REINFORCE KEY CONCEPTS

Terms and Definitions

Select the correct term from the following list and write the corresponding letter in the blank next to the statement.

A. Abortifacient
B. Benign
C. Depot
D. Fertilization
E. Gametes
F. Negative feedback
G. Palliative
H. Spermicide
I. Teratogen

_____ 1. An area of the body where a substance can accumulate or be stored for later distribution

_____ 2. Any agent that causes abnormal embryonic or fetal development

_____ 3. Something that brings relief but does not cure

_____ 4. Any treatment that causes abortion of a fetus

_____ 5. The process by which a sperm unites with an ovum

_____ 6. An agent that kills sperm

_____ 7. A self-regulating mechanism in which the output of a system has input or control on the process; in this case, the stimulus results in reactions that reduce the effects of the stimulus

_____ 8. A condition, tumor, or growth that is not cancerous and therefore will not metastasize

_____ 9. Sex cells, or ova and sperm

Select the correct term from the following list and write the corresponding letter in the blank next to the statement.

A. Endometrium
B. Estrogen
C. Fallopian tube
D. Mammary gland
E. Menopause
F. Menses
G. Oocyte
H. Ovaries
I. Pelvic inflammatory disease (PID)
J. Progesterone
K. Uterus

_____ 10. The mucous membrane lining the inner wall or layer of the uterus

_____ 11. The female reproductive germ cell, more commonly known as an egg

_____ 12. Cessation of menstruation; a natural phenomenon in which a woman passes from a reproductive state to a nonreproductive state

_____ 13. The female reproductive organs in which ova, or eggs, are produced

_____ 14. The organ in the lower abdomen of a woman where gestation of a fetus occurs

_____ 15. Any of a group of anabolic sex hormones that promote the development and maintenance of female sexual characteristics

_____ 16. The time of menstruation

_____ 17. The milk-producing gland of women

_____ 18. An anabolic sex hormone that stimulates the uterus to prepare for pregnancy

_____ 19. Inflammation of the female genital tract, accompanied by fever and lower abdominal pain

_____ 20. A narrow tube that connects the ovary to the uterus

Select the correct term from the following list and write the corresponding letter in the blank next to the statement.

A. Androgen
B. Benign prostatic hyperplasia (BPH)
C. Erectile dysfunction (ED)
D. Nocturia
E. Prostate
F. Sperm
G. Spermatogenesis
H. Testes
I. Testosterone

_____ 21. The male reproductive germ cell

_____ 22. Enlargement of the prostate

_____ 23. A gland surrounding the neck of the bladder in males that produces a fluid component of semen

_____ 24. An anabolic sex hormone produced in the testes that stimulates the development of male sexual characteristics

_____ 25. Male sex hormone

_____ 26. The male reproductive organs that produce sperm

_____ 27. Urination at night

_____ 28. Inability of a man to maintain an erection sufficient for satisfying sexual activity

_____ 29. The development of sperm in the testes

True or False

Write T or F next to each statement.

_____ 1. The reproductive system is not interdependent with other body systems.

_____ 2. The gonads provide characteristics of both males and females.

_____ 3. Enzymes largely control the functions of the reproductive system.

_____ 4. The hypothalamus can distinguish between natural and synthetic hormones.

_____ 5. Synthetic progestins are used more frequently than natural forms because synthetic forms are more effective.

_____ 6. Hormone treatment is the most common treatment for infertility.

_____ 7. Concurrent use of oral contraceptives and cigarette smoking decreases the risk of serious cardiovascular effects.

_____ 8. Natural testosterone used for medicinal purposes is obtained from the testes of bulls.

_____ 9. Hormone therapy is the most common medical treatment for prostate cancer.

_____ 10. Oral birth control or contraceptive gels can protect against STDs.

Female Reproductive System
Identify each component in this system and enter the term next to the corresponding number.

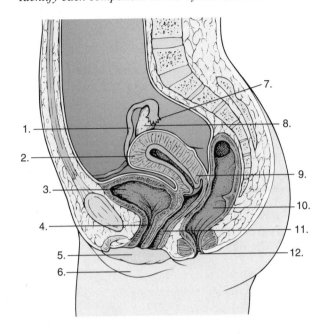

1. _____

2. _____

3. _____

4. _____

5. _____

6. _____

7. _____

8. _____

9. _____

10. _____

11. _____

12. _____

Male Reproductive System
Identify each component in this system and enter the term next to the corresponding number.

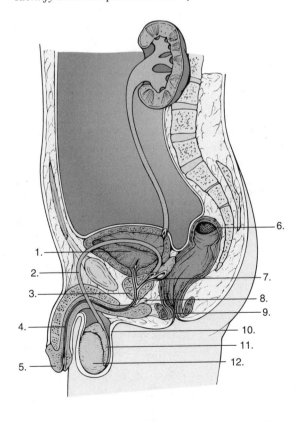

1. _____

2. _____

3. _____

4. _____

5. _____

6. _____

7. _____

8. _____

9. _____

10. _____

11. _____

12. _____

343

Multiple Choice

Complete each question by circling the best answer.

1. The primary oral estrogen products in use clinically

   are conjugated estrogens and _____.
   A. medroxyprogesterone
   B. progestin
   C. androgen
   D. estradiol

2. Because of the abuse potential of androgen products, the Drug Enforcement Administration (DEA) placed

   these products on the _____ list of controlled medications.
   A. Schedule II
   B. Schedule III
   C. Schedule IV
   D. Schedule V

3. The most abundant androgen is:
   A. Estrogen
   B. Testosterone
   C. Progesterone
   D. Inhibin

4. Oral contraceptives are formulated in which of the following combinations?
   A. Monophasic
   B. Biphasic
   C. Triphasic
   D. All the above

5. The goal of treatment for benign prostatic hypertrophy is to:
   A. Relieve hesitancy of urination
   B. Decrease nocturia
   C. Prevent the development of urinary tract infections
   D. All the above

6. Which of the following is used to treat abnormal uterine bleeding?
   A. Prometrium (progesterone)
   B. Uroxatral (alfuzosin)
   C. Androderm (testosterone)
   D. Flagyl (metronidazole)

7. For the treatment of oligospermia, which of the following can be used?
   A. Proscar (finasteride)
   B. Avodart (dutasteride)
   C. Clomid (clomiphene)
   D. Mirena (levonorgestrel)

8. Palliative treatment of metastatic breast cancer may include:
   A. Methitest (methyltestosterone)
   B. Menest (esterified estrogen)
   C. Nexplanon (etonogestrel)
   D. Lupron depot (leuprolide)

9. For osteoporosis prophylaxis, which of the following can be used?
   A. Zoladex (goserelin)
   B. Premarin (conjugated estrogens)
   C. Methitest (methyltestosterone)
   D. Provera (medroxyprogesterone)

10. The drug _____ is a recent medication used for the treatment of hepatitis C.
    A. Valtrex (valacyclovir)
    B. Invirase (saquinavir)
    C. Harvoni (ledipasvir/sofosbuvir)
    D. Videx (didanosine)

Fill in the Blanks

Answer each question by completing the statement in the space provided.

1. Combination oral _____ may consist of estrogen and progestin to inhibit ovulation.

2. Some of the combination oral contraceptive _____ include thromboembolism, myocardial infarction, and stroke.

3. Barrier devices are _____ methods of birth control.

4. Mifepristone acts as an _____ to progesterone and prevents the maintenance of the pregnancy.

5. HRT may _____ a women's risk of developing breast cancer, stroke, blood clots, and heart disease.

6. When using testosterone gel products, it is important to _____ the application site and not hold small children where transfer of the testosterone may occur.

7. Finasteride is also available in a 1-mg dose under the brand name _____ for the treatment of male pattern baldness.

8. Because 5-alpha reductase inhibitors may cause birth defects, a woman who is pregnant or trying to become pregnant should _____ contact with crushed or broken tablets because the active drug can penetrate through the skin.

9. Patients taking _____ should not take sildenafil or related drugs concurrently because of the potential for dangerous decreases in blood pressure that can occur upon combination.

10. If untreated, some STDs can cause _____ sterility, blindness, and even death.

Matching

Match the following trade and generic drug names.

_____ 1. Proscar

_____ 2. Flomax

_____ 3. Premarin

_____ 4. Viramune

_____ 5. Provera

_____ 6. Muse

_____ 7. Ortho Tri-Cyclen

_____ 8. Zerit

_____ 9. Lupron Depot

_____ 10. Viagra

_____ 11. Estrace

_____ 12. Ortho Evra

_____ 13. Prometrium

_____ 14. Uroxatral

_____ 15. Methitest

A. conjugated estrogens
B. nevirapine
C. finasteride
D. medroxyprogesterone
E. tamsulosin
F. stavudine
G. sildenafil
H. leuprolide
I. alfuzosin
J. ethinyl estradiol/norgestimate
K. progesterone
L. methyltestosterone
M. estradiol
N. alprostadil
O. ethinyl estradiol/norelgestromin

Match the following drugs with their indication.

_____ 16. Lupron (leuprolide)

_____ 17. Clomid (clomiphene)

_____ 18. Valtrex (valacyclovir)

_____ 19. Prempro (conjugated estrogens and medroxyprogesterone)

_____ 20. Enpresse (ethinyl estradiol/levonorgestrel)

_____ 21. Epivir (lamivudine)

_____ 22. Vibramycin (doxycycline)

_____ 23. AndroGel (testosterone)

_____ 24. Tyzeka (telbivudine)

_____ 25. Cardura (doxazosin)

_____ 26. Caverject (alprostadil)

_____ 27. Zoladex (goserelin)

_____ 28. Pegasys (interferon alfa-2a pegylated)

_____ 29. Android (methyltestosterone)

_____ 30. Cialis (tadalafil)

A. Androgen supplement
B. Oral contraceptive
C. Endometriosis
D. Breast cancer
E. Pelvic inflammatory disease
F. Infertility
G. Prostate cancer
H. Benign prostatic hypertrophy
I. Erectile dysfunction
J. Hormone replacement therapy
K. Sexually transmitted disease
L. HIV
M. Hepatitis B and C

Short Answer

Reply to each question based on what you have learned in the chapter.

1. List the available dosage forms of estrogen.

_____

_____

2. List six types of non-oral contraceptives and their available dosage forms.

_____

_____

3. List six types of androgens and their available dosage forms.

_____

_____

4. List two drug classes used to treat benign prostatic hypertrophy (BPH).

_____

_____

5. List the pregnancy category for all estrogens.

_____

6. List the drug classifications with an example used to treat HIV and AIDS.

_____

_____

_____

_____

Research Activities

Follow the instructions given in each exercise and provide a response.

1. Access the website *https://www.cdc.gov/vaccines/ vpd/hpv/public/index.htm* and read about the CDC recommendations for human papillomavirus (HPV) vaccinations for young adolescents.

    A. How many shots of the HPV vaccine does the CDC recommend for 11- to 12-year-olds?

    B. How many shots of the HPV vaccine does the CDC recommend for teens and young adults who start the HPV vaccine series later, at ages 15 through 26 years?

    C. List the vaccines available to protect against HPV.

2. Access the website *http://www.nlm.nih.gov/medlineplus/ ency/article/000369.htm* and read about polycystic ovarian syndrome (PCOS).

    A. What are the symptoms of PCOS?

    B. What health conditions are common in women with PCOS?

    C. What drug therapy is used to help treat the symptoms of PCOS?

REFLECT CRITICALLY

Critical Thinking

Reply to each question based on what you have learned in the chapter.

1. Women have been told for many years that when menopause occurs, they will need hormonal replacement therapy (HRT). However, recently released information indicates that long-term HRT is more harmful than beneficial. If you were the pharmacist, what advice would you give women on this subject?

2. Birth control has been taught in middle schools and high schools for many years to curb teen pregnancy. Why is the rate of teen pregnancy still high?

3. Propecia was approved by the Food and Drug Administration (FDA) for the treatment of hair loss. The active ingredient in Propecia is finasteride, which is the same drug used to treat benign prostatic hypertrophy, under the brand name Proscar. What is the difference in strength between Propecia and Proscar, and what are the side effects of finasteride?

RELATE TO PRACTICE

Lab Scenarios
Therapeutic Agents for the Reproductive System

Objective: To review with the pharmacy technician terms associated with the organs of the reproductive system and review the brand and generic names, indications, dosage forms, routes of administration, and recommended daily dosage of medications used to treat disorders of the reproductive system

References:
https://www.cdc.gov/nchs/fastats/contraceptive.htm
https://www.cdc.gov/hiv/statistics/overview/index.html
https://www.cdc.gov/std/hpv/stdfact-hpv.htm

Lab Activity #24.1: Define the following terms associated with the reproductive system.

Equipment needed:
- Medical dictionary
- Pencil/pen

Time needed to complete this activity: 30 minutes

1. Amenorrhea _____

2. Anabolic steroid _____

3. Dysfunctional uterine bleeding (DUB) _____

4. Dysmenorrhea _____

5. Endometriosis _____

6. Hypogonadism _____

7. Hysterectomy _____

8. Infertility _____

9. Kallmann's syndrome _____

10. Klinefelter's syndrome _____

11. Polycystic ovarian syndrome (PCOS) _____

12. Pregnancy _____

13. Premenstrual syndrome (PMS) _____

14. Salpingitis _____

15. Stein-Leventhal syndrome _____

16. Tubal ligation _____

17. Vasectomy _____

18. Vaginitis _____

Lab Activity #24.2: Using a drug reference book, identify the brand name, drug classification, indication, dosage forms, routes of administration, and recommended daily dosage of the *most common* medications used to treat conditions affecting the reproductive system.

Equipment needed:
- *Drug Facts & Comparisons* or *Physicians' Desk Reference*
- Pencil/pen

Time needed to complete this activity: 60 minutes

Generic Name	Brand Name	Classification	Indication(s)	Dose Form(s)	Route(s)	Recommended Daily Dosage	Auxiliary Label(s)
Acyclovir							
Alfuzosin							
Anastrozole							

Generic Name	Brand Name	Classification	Indication(s)	Dose Form(s)	Route(s)	Recommended Daily Dosage	Auxiliary Label(s)
Clindamycin							
Dutasteride							
Estradiol							
Estrogens, conjugated							
Ethinyl Estradiol/ Desogestrel							
Ethinyl Estradiol/ Drospirenone							
Ethinyl Estradiol/ Levonorgestrel							
Ethinyl Estradiol/ Norethindrone							
Ethinyl Estradiol/ Norgestimate							
Finasteride							
Fluconazole							
Tamsulosin HCl							
Testosterone							
Valacyclovir							

Using Therapeutic Agents for the Reproductive System

Objective: To review with the pharmacy technician dosage calculations and extemporaneous (non-sterile) compounding.

Lab Activity #24.3: Compounding a cream. Testosterone is on the NIOSH hazardous drug list and should therefore follow USP <800> guidelines when compounding in addition to USP <795> guidelines.

Prepare 1 oz of the following formula:

Testosterone	60 mg
Glycerin	qs
Dermabase cream	qs 30 g

Equipment needed:
- Calculator
- Pen
- Disinfecting agent/cleanser
- Sink with running hot and cold water
- Lint-free paper towels
- Personal protective equipment (PPE)
- Weighing boats or weighing papers
- Electronic balance or torsion balance with metric weights
- Spatulas
- Mortar card
- Ointment slab, parchment paper, or glass mortar and pestle
- Testosterone powder
- Glycerin
- Dermabase cream
- 1-oz ointment jar or tube for dispensing
- Label
- Auxiliary labels (including hazardous drug labels)
- Zippered plastic storage bag (if desired)

Procedure
1. Perform the necessary calculations for the prescription.
2. Gather all necessary supplies.
3. Ensure that equipment, supplies, and compounding area are clean and disinfected.
4. Organize materials on workbench.
5. Double check recipe and calculations.
6. Wash hands and dry thoroughly.
7. Put on PPE for compounding a hazardous drug.
8. Weigh testosterone powder on electronic balance or torsion balance inside approved hood for compounding with hazardous drugs.
9. Levigate testosterone powder with a few drops of glycerin to form a smooth paste.
10. Using geometric dilution and **S** pattern technique, incorporate Dermabase cream; qs to 30 g.
11. Check product for uniformity and appearance.
12. Using a zippered plastic storage bag, package the cream ensuring pharmaceutical elegance and weigh final packaged product.
13. Label product with all necessary information, including the levigating agent and auxiliary labels.
14. Document procedure and all necessary information on compounding log and controlled substance log.
15. Clean equipment and put away.
16. Clean work area.

Packaging: light-resistant container
Labeling: For external use only. Use only as directed. HD label warning.
BUD: Use USP <795> guidelines to determine BUD
Storage: Room temperature

Time needed to complete this activity: 45 minutes

Pharmacy Compounding Log					
Drug Name	**Manufacture**	**Mfg. Lot Number**	**Mfg. Expiration Date**	**Quantity Weighed/Measured**	**Technician Initials**

BUD assigned: _____

25 Therapeutic Agents for the Immune System

ASHP ACCREDITATION STANDARDS FOR PHARMACY TECHNICIAN EDUCATION AND TRAINING PROGRAMS

Standard 2.4: Describe wellness promotion and disease prevention concepts.
Standard 2.5: Demonstrate basic knowledge of anatomy, physiology and pharmacology, and medical terminology relevant to the pharmacy technician's role.
Standard 3.21: Explain accepted procedures in delivery and documentation of immunizations.
Standard 5.1: Describe and apply state and federal laws pertaining to processing, handling, and dispensing of medications including controlled substances.

REINFORCE KEY CONCEPTS

Terms and Definitions

Select the correct term from the following list and write the corresponding letter in the blank next to the statement.

A. Attenuated
B. Biological response modifier (BRM)
C. Hashimoto thyroiditis
D. Immunization
E. Juvenile rheumatoid arthritis (JRA)
F. Rheumatoid arthritis (RA)
G. Systemic lupus erythematosus (SLE)
H. Toxoids
I. Transplant rejection
J. Vaccine
K. Virion
L. Virus

_____ 1. A progressive degenerative and crippling autoimmune joint disease

_____ 2. An autoimmune disease leading to hypothyroidism

_____ 3. An immune response after tissue or organ transplantation

_____ 4. A virus particle

_____ 5. Rheumatoid arthritis that affects children

_____ 6. A term that describes an altered or weakened live vaccine made from the disease organism against which the vaccine protects

_____ 7. Vaccines in which toxins have been rendered harmless but still evoke an antigenic response, improving immunity against active toxins at some future date

_____ 8. A biological preparation that improves immunity to a particular disease by invoking an immune response and a "memory" of the response for future use

_____ 9. An autoimmune inflammatory disease of connective tissue with variable features, including fever, weakness, fatigue, and other systemic manifestations

_____ 10. An agent used to modify the body's immune response

_____ 11. A microscopic, nonliving organism that replicates exclusively inside the host's cell using parts of the host cell, including DNA, ribosomes, and proteins

_____ 12. The act of conferring immunity, such as with vaccination

Select the correct term from the following list and write the corresponding letter in the blank next to the statement.

A. Anaphylaxis
B. Hematopoiesis
C. Humoral immunity
D. Immunity
E. Inflammation
F. Innate immunity
G. Spleen
H. Systemic
I. Vasodilation

_____ 13. Natural immunity

_____ 14. An infection resistance type caused by the body's immune response after exposure to antigens or vaccine administration

_____ 15. Widening of the vasculature, leading to increased blood flow

_____ 16. Pertaining to the entire organism; "widespread" in contrast to "local"

_____ 17. The formation of blood cells

_____ 18. A localized physical condition associated with red, swollen, hot, and often painful tissue

_____ 19. The immune response mediated by antibodies

_____ 20. A lymphatic organ involved in blood cell production and removal as well as lymphocyte storage

_____ 21. An extreme, potentially life-threatening allergic reaction

Select the correct term from the following list and write the corresponding letter in the blank next to the statement.

A. Antibodies
B. Antigen
C. Antigen-presenting cell (APC)
D. Cytokine
E. Immunoglobulin
F. Leukocyte
G. Lymph node
H. Lymphocyte
I. Monocyte
J. Phagocyte
K. Plasma cell

_____ 22. A structure that consists of many small, oval nodules that filter lymphatic fluid and fight infection, the site of lymphocyte, monocyte, and plasma cell production

_____ 23. Complex molecules (immunoglobulins) made in response an antigen's presence that neutralize a foreign substance's effect

_____ 24. A white blood cell (WBC)

_____ 25. A protein that signals cells of the immune system

_____ 26. A cell of the immune system that engulfs cells, debris, and antigens

_____ 27. An antibody

_____ 28. A mononuclear leukocyte found in the blood, lymph, and lymphoid tissues

_____ 29. A cell of the immune system that secretes antibodies

_____ 30. A substance that prompts antibody production, resulting in an immune response

_____ 31. A phagocytic leukocyte

_____ 32. An immune system cell that presents antigens to lymphocytes to activate an immune response

True or False

Write T or F next to each statement.

_____ 1. The body has a built-in defense mechanism that helps protect it from invading organisms.

_____ 2. The thymus is much larger in adults than in children.

_____ 3. There are two types of immunity, inactive and passive.

_____ 4. Inflammation is a necessary response to injury.

_____ 5. Thyroid hormone replacement agents need to be taken for life due to the chronic nature of the condition.

_____ 6. Many hospitals require proof of childhood immunizations before hiring technicians or providing externships to technician students.

_____ 7. A vaccine is available for tuberculosis and is used in the United States because it guarantees immunity.

352

8. The two most common vaccines are activated and live-attenuated vaccines.

9. Immunizations for diseases caused by a parasite, such as malaria, and fungal infections have been developed and are available.

10. Most vaccines should be kept in the refrigerator.

System Identifier

Identify each component of the lymphatic system and enter the term next to the corresponding number.

1. _____

2. _____

3. _____

4. _____

5. _____

6. _____

Multiple Choice

Complete each question by circling the best answer.

1. All the following can be used as a treatment for systemic lupus erythematosus (SLE) *except*:
   A. Gengraf (cyclosporine)
   B. Trexall (methotrexate)
   C. Tapazole (methimazole)
   D. Benlysta (belimumab)

2. Which of the following may be given to help treat rheumatoid arthritis and juvenile rheumatoid arthritis?
   A. propylthiouracil
   B. Orencia (abatacept)
   C. Tapazole (methimazole)
   D. Rapamune (sirolimus)

3. Therapy for Graves's disease includes:
   A. propylthiouracil
   B. radioactive iodine
   C. Tapazole (methimazole)
   D. All of the above

4. To help prevent kidney transplant rejection, _____ can be given intravenously every four weeks.
   A. Nulojix (belatacept)
   B. Tysabri (natalizumab)
   C. Rapamune (sirolimus)
   D. Copaxone (glatiramer)

5. Varicella, MMR, and hepatitis B are all examples of which type of vaccine?
   A. Immune globulin
   B. Antivenins
   C. Viral
   D. Toxoids

6. _____ is a conjugated vaccine in which bacterial cells that have been altered and mixed with toxoids to increase their overall effectiveness.
   A. Rabies
   B. Tetanus and diphtheria
   C. Polio
   D. Japanese encephalitis

7. _____ is a subunit vaccine that is grown in yeast cells and then is given as a vaccine.
   A. Hepatitis B
   B. Influenza
   C. Yellow fever
   D. Rotavirus

8. Which of the following is an acellular vaccine?
   A. Pertussis
   B. Tetanus
   C. Diphtheria
   D. Varicella

9. _____ is a newer type of vaccine that is based on using an antibody that is shaped like the antigen, which can make it possible to kill deadly viruses such as human immunodeficiency virus.
   A. Transplant vaccine
   B. Subunit vaccine
   C. Antiidiotypic vaccine
   D. Acellular vaccine

10. To help treat multiple sclerosis, _____ can be given once weekly by intramuscular injection.
   A. Campath (alemtuzumab)
   B. Rebif (interferon beta-1a)
   C. Benlysta (belimumab)
   D. Avonex (interferon beta-1a)

11. Which of the following medications can be taken for prophylaxis of kidney transplant rejection?
   A. Rapamune (sirolimus)
   B. Orencia (abatacept)
   C. Tapazole (methimazole)
   D. Cimzia (certolizumab pegol)

12. Drug therapy for rheumatoid arthritis includes all the following medications *except*
   A. Humira (adalimumab)
   B. Benlysta (belimumab)
   C. Trexall (methotrexate)
   D. Enbrel (etanercept)

Fill in the Blanks

Answer each question by completing the statement in the space provided.

1. Mast cells contain _____, which they release during an allergic response.

Matching

Match the following trade and generic drug names.

_____ 1. CellCept

_____ 2. Imuran

_____ 3. Prograf

_____ 4. Sandimmune

_____ 5. Rapamune

_____ 6. Copaxone

_____ 7. Humira

_____ 8. Orencia

_____ 9. Avonex

_____ 10. Enbrel

A. glatiramer
B. interferon beta-1a
C. tacrolimus
D. mycophenolate
E. etanercept
F. adalimumab
G. azathioprine
H. abatacept
I. sirolimus
J. cyclosporine

2. Individuals who know they can suffer anaphylactic shock from a bee sting or other allergic reaction should always carry an _____ autoinjector in case they are stung or have an allergic exposure.

3. Treatment approaches to rheumatoid arthritis (RA) target both symptomatic management and _____ of joint destruction and disability.

4. Physicians often prescribe _____ for Hashimoto's thyroiditis because of its ease of dosing.

5. To avoid _____ rejection, health providers use immunosuppressive drugs to suppress the immune system and keep the organ viable.

6. The _____ contains important information about the vaccine and its potential side effects and must be available by law for certain vaccinations.

7. The disadvantage of using killed or inactive _____ in a vaccine is that booster shots are needed to maintain a sufficient level of antibodies to prevent disease.

8. Tetanus booster immunizations should be given every _____ years throughout a person's lifetime.

9. The varicella vaccine should be kept _____ until the time of use.

10. Antivenins counteract _____ from creatures such as snakes and spiders.

Match the following vaccine with their availability as a live or inactivated vaccine.

_____ 11. Adenovirus

_____ 12. Anthrax

_____ 13. DTaP

_____ 14. *Haemophilus influenzae* type b

_____ 15. Hepatitis A

_____ 16. Hepatitis B

_____ 17. Herpes zoster (Zostavax)

_____ 18. Herpes zoster (Shingrix)

_____ 19. Human papillomavirus

_____ 20. Measles, mumps, rubella (MMR)

_____ 21. Polio

_____ 22. Rabies

_____ 23. Rotavirus

_____ 24. Varicella

_____ 25. Yellow fever

A. Live
B. Inactivated
C. Non-live recombinant

Short Answer

Reply to each question based on what you have learned in the chapter.

1. List the vaccine available for herpes zoster (shingles) and who may receive the vaccine.

   _____

   _____

2. List three types of vaccines for meningitis and who may receive each type.

   _____

   _____

   _____

3. List two types of vaccines for pneumonia and who may receive each type.

   _____

   _____

4. List the vaccine(s) that are recommended for those in the military.

   _____

   _____

5. List the CDC guidelines for refrigerator temperature for storage of vaccines.

   _____

6. List the antivenins for the black widow spider and rattle snake venom.

   _____

   _____

355

Research Activities

Follow the instructions given in each exercise and provide a response.

1. Access the website *http://wwwnc.cdc.gov/travel/*.

   A. Choose a country to travel to and list the vaccines you will need to receive before going on your trip.

   B. Choose one of the Travel Health Notices posted. List the necessary precautions you would need to take if you were planning to travel there.

2. Access the website *http://www.cdc.gov/vaccines/vac-gen/shortages/default.htm*. List any vaccine delay or shortage. For each one listed, what is the anticipated date of availability?

3. Access the website *https://www2a.cdc.gov/vaccines/statevaccsApp/default.asp*.

   A. What vaccinations does your state require hospital employees to have?

   B. What vaccinations does your state require hospital inpatients to be offered?

   C. What vaccinations does your state require ambulatory care employees to have?

D. Does your state allow for opting out of receiving vaccinations? If so, in what circumstances may one opt out?

REFLECT CRITICALLY

Critical Thinking

Reply to each question based on what you have learned in the chapter.

1. Human immunodeficiency virus (HIV) infection can be a devastating disease. What type of lymphocyte is most important for patients with HIV infection? Why?

2. In the United States, sanitization and hygiene are stressed, yet people still frequently become ill. Does constant sanitization bring about a healthier immune system or does it weaken it?

3. The World Health Organization (WHO) has been working tirelessly to eradicate infectious diseases throughout the world, with much success. What would happen to the planet's population if all infectious diseases were eradicated and vaccinations were not needed?

4. Many people decide every year to not receive the flu vaccine because "they always get the flu when they get the vaccine." What could you say to help convince them that they are unable to get the flu from the vaccine? List reasons why they may still come down with the flu even though they received the vaccine.

356

Lab Scenarios

Therapeutic Agents for the Immune System

Objective: To review with the pharmacy technician terms associated with the components of the immune system and review the brand and generic names, indications, dosage forms, routes of administration, and recommended daily dosage of medications used to treat disorders of the immune system

---

DID YOU KNOW?

- Not all children between the ages of 19 and 35 months have received the necessary vaccinations: 83% received diphtheria, tetanus, and pertussis vaccine; 93% received the polio vaccine; 92% received the MMR vaccine; 91% received the varicella vaccine.
- 1.5 million adults suffer from rheumatoid arthritis, with women two to three times as likely to be affected than men.
- Juvenile arthritis is prevalent around the world affecting two children per 1000.
- Women are at greater risk for developing systemic lupus erythematosus between the age of 15 to 44, with 15% to 20% of the cases being diagnosed before the age of 18.

References:

https://www.arthritis.org/getmedia/e1256607-fa87-4593-aa8a-8db4f291072a/2019-abtn-final-march-2019.pdf
https://www.cdc.gov/nchs/fastats/immunize.htm

Lab Activity #25.1: Define the following terms associated with the immune system.

Equipment needed:
- Medical dictionary
- Pencil/pen

Time needed to complete this activity: 30 minutes

1. Acquired immunity _____

2. Autoimmune disease _____

3. Hypersensitivity _____

4. Immunodeficiency _____

5. Immunosuppression _____

6. Multiple sclerosis (MS) _____

7. Severe combined immunodeficiency

_____

Lab Activity #25.2: Using a drug reference book, identify the generic name, drug classification, indications, dosage forms, routes of administration, and recommended daily dosage of the *most common* medications used to treat conditions affecting the immune system.

Equipment needed:
- *Drug Facts & Comparisons* or *Physicians' Desk Reference*
- Pencil/pen

Time needed to complete this activity: 60 minutes

Generic Name	Brand Name	Classification	Indications(s)	Dosage Form(s)	Route(s)	Recommended Daily Dosage	Auxiliary Label(s)
Abatacept							
Adalimumab							
Anakinra							
Azathioprine							

Continued

Generic Name	Brand Name	Classification	Indications(s)	Dosage Form(s)	Route(s)	Recommended Daily Dosage	Auxiliary Label(s)
Belatacept							
Belimumab							
Certolizumab							
Cyclosporine							
Dexamethasone							
Etanercept							
Everolimus							
Glatiramer acetate							
Golimumab							
Hydroxychloroquine sulfate							
Infliximab							
Interferon beta-1b							
Interferon beta-1a							
Methotrexate							
Mycophenolate mofetil							

Chapter 25 Therapeutic Agents for the Immune System

Generic Name	Brand Name	Classification	Indications(s)	Dosage Form(s)	Route(s)	Recommended Daily Dosage	Auxiliary Label(s)
Natalizumab							
Prednisolone							
Prednisone							
Rituximab							
Sirolimus							
Tacrolimus							

Using Therapeutic Agents for the Immune System

Objective: To introduce the pharmacy technician to the use of vaccines in the practice of pharmacy

Lab Activity #25.3: Using the Centers for Disease Control and Prevention website, *https://www.cdc.gov/flu*, answer the following questions regarding seasonal influenza.

Equipment needed:
■ Computer with Internet connection
■ Paper
■ Pencil/pen

Time needed to complete this activity: 45 minutes

1. Who should be vaccinated for seasonal influenza?

   _____

   _____

   _____

2. What are some of the symptoms of seasonal influenza?

   _____

   _____

   _____

3. Who is at risk for contracting the flu?

   _____

   _____

   _____

4. How does the flu spread from individual to individual?

   _____

   _____

   _____

   _____

5. What are three ways to protect one from getting seasonal influenza?

   _____

   _____

   _____

   _____

6. What is the composition of the current flu vaccine?

_____

_____

_____

7. At what temperature should the flu vaccine be stored?

_____

_____

_____

8. Which month do we experience the greatest number of cases of the flu?

_____

9. What antiviral medications may be used in the treatment of seasonal influenza?

_____

10. Complete the following table:

Trade Name	Manufacturer	Presentation	Mercury Content	Age Group	Number of Doses	Route of Administration	Storage Requirement
Fluzone Quadrivalent							
Fluzone High-Dose Trivalent							
Fluzone Intradermal Quadrivalent							
Fluvirin Trivalent							
Fluarix Quadrivalent							
FluLaval Quadrivalent							

360

Trade Name	Manufacturer	Presentation	Mercury Content	Age Group	Number of Doses	Route of Administration	Storage Requirement
Fluad Trivalent							
Flubok Trivalent							
Flucelvax Quadrivalent							
FluMist							
Afluria Quadrivalent							
Afluria Trivalent							

11. A 66-year-old female patient comes to your pharmacy requesting a flu vaccine. Which flu vaccine(s) could the patient receive?

_____

12. A 34-year-old male patient comes to your pharmacy requesting a flu vaccine. He informs you he is allergic to eggs. Which vaccine(s) could the patient received?

_____

13. A 17-year-old female patient comes to your pharmacy with his parent requesting a flu vaccine. The parent informs you she is allergic to eggs. Which vaccine(s) could the patient receive?

_____

14. Visit the website *https://www.cdc.gov/vaccines/hcp/vis/current-vis.html* and locate the VIS required to give the patient when receiving the flu vaccine. Where can a patient report an adverse reaction to the vaccine?

_____

Objective: Obtain information on immunization training requirements within your state.

Lab Activity #25.4: Use the Internet to research information on the criteria to immunize patients in your state at a community pharmacy and complete the following table.

Equipment needed:
■ Computer with Internet connection
■ Pencil/pen

Time needed to complete this activity: 30 minutes

What is the name of your state?	
Who may immunize pharmacy patients?	
What immunizations may they perform?	
What age group may be immunized at the pharmacy? List any restrictions or special circumstances.	
Describe the training required to be able to immunize a patient.	
Does an individual require clinical training before being permitted to immunize patients?	
Does an individual need to register with a regulatory agency in the state? If yes, which agency?	
Does an individual need to be licensed to immunize patients?	
What does it cost to be able to immunize patients?	
Does an individual need continuing education for the renewal of his or her registration or license? If so, how many CEUs are needed annually?	

Objective: Retail pharmacy visit.

Lab Activity #25.5: Visit a retail pharmacy that offers flu shots or other immunizations to their patients. Ask for a copy of the paperwork that the patient must fill out before receiving an immunization.

Equipment needed:
- None

Time needed to complete this activity: 30 minutes

1. Compare and contrast the information found on the sheet with other members of your class. What is the same? What is different?

   _____

   _____

   _____

   _____

2. Does medical or prescription drug coverage pay for the immunization?

   _____

   _____

   _____

3. What documentation must the pharmacy keep and for how long?

   _____

   _____

   _____

Lab Activity #25.6: Use the Centers for Disease Control and Prevention (CDC) website *https://www.cdc.gov/vaccines/* to identify the generic name, indications, contraindications, adverse effects, and the routes of administration of the vaccines listed in the following table.

Equipment needed:
- Computer with Internet connection
- Pencil/pen

Time needed to complete this activity: 60 minutes

Brand (Trade) Name	Generic Name	Indication	List Two Contraindications	List Five Adverse Effects	Routes of Administration	Storage Requirements	Can It Be Administered at the Pharmacy?
Adacel							
BioThrax							
Boostrix							
Daptacel							
Dryvax							
Engerix-B							
Gardasil							
Havrix							
Imovax Rabies							
Infanrix							
IPOL							
Ixiaro							
JE-VAX							
Kinrix							

Continued

Chapter **25** **Therapeutic Agents for the Immune System**

Brand (Trade) Name	Generic Name	Indication	List Two Contraindications	List Five Adverse Effects	Routes of Administration	Storage Requirements	Can It Be Administered at the Pharmacy?
Menactra							
Menomune							
Menveo							
M-M-R II							
Pediarix							
Pentacel							
Pneumovax 23							
Prevnar							
ProQuad							
Recombivax HB							
Rotarix							
Shingrix							
Twinrix							
Varivax							

Brand (Trade) Name	Generic Name	Indication	List Two Contraindications	List Five Adverse Effects	Routes of Administration	Storage Requirements	Can It Be Adminis- tered at the Pharmacy?
Vivotif							
YF-Vax							
Zostavax							

26 Therapeutic Agents for the Eyes, Ears, Nose, and Throat

ASHP ACCREDITATION STANDARDS FOR PHARMACY TECHNICIAN EDUCATION AND TRAINING PROGRAMS

Standard 2.5: Demonstrate basic knowledge of anatomy, physiology and pharmacology, and medical terminology relevant to the pharmacy technician's role.

Standard 3.1: Assist pharmacists in collecting, organizing, and recording demographic and clinical information for the Pharmacists; Patient Care Process.

Standard 3.2: Receive, process, and prepare prescriptions/medication orders for completeness, accuracy, and authenticity to ensure safety.

Standard 5.1: Describe and apply state and federal laws pertaining to processing, handling, and dispensing of medications including controlled substances.

REINFORCE KEY CONCEPTS

Terms and Definitions

Select the correct term from the following list and write the corresponding letter in the blank next to the statement.

A. Bactericidal
B. Bacteriostatic
C. Carbonic anhydrase
D. Fungicidal
E. Miosis
F. Mydriasis
G. Ophthalmic
H. Otic
I. Sympathomimetic

_____ 1. Inhibits bacterial cell growth

_____ 2. Able to destroy or inhibit the growth of fungi

_____ 3. Dilation of the pupil

_____ 4. Pertaining to the ear

_____ 5. Causes bacterial cell death

_____ 6. Producing physiological effects resembling those caused by the sympathetic nervous system

_____ 7. Pertaining to the eye

_____ 8. Contraction of the pupil

_____ 9. An enzyme that converts carbonic acid into carbon dioxide and water

Select the correct term from the following list and write the corresponding letter in the blank next to the statement.

A. Cerumen
B. Exudate
C. Glomerulonephritis
D. Intraocular pressure (IOP)
E. Myopia
F. Ototoxicity
G. Rheumatic fever
H. Tinnitus

_____ 10. Earwax

_____ 11. A noncontagious acute fever marked by inflammation and pain in the joints

_____ 12. Nearsightedness

_____ 13. Acute inflammation of the kidney, typically caused by an immune response

_____ 14. Ringing or buzzing in the ears

_____ 15. The pressure exerted by the fluids inside the eyeball

_____ 16. Toxic effects on the organs of hearing or balance or the auditory nerve

_____ 17. A mass of cells and fluid that has seeped out of blood vessels because of inflammation

366

Select the correct term from the following list and write the corresponding letter in the blank next to the statement.

A. Auditory canal
B. Auditory ossicles
C. Auricle
D. Eustachian tube
E. Larynx
F. Pharynx
G. Tympanic membrane

_____ 18. The outer projecting portion of the ear

_____ 19. The membrane-lined cavity behind the nose and mouth that connects them to the esophagus

_____ 20. A 1-inch segment of the tube that extends from the external ear to the middle ear

_____ 21. A structure in the middle ear that connects with the nasopharynx (throat); it equalizes pressure between the outside air and middle ear and drains mucus

_____ 22. A thin membrane that separates the external ear from the middle ear; also known as the eardrum

_____ 23. Small bones of the middle ear that transmit sound from the eardrum to the inner ear

_____ 24. A hollow muscular organ that forms an air passage to the lungs and holds the vocal cords

Select the correct term from the following list and write the corresponding letter in the blank next to the statement.

A. Aqueous humor
B. Ciliary body
C. Conjunctiva
D. Cornea
E. Iris
F. Lacrimal fluid
G. Lens
H. Orbit
I. Pupil
J. Retina
K. Sclera
L. Vitreous humor

_____ 25. The transparent tissue covering the anterior portion of the eye

_____ 26. The white of the eyes

_____ 27. The part of the eye that connects the iris to the choroid

_____ 28. The eye socket

_____ 29. The fluid in the eye that cleans and lubricates the eyes

_____ 30. A gel-like substance that fills the posterior cavity of the eye between the lens and retina; it helps maintain the shape of the eye

_____ 31. The fluid found in the anterior chamber of the eye, in front of the lens

_____ 32. The circular opening in the iris that allows light to enter

_____ 33. The colored part of the eye seen through the cornea; it consists of smooth muscles that regulate pupil size

_____ 34. The innermost layer of the eye; a complex structure considered part of the CNS; contains photoreceptors that transmit impulses to the optic nerve, in addition to the macula lutea

_____ 35. The transparent protective mucous membrane that lines the underside of the eyelid

_____ 36. Flexible, clear tissue that focuses images

True or False

Write T or F next to each statement.

_____ 1. Keeping eye solutions sterile is imperative because foreign objects instilled into the eyes can cause damage or infection.

_____ 2. Fungal conjunctivitis is very common.

_____ 3. The best way to avoid conjunctivitis is by washing hands before touching eyes.

_____ 4. Patients should not remove contact lenses before instilling most medications.

_____ 5. Glaucoma can cause blindness.

_____ 6. The human ear is only responsible for hearing, balance, and equilibrium.

_____ 7. Antibiotics are effective against viral ear infections.

_____ 8. Otic medicines can be used in eyes because they are sterile.

367

9. Individuals who use saline irrigations to treat sinusitis should use sterile or bottled water to prepare the saline rinse.

_____ 10. An ophthalmic medication is commonly prescribed to treat an otic condition.

System Identifier

Identify the components of the eye and eyelid and enter the term next to the corresponding number.

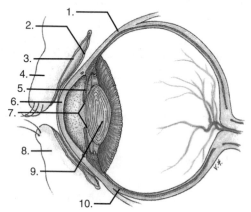

From Potter PA, Perry AG: Fundamentals of nursing, ed 8, St Louis, 2013, Mosby

1. _____
2. _____
3. _____
4. _____
5. _____
6. _____
7. _____
8. _____
9. _____
10. _____

Identify the components of the ear *and enter the term next to the corresponding number.*

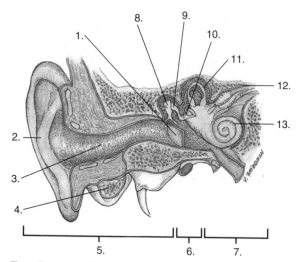

From Potter PA, Perry AG: Fundamentals of nursing, ed 8, St Louis, 2013, Mosby

1. _____
2. _____
3. _____
4. _____
5. _____
6. _____
7. _____
8. _____
9. _____
10. _____
11. _____
12. _____
13. _____

Multiple Choice

Complete each question by circling the best answer.

1. A person who is trained to perform an eye examination is called an:
   A. Optician
   B. Optometrist
   C. Optimist
   D. Ophthalmologist

2. Agents indicated for the treatment of glaucoma include all the following *except*:
   A. Miostat (carbachol)
   B. Xalatan (latanoprost)
   C. Azopt (brinzolamide)
   D. Bleph-10 (sulfacetamide)

3. Glaucoma is caused by:
   A. Viral infections
   B. Bacterial infections
   C. Increased pressure within the eye
   D. Allergies

4. Which of the following is *not* a cause of conjunctivitis?
   A. Virus
   B. Bacterial infections
   C. Postoperative ocular inflammation
   D. Allergies

5. Which drug would be indicated for allergic conjunctivitis?
   A. Patanol (olopatadine)
   B. Tobrex (tobramycin)
   C. Travatan (travoprost)
   D. Isopto-Carpine (pilocarpine)

6. Xalatan should be stored in the refrigerator until opened and, once opened, it may be stored at room temperature for _____
   A. 2 weeks
   B. 4 weeks
   C. 6 weeks
   D. 6 months

7. Which of the following is a prescription product that can alleviate chronic dry eyes caused by inflammation?
   A. Restasis (cyclosporine)
   B. Betoptic-S (betaxolol)
   C. Alphagan P (brimonidine)
   D. Visine (tetrahydrozoline)

8. Which of the following is used for the treatment of allergy symptoms?
   A. Restasis (cyclosporine)
   B. Betagan (levobunolol)
   C. Azopt (brinzolamide)
   D. Chlor-Trimeton (chlorpheniramine)

9. Which of the following anti-infectives is associated with ototoxicity?
   A. vancomycin
   B. azithromycin
   C. amoxicillin
   D. sulfacetamide

10. Which of the following is used to treat fungal infections?
    A. Viroptic (trifluridine)
    B. Natacyn (natamycin)
    C. Polytrim (polymyxin B/trimethoprim)
    D. Vigamox (moxifloxacin)

Fill in the Blanks

Answer each question by completing the statement in the space provided.

1. Health providers use mast cell stabilizers, antihistamines, and decongestants for _____ _____ treatment.

2. Corticosteroids relieve _____ from infection, allergies, or injury.

3. Viruses, bacteria, fungi, or allergies cause _____, an acute conjunctival inflammation known as "pink eye."

4. The three most common _____ eye infections are herpes simplex, keratitis, and viral conjunctivitis.

5. Drugs that reduce aqueous humor or IOP help _____ patients.

6. Aminoglycosides in high doses for extended periods are notable for _____.

7. Using ophthalmic agents in the ear is acceptable because ophthalmic preparations are _____

8. The prognosis for bacterial sinusitis is good with _____ therapy, rest, and hydration.

9. Amoxicillin is a first-line therapy for bacterial sinusitis because of low cost and a _____ antimicrobial spectrum.

10. Streptococcal tonsillopharyngitis (strep throat) is a bacterial throat infection associated with an abrupt onset of throat pain, fever, and exudate from the tonsils that can be treated with _____

Matching

Match the following trade and generic drug names.

_____ 1. Trusopt

_____ 2. Xalatan

_____ 3. Voltaren Ophtha

_____ 4. Travatan Z

_____ 5. Tobrex

_____ 6. Alphagan P

_____ 7. Timoptic

_____ 8. Zymaxid

_____ 9. Neo-Synephrine

_____ 10. Allegra

A. latanoprost
B. travoprost
C. tobramycin
D. dorzolamide
E. diclofenac
F. phenylephrine
G. gatifloxacin
H. fexofenadine
I. brimonidine
J. timolol

Match the following medications or products with the conditions they treat.

_____ 11. Boro-Packs (acetic acid/aluminum acetate)

_____ 12. Zaditor (ketotifen)

_____ 13. Auraphene-B (carbamide peroxide)

_____ 14. erythromycin

_____ 15. Ceftin (cefuroxime)

A. Allergy of the eyes
B. Otitis media
C. Eye infection
D. Ear wax removal
E. Swimmer's ear

Match the following medications with their drug classification.

_____ 16. Lumigan (bimatoprost)

_____ 17. Betagan (levobunolol)

_____ 18. Azopt (brinzolamide)

_____ 19. Viroptic (trifluridine)

_____ 20. PredForte (prednisolone)

_____ 21. Isopto Carpine (pilocarpine)

_____ 22. Opticrom (cromolyn)

_____ 23. Acular (ketorolac)

_____ 24. Genoptic (gentamicin)

_____ 25. Afrin (oxymetazoline)

A. Antiviral
B. Cholinergic agonist
C. Beta-adrenergic blocker
D. Mast cell stabilizer
E. NSAID
F. Prostaglandin agonist
G. Aminoglycoside antibiotic
H. Corticosteroid
I. Adrenergic agonist
J. Carbonic anhydrase inhibitor

Short Answer

Reply to each question based on what you have learned in the chapter.

1. List two ways those with allergies can minimize symptoms without drug therapy.

   _____

   _____

2. List the side effects of ophthalmic antiviral medications.

   _____

   _____

3. List several ways to help avoid conjunctivitis.

   _____

   _____

4. List available ophthalmic dosage forms for treating glaucoma.

   _____

   _____

5. List five drug classifications that treat glaucoma.

   _____

   _____

6. In addition to anti-infectives, list other types of medications that may be used to treat the symptoms of otitis media.

   _____

   _____

7. In addition to antibiotic therapy, list other medications that can be used for symptom management of bacterial sinusitis.

   _____

   _____

Research Activities

Follow the instructions given in each exercise and provide a response.

1. Visit a local pharmacy and locate the eye- and ear-care sections.

   A. What is the active ingredient in most OTC eye drops?

   B. What is the active ingredient in most OTC ear drops?

   C. What is the active ingredient in nasal saline spray?

2. Access the website *http://www.glaucoma.org/research/*. What are the latest developments in the treatment of glaucoma?

REFLECT CRITICALLY

Critical Thinking

Reply to each question based on what you have learned in the chapter.

1. You have been working in the intravenous (IV) room all day and your eyes are feeling very dry. What is the reason for your "dry eyes" and what can you do to resolve the situation?

2. Night blindness is often caused by a lack of vitamin A. What food(s) can you eat to help prevent night blindness?

3. Your child came home from school with "pink eye." How can you prevent yourself from getting this contagious eye infection?

4. Why is sodium chloride (NaCl) an ingredient in every artificial tear product?

5. How is having an inner ear infection different from having a middle ear infection?

RELATE TO PRACTICE

Lab Scenarios
Therapeutic Agents for the Eyes, Ears, Nose, and Throat

Objective: To review with the pharmacy technician terms associated with the eyes, ears, nose, and throat and review the brand and generic names, indications, dosage forms, routes of administration, and recommended daily dosage of medications used to treat disorders affecting the eyes, ears, nose, and throat.

DID YOU KNOW?

- Glaucoma is the leading cause of blindness in the United States and second-leading cause in the world.
- Approximately 3 million Americans have glaucoma and are not aware of it.
- More than 10 million physician visits are made yearly for glaucoma.

Reference:
https://www.glaucoma.org/glaucoma/glaucoma-facts-and-stats.php

Lab Activity #26.1: Define the following terms associated with the eyes, ears, nose, and throat.

Equipment needed:
- Medical dictionary
- Pencil/pen

Time needed to complete this activity: 30 minutes

1. Auralgia _____

2. Blepharitis _____

3. Closed-angle glaucoma _____

4. Conjunctivitis _____

5. Cytomegalovirus _____

6. Herpes simplex keratitis _____

7. Herpes zoster ophthalmicus _____

8. Iritis _____

9. Keratitis _____

10. Ocular toxoplasmosis _____

11. Open-angle glaucoma _____

12. Otalgia _____

13. Otitis externa _____

14. Otitis media _____

15. Otorrhea _____

16. Otosclerosis _____

17. Photopsia _____

18. Stye _____

19. Uveitis _____

20. Vertigo _____

Lab Activity #26.2: Using a drug reference book, identify the generic name, drug classification, indications, dosage forms, routes of administration, and recommended daily dosage of the *most common* medications used to treat conditions affecting the eyes, ears, nose, and throat.

Equipment needed:
- *Drug Facts & Comparisons* or *Physicians' Desk Reference*
- Pencil/pen

Time needed to complete this activity: 60 minutes

Generic Name	Brand (Trade) Name	Classification	Indication	Dosage Forms Available	Routes of Administration	Recommended Daily Dosage	Auxiliary Label(s)
Amoxicillin							
Amoxicillin/Clavulanate potassium							
Antipyrine/benzocaine							
Azithromycin							
Bimatoprost							
Brimonidine							
Cefdinir							
Ciprofloxacin							
Cyclosporine							
Dorzolamide							
Latanoprost							
Olopatadine							
Scopolamine							

Continued

Generic Name	Brand (Trade) Name	Classification	Indication	Dosage Forms Available	Routes of Administration	Recommended Daily Dosage	Auxiliary Label(s)
Timolol							
Tobramycin/dexa-methasone							
Travoprost							

Using Therapeutic Agents for the Eyes, Ears, Nose, and Throat

Objective: To review with the pharmacy technician prescription orders, dosage calculations, and reconstituting a solid

Lab Activity #26.3: Answer the questions based on the prescription orders for each question.

Equipment needed:
- *Drug Facts and Comparisons* or *Physician's Desk Reference*
- Pencil/pen
- Calculator

Time needed to complete this activity: 30 minutes

The following are approved DAW codes:
- DAW 0: no product selection indicated
- DAW 1: substitution not allowed by provider
- DAW 2: substitution allowed: patient requested product dispensed
- DAW 3: substitution allowed: pharmacist selected product dispensed
- DAW 4: substitution allowed: generic drug not in stock
- DAW 5: substitution allowed: brand drug dispensed as generic
- DAW 6: override
- DAW 7: substitution not allowed: brand drug mandated by law
- DAW 8: substitution allowed: generic drug not available in marketplace
- DAW 9: other

1. Rx 1:
   Ciloxan Ophthalmic Solution, 10 mL
   gtts i to ii ou q2h while awake ×2d, gtts i to ii q4h while awake ×5d

   A. How much will be dispensed (use metric quantities)?

   _____

   B. How many days will the medication last?

   _____

   C. How many refills are permitted on the prescription?

   _____

   D. What DAW code will be used?

   _____

   E. Write directions as they would appear on the medication label.

   _____

   _____

   F. What auxiliary label(s) should be affixed to the medication label?

   _____

   _____

   _____

2. Rx 2:
   A/B Otic Solution, 10 mL
   gtts iii to v q2h prn p
   Ref:

   A. How much will be dispensed (use metric quantities)?

   _____

   B. How many days will the medication last?

   _____

   C. How many refills are permitted on the prescription?

   _____

   D. What DAW code will be used?

   _____

   E. Write directions as they would appear on the medication label.

   _____

   _____

   F. What auxiliary label(s) should be affixed to the medication label?

   _____

   _____

   _____

3. Rx 3:
   Vigamox, 3 mL
   gtts i os tid x7d
   Ref:

   A. How much will be dispensed (use metric quantities)?

   _____

   B. How many days will the medication last?

   _____

   C. How many refills are permitted on the prescription?

   _____

   D. What DAW code will be used?

   _____

E. Write directions as they would appear on the medication label.

_____

_____

F. What auxiliary label(s) should be affixed to the medication label?

_____

_____

_____

4. Rx 4:
   Ocuflox ophthalmic solution, 5 mL
   i – ii gtts ou q2-4h x2 days, then qid x5 days
   Ref:

   A. How much will be dispensed (use metric quantities)?

   _____

   B. How many days will the medication last?

   _____

   C. How many refills are permitted on the prescription?

   _____

   D. What DAW code will be used?

   _____

   E. Write directions as they would appear on the medication label.

   _____

   _____

   F. What auxiliary label(s) should be affixed to the medication label?

   _____

   _____

   _____

5. Rx 5:
   Azopt 1% ophthalmic suspension, 2.5 mL
   gtt i od tid
   Ref ×2

   A. How much will be dispensed (use metric quantities)?

   _____

   B. How many days will the medication last?

   _____

   C. How many refills are permitted on the prescription?

   _____

   D. What DAW code will be used?

   _____

   E. Write directions as they would appear on the medication label.

   _____

   _____

   F. What auxiliary label(s) should be affixed to the medication label?

   _____

   _____

   _____

6. Rx 6:
   Lumigan 0.03% ophthalmic solution, 2.5 mL
   gtt i ou qpm
   Ref ×1

   A. How much will be dispensed (use metric quantities)?

   _____

   B. How many days will the medication last?

   _____

   C. How many refills are permitted on the prescription?

   _____

   D. What DAW code will be used?

   _____

E. Write directions as they would appear on the medication label.

   _____

   _____

F. What auxiliary label(s) should be affixed to the medication label?

   _____

   _____

   _____

7. Rx 7:
   Emadine, 5 mL
   gtt i ou up to 4x/day
   Ref ×5

   A. How much will be dispensed (use metric quantities)?

   _____

   B. How many days will the medication last?

   _____

   C. How many refills are permitted on the prescription?

   _____

   D. What DAW code will be used?

   _____

   E. Write directions as they would appear on the medication label.

   _____

   _____

   F. What auxiliary label(s) should be affixed to the medication label?

   _____

   _____

   _____

8. Rx 8:
   Timoptic ophthalmic solution, 10 mL
   gtt i ou bid
   Ref ×3

   A. How much will be dispensed (use metric quantities)?

   _____

   B. How many days will the medication last?

   _____

   C. How many refills are permitted on the prescription?

   _____

   D. What DAW code will be used?

   _____

   E. Write directions as they would appear on the medication label.

   _____

   _____

   F. What auxiliary label(s) should be affixed to the medication label?

   _____

   _____

9. Rx 9:
   Genoptic, 5 mL
   gtt ii ou q4h
   Ref:

   A. How much will be dispensed (use metric quantities)?

   _____

   B. How many days will the medication last?

   _____

   C. How many refills are permitted on the prescription?

   _____

   D. What DAW code will be used?

   _____

E. Write directions as they would appear on the medication label.

   _____

   _____

F. What auxiliary label(s) should be affixed to the medication label?

   _____

   _____

10. Rx 10:
    Xalatan, 2.5 mL
    gtt i ou qpm
    Ref ×6
    Patient Has Requested Brand Name

    A. How much will be dispensed (use metric quantities)?

    _____

    B. How many days will the medication last?

    _____

    C. How many refills are permitted on the prescription?

    _____

    D. What DAW code will be used?

    _____

    E. Write directions as they would appear on the medication label.

    _____

    _____

    F. Where should this medication be stored?

    _____

    G. What auxiliary label(s) should be affixed to the medication label?

    _____

    _____

Lab Activity #26.4: Reconstituting an antibiotic.

Equipment needed:
- Pen
- Calculator

Time needed to complete this activity: 20 minutes

Answer the questions based on the following prescription order:

Dr. Jack Davidson
2145 Main Street
St. Louis, MO 63144
314-987-0100

Name: Daniel Davis   Date: July 16, 202X

Address: 210 Anywhere St., St. Louis, MO   DOB: May 20, 2012

Rx: Amoxicillin Suspension
         200 mg bid × 10d for ear infection

Refills: none   Jack Davidson, MD

                                                     DEA no _____

---

1. You have the following in stock at your pharmacy, which one should you choose?

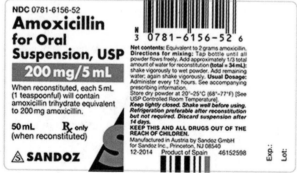

A.

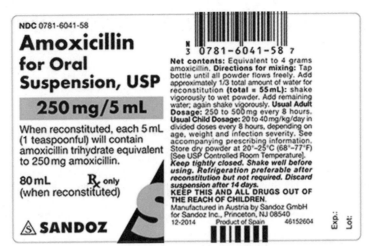

B.

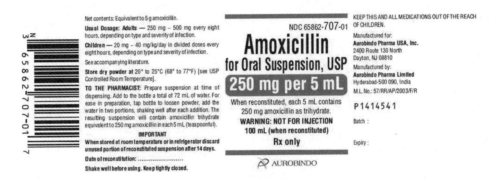

C.

2. How many milliliters of amoxicillin 250 mg/5 mL suspension will the patient take at each dose?

_____

3. How many milliliters of water are necessary to reconstitute this medication?

_____

4. How should this medication be stored after reconstitution?

_____

5. After how many days should this medication be discarded after reconstitution?

_____

6. What auxiliary labels should be placed on the medication?

_____

Chapter **26** **Therapeutic Agents for the Eyes, Ears, Nose, and Throat**

27 Therapeutic Agents for the Dermatologic System

ASHP ACCREDITATION STANDARDS FOR PHARMACY TECHNICIAN EDUCATION AND TRAINING PROGRAMS

Standard 2.5: Demonstrate basic knowledge of anatomy, physiology and pharmacology, and medical terminology relevant to the pharmacy technician's role.

Standard 3.1: Assist pharmacists in collecting, organizing, and recording demographic and clinical information for the Pharmacists; Patient Care Process.

Standard 3.2: Receive, process, and prepare prescriptions/medication orders for completeness, accuracy, and authenticity to ensure safety.

Standard 3.16: Prepare simple non-sterile medications per applicable USP chapters (e.g., reconstitution, basic ointments and creams).

Standard 3.17: Assist pharmacists in preparing medications requiring compounding of non-sterile products.

Standard 5.1: Describe and apply state and federal laws pertaining to processing, handling, and dispensing of medications including controlled substances.

REINFORCE KEY CONCEPTS

Terms and Definitions

Select the correct term from the following list and write the corresponding letter in the blank next to the statement.

A. Acne vulgaris
B. Alopecia
C. Eczema
D. Hirsutism
E. Onychomycosis
F. Pruritus
G. Perspiration
H. Urticaria
I. Xerosis

_____ 1. A fungal infection of the fingernails or toenails

_____ 2. Commonly known as pimples, acne occurs when the skin pores clog with oil or bacteria

_____ 3. Itching

_____ 4. Partial or complete absence of hair from body areas where it usually grows, baldness

_____ 5. The process of sweating

_____ 6. A condition in which patches of skin become rough and inflamed

_____ 7. Red welts that arise on the surface of the skin; they are often attributable to an allergic reaction but may have nonallergic causes; also known as hives

_____ 8. Abnormal growth of hair on a person's face and body

_____ 9. Abnormal dryness of the skin, eyes, or mucous membranes

Select the correct term from the following list and write the corresponding letter in the blank next to the statement.

A. Dermis
B. Eschar
C. Epidermis
D. Exfoliation
E. Hypodermis
F. Melanin
G. Sebaceous glands
H. Subcutaneous layer

_____ 10. The deepest layer of the skin, consisting of fat cells and collagen; it protects the body and conserves heat

_____ 11. Outermost skin layer composed of the stratum corneum, or horny layer, the keratinocytes (squamous cells), and the basal layer; contains melanin

_____ 12. A dark brown to black pigment found in the hair, skin, and iris of the eye

_____ 13. A slough produced by a thermal burn, by application of a corrosive, or by gangrene

_____ 14. Subcutaneous tissue

380

_____ 15. A thick layer of connective tissue that contains collagen

_____ 16. The peeling off of dead skin

_____ 17. Skin glands responsible for the secretion of oil called sebum

Select the correct term from the following list and write the corresponding letter in the blank next to the statement.

A. Antiseptics
B. Comedones
C. Emollient
D. Head louse
E. Keratolytics
F. Metastasize
G. Nodules
H. Papules
I. Pustules
J. Seborrhea
K. Sebum
L. Sweat glands

_____ 18. A preparation that softens the skin

_____ 19. Small blisters or pimples on the skin containing pus

_____ 20. Drugs that cause shedding of the outer layer of the skin

_____ 21. Glands in the dermis that are activated by an increase in body temperature to cool the body

_____ 22. Small swellings or aggregations of cells in the body

_____ 23. Substances that slow or stop microorganism growth on surfaces such as skin

_____ 24. An oily/waxy substance that lubricates the skin and retains water to provide moisture

_____ 25. A louse that infests the scalp and hair of the human head

_____ 26. Excessive discharge of sebum from the sebaceous glands

_____ 27. With regard to cancer, to spread from the place of origin as a primary tumor to distant locations in the body

_____ 28. Small, raised, solid pimples on the skin

_____ 29. Blackheads, plugs of keratin and sebum in hair follicles blackened at the surface

True or False

Write T or F next to each statement.

_____ 1. The skin is one of the smallest organs in the body.

_____ 2. The lunula is the small white portion at the tip of the nail.

_____ 3. Psoriasis is an uncommon and infectious inflammatory skin disorder.

_____ 4. Phototherapy may be used as treatment for psoriasis.

_____ 5. Chickenpox is a contagious disease and may cause serious complications in young children.

_____ 6. Patients with first-degree burns can treat their burn at home.

_____ 7. Warts are not contagious.

_____ 8. With skin cancers, the outcome is good if detected early.

_____ 9. Lice does not transfer easily from hairbrushes and hats.

_____ 10. Onychomycosis treatment depends on the infection severity and number of affected nails.

System Identifier

Label the following parts of the skin.

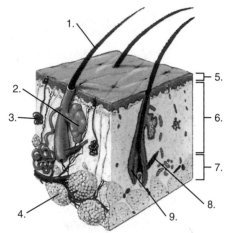

From Damjanov I: *Pathology for the health professions*, ed 4, Philadelphia, 2011, Saunders.

1. _____

2. _____

3. _____

4. _____

5. _____

6. _____

7. _____

8. _____

9. _____

Multiple Choice

Complete each question by circling the best answer.

1. The function of the skin is to protect the body against heat, cold, light, dehydration, and:
   A. sunburn
   B. injuries
   C. infection
   D. broken bones

2. OTC medications can relieve some issues with all the following *except*:
   A. Acne
   B. Impetigo
   C. Hives
   D. Sunburn

3. Mild acne most often responds to _____, which helps dry the skin.
   A. salicylic acids
   B. Retin-A (tretinoin)
   C. tetracycline
   D. Clearplex V (benzoyl peroxide)

4. The iPLEDGE program is aimed at preventing pregnancy during the use of _____ products.
   A. tetracycline
   B. Retin-A (tretinoin)
   C. Benadryl (diphenhydramine)
   D. Accutane (isotretinoin)

5. _____ are used to treat the symptoms of urticaria.
   A. Decongestants
   B. Antihistamines
   C. Sunscreens
   D. NSAIDS

6. Psoriasis patients who have developed arthritic symptoms are often prescribed:
   A. Trexall (methotrexate)
   B. NSAIDS
   C. sulfasalazine
   D. All the above

7. Treatment for herpes zoster includes:
   A. neomycin
   B. Valtrex (valacyclovir)
   C. Lotrimin (clotrimazole)
   D. Diprolene (betamethasone)

8. Treatment for plantar warts includes:
   A. Clearplex V (benzoyl peroxide)
   B. Nix (permethrin)
   C. Compound W (salicylic acid)
   D. Synalar (fluocinolone)

9. Impetigo can be treated with:
   A. Bactroban (mupirocin)
   B. Carac (fluorouracil)
   C. Theraplex T (coal tar)
   D. Cortizone (hydrocortisone)

10. The topical antimetabolite, _____, inhibits cancer cells from synthesizing DNA and is used to treat basal cell and squamous cell cancers on the surface of the skin.
    A. Efudex (fluorouracil)
    B. Azelex (azelaic acid)
    C. Protopic (tacrolimus)
    D. Zithranol (anthralin)

Fill in the Blanks

Answer each question by completing the statement in the space provided.

1. The most effective nondrug _____ treatment is keeping skin clean and bacteria free by using cleansing agents that reduce sebum production and exfoliate dead skin cells.

2. The oral retinoids, _____, is reserved for severe acne.

3. Applying a cold, wet compress can help alleviate the _____ that accompanies hives.

4. If the patient needs an antihistamine, oral _____ can dramatically reduce the appearance of hives and itching.

5. The use of _____ creams or ointments can help protect against xerosis.

6. Currently _____ has no cure, and patients require constant treatment to prevent outbreaks.

7. In most cases the prognosis for a tinea infection is good with _____ and the feet are kept clean and dry.

8. Impetigo is a highly _____ condition caused by streptococcal organisms, or *Staphylococcus aureus*.

9. The three main types of _____ cancer are melanoma, squamous cell cancer, and basal cell cancer.

10. If a fungal infection becomes _____, a doctor may prescribe oral agents such as ketoconazole or fluconazole.

Matching

Match the trade and generic drug names.

_____ 1. Bactroban

_____ 2. Lamisil

_____ 3. Nizoral

_____ 4. Temovate

_____ 5. Retin-A Micro

_____ 6. Clindagel

_____ 7. Cutivate

_____ 8. Topicort

_____ 9. Stelara

_____ 10. Nystop

A. clobetasol propionate
B. terbinafine
C. nystatin
D. ustekinumab
E. tretinoin
F. clindamycin
G. mupirocin
H. fluticasone propionate
I. ketoconazole
J. desoximetasone

Match the drugs with their indications.

_____ 11. Silvadene (silver sulfadiazine)

_____ 12. Elidel (pimecrolimus)

_____ 13. Desenex (miconazole)

_____ 14. Claravis (isotretinoin)

_____ 15. Remicade (infliximab)

_____ 16. Altabax (retapamulin)

_____ 17. Efudex (fluorouracil)

A. Antifungal
B. Psoriasis
C. Antibacterial
D. Burn wound infections
E. Acne
F. Eczema
G. Skin cancer

Short Answer

Reply to each question based on what you have learned in the chapter.

1. List three common skin conditions that can be self-managed with OTC products.

   _____

   _____

2. List two topical agents that can be used to help treat mild acne and describe how they work.

   _____

   _____

3. List the antihistamine frequently used to treat urticaria and its common side effects.

   _____

   _____

4. List two drug classifications frequently used to treat pruritus.

   _____

   _____

5. List three modalities of psoriasis treatment.

   _____

   _____

6. List two medications used for the treatment burns.

   _____

   _____

7. List one over-the-counter treatment for warts.

   _____

8. List two over-the-counter medications used for the treatment of athlete's foot.

   _____

   _____

9. List two medications used for the treatment of impetigo.

   _____

   _____

10. List two prescription treatments for resistant cases of lice.

    _____

    _____

11. List two medications used for the treatment of shingles.

    _____

    _____

Research Activities

Follow the instructions given in each exercise and provide a response.

1. Access the website *https://www.ipledgeprogram.com/ PrescriberInformation.aspx.*

   A. What are the isotretinoin prescribing requirements for females and males?

   B. What are the requirements for pharmacists when dispensing isotretinoin?

   C. As a pharmacy technician, how can you help the pharmacist meet the necessary requirements to dispense isotretinoin?

2. Access the website *http://www.mayoclinic.org/diseases-conditions/burns/basics/treatment/con-20035028.*

   A. What treatments can be used to encourage healing in a burn?

   B. Which treatments would come from the pharmacy department?

REFLECT CRITICALLY

Critical Thinking

Reply to each question based on what you have learned in the chapter.

1. Jamie is a pharmacy technician in a local retail store. A patient is complaining that her skin condition is worsening while using the prescribed antibacterial agent. Jamie directs the patient to the pharmacist for counseling. What will the pharmacist most likely tell the patient?

2. A patient is prescribed a corticosteroid ointment for psoriasis. Describe some of the possible side effects, especially if used long term.

3. Cathy goes to the doctor shortly after giving birth and returning home from the hospital. Cathy is complaining of vaginal itching. On further questioning, Cathy reveals that the newborn has "white spots" in her mouth. What do you suspect may be the problem, and what might be prescribed?

4. Gus is a pharmacy technician in a specialty hospital. A patient is brought in with multiple severe burns. What special precautions would Gus need to observe when preparing medication for this patient?

RELATE TO PRACTICE

Lab Scenarios

Therapeutic Agents for the Dermatologic System

Objective: To review with the pharmacy technician terms associated with the dermatologic system and review the brand and generic names, indications, dosage forms, routes of administration, auxiliary labels, and daily dosage of medications used to treat disorders of the dermatologic system

---

DID YOU KNOW?

- Acne is the most common skin condition, affecting approximately 50 million Americans.
- Atopic dermatitis affects up to 25% of children and 2–3% of adults.
- Approximately 7.5 million Americans have psoriasis.
- An estimated $51.7 billion to $63.2 billion are spent on the treatment of psoriasis.
- Skin cancer is the most common cancer affecting Americans.
- Approximately 9,500 Americans are diagnosed with skin cancer every day.

Reference:
https://www.aad.org/media/stats-numbers

Lab Activity #27.1: Define the following terms associated with the dermatologic system.

   Equipment Needed:
- Medical dictionary
- Pencil/pen

   Time needed to complete this activity: 30 minutes

1. Acne _____

2. Allergy _____

3. Blister _____

4. Candidiasis _____

5. Cysts _____

6. Decubitus ulcer _____

7. Dermatitis _____

8. Fungus _____

9. Mycoses _____

10. Petechiae _____

11. Psoriasis _____

12. Ringworm _____

13. Rosacea _____

14. Scabies _____

15. Tinea capitis _____

16. Tinea manus _____

17. Tinea pedis _____

18. Tinea unguium _____

19. Urticaria _____

20. Wheal _____

Lab Activity #27.2: Using a drug reference book, identify the generic name, drug classification, indications, dosage forms, routes of administration, and daily dosage of the *most common* medications used to treat conditions affecting the dermatologic system.

Equipment needed:
- *Drug Facts & Comparisons* or *Physicians' Desk Reference*
- Pencil/pen

Time needed to complete this activity: 60 minutes

Generic name	Brand Name	Classification	Indication(s)	Dosage Form(s)	Route(s)	Recommended Daily Dosage	Auxiliary Label(s)
Adapalene							
Azelaic acid							
Betamethasone							
Calcipotriene							
Clindamycin topical							
Desoximetasone							
Doxycycline							
Fluocinonide							
Golimumab							

Generic name	Brand Name	Classification	Indication(s)	Dosage Form(s)	Route(s)	Recommended Daily Dosage	Auxiliary Label(s)
Infliximab							
Isotretinoin							
Ketoconazole							
Lindane							
Malathion							
Minocycline							
Mupirocin							
Retapamulin							
Silver sulfadiazine							
Tacrolimus							
Tazarotene							
Terbinafine							
Tetracycline							
Tretinoin							
Triamcinolone							
Ustekinumab							

Chapter **27** **Therapeutic Agents for the Dermatologic System**

Using Therapeutic Agents for the Dermatologic System

Objective: To review with the pharmacy technician prescription orders, dosage calculations, and extemporaneous (nonsterile) compounding

Lab Activity #27.3: Answer the questions based on the prescription orders for each question.

Equipment needed:
- *Drug Facts and Comparisons* or *Physician's Desk Reference*
- Pencil/pen
- Calculator

Time needed to complete this activity: 15 minutes

The following are approved DAW codes:
- DAW 0: no product selection indicated
- DAW 1: substitution not allowed by provider
- DAW 2: substitution allowed: patient requested product dispensed
- DAW 3: substitution allowed: pharmacist selected product dispensed
- DAW 4: substitution allowed: generic drug not in stock
- DAW 5: substitution allowed: brand drug dispensed as generic
- DAW 6: override
- DAW 7: substitution not allowed: brand drug mandated by law
- DAW 8: substitution allowed: generic drug not available in marketplace
- DAW 9: other

---

1. Rx 1:
   Clindagel 30 g
   app once daily
   Ref ×1

   A. How much will be dispensed (use metric quantities)?

   _____

   B. How many days will the medication last?

   _____

   C. How many refills are permitted on the prescription?

   _____

   D. What DAW code will be used?

   _____

E. Write directions as they would appear on the medication label.

_____

_____

F. What auxiliary label(s) should be affixed to the medication label?

_____

_____

_____

2. Rx 2:
   Minocin 50 mg 1-month supply
   i cap q12h
   Ref ×5

   A. How much will be dispensed?

   _____

   B. How many days will the medication last?

   _____

   C. How many refills are permitted on the prescription?

   _____

   D. What DAW code will be used?

   _____

   E. Write directions as they would appear on the medication label.

   _____

   _____

   F. What auxiliary label(s) should be affixed to the medication label?

   _____

   _____

3. Rx 3:
   Erygel, 30 g
   app twice daily
   Ref ×2
   Patient wants brand name

   A. How much will be dispensed (use metric quantities)?

   _____

   B. How many days will the medication last?

   _____

   C. How many refills are permitted on the prescription?

   _____

   D. What DAW code will be used?

   _____

   E. Write directions as they would appear on the medication label.

   _____

   _____

   F. What auxiliary label(s) should be affixed to the medication label?

   _____

   _____

   _____

4. Rx 4:
   Altabax ung, 30g
   app affected area BID ×5d
   Ref: 0
   Brand Medically Necessary

   A. How much will be dispensed (use metric quantities)?

   _____

   B. How many days will the medication last?

   _____

   C. How many refills are permitted on the prescription?

   _____

   D. What DAW code will be used?

   _____

   E. Write directions as they would appear on the medication label.

   _____

   _____

   F. What auxiliary label(s) should be affixed to the medication label?

   _____

   _____

   _____

5. Rx 5:
   Temovate ung, 45 g
   app affected area bid utd ×2 weeks
   Ref: 0

   A. How much will be dispensed (use metric quantities)?

   _____

   B. How many days will the medication last?

   _____

   C. How many refills are permitted on the prescription?

   _____

   D. What DAW code will be used?

   _____

   E. Write directions as they would appear on the medication label.

   _____

   _____

   F. What auxiliary label(s) should be affixed to the medication label?

   _____

   _____

   _____

Chapter **27 Therapeutic Agents for the Dermatologic System**

6. Rx 6:
   Triderm 0.1%, 80 g
   app affected bid to qid
   Ref: 0

   A. How much will be dispensed (use metric quantities)?

   _____

   B. How many days will the medication last?

   _____

   C. How many refills are permitted on the prescription?

   _____

   D. What DAW code will be used?

   _____

   E. Write directions as they would appear on the medication label.

   _____

   _____

   F. What auxiliary label(s) should be affixed to the medication label?

   _____

   _____

   _____

7. Rx 7:
   Lamisil 250 mg #30
   i tab daily
   Ref ×3
   Generic is not available in your pharmacy

   A. How much will be dispensed?

   _____

   B. How many days will the medication last?

   _____

   C. How many refills are permitted on the prescription?

   _____

D. What DAW code will be used?

_____

E. Write directions as they would appear on the medication label.

_____

_____

F. What auxiliary label(s) should be affixed to the medication label?

_____

_____

_____

8. Rx 8:
   Ketoconazole shampoo, 120 mL
   app shampoo 2×/week ×4 weeks
   Ref:

   A. How much will be dispensed (use metric quantities)?

   _____

   B. How many days will the medication last?

   _____

   C. How many refills are permitted on the prescription?

   _____

   D. What DAW code will be used?

   _____

   E. Write directions as they would appear on the medication label.

   _____

   _____

   F. What auxiliary label(s) should be affixed to the medication label?

   _____

   _____

9. Rx 9:
   Enbrel (1 carton)
   50 mg weekly
   Ref ×3

   A. How much will be dispensed (use metric quantities)?

   _____

   B. How many days will the medication last?

   _____

   C. How many refills are permitted on the prescription?

   _____

   D. What DAW code will be used?

   _____

   E. Write directions as they would appear on the medication label.

   _____

   _____

   F. Where should this medication be stored?

   _____

   G. What auxiliary label(s) should be affixed to the medication label?

   _____

   _____

   _____

10. Rx 10:
    Elidel cream, 60 g
    app to affected area BID
    Ref ×0

    A. How much will be dispensed (use metric quantities)?

    _____

    B. How many days will the medication last?

    _____

C. How many refills are permitted on the prescription?

_____

D. What DAW code will be used?

_____

E. Write directions as they would appear on the medication label.

_____

_____

F. What auxiliary label(s) should be affixed to the medication label?

_____

_____

_____

Lab Activity #27.4: Calculate the quantity of the ingredients needed to prepare the following topical medications.

Equipment needed:
- Calculator
- Pencil/pen
- Paper

Time needed to complete this activity: 30 minutes

1. You are to prepare 2 oz of 1% hydrocortisone cream from 2.5% hydrocortisone cream and 0.25% hydrocortisone cream. How many grams of each ingredient will you need?

   2.5% hydrocortisone cream: _____

   0.25% hydrocortisone cream: _____

2. You are to prepare an ointment containing 20% coal tar from 1200 g of 5% coal tar ointment and concentrated coal tar. How many grams of coal tar should be added to the 1200 g of 5% coal tar ointment to prepare a 20% coal tar ointment?

   Coal tar: _____

3. You are to prepare 6 oz of deltasone cream 0.025%. How many grams of deltasone will you need?

   Deltasone: _____

4. You have 6 oz of 0.1% betamethasone cream in stock. To prepare a 0.05% betamethasone cream you will have to dilute your stock. How many grams of diluent cream will you need to add to prepare 0.05% betamethasone cream?

Diluent cream: _____

5. You are to prepare 4 oz of a 4% zinc oxide ointment. How many grams of zinc oxide will you need?

Zinc oxide: _____

Lab Activity #27.5: Compounding a paste.

Prepare 2 ounces of the following formula:

Zinc oxide	7.5 g
Cornstarch	7.5 g
Glycerin	qs
White petrolatum	15 g

Equipment needed:
- Calculator
- Pen
- Disinfecting agent/cleanser
- Sink with running hot and cold water
- Lint-free paper towels
- Personal protective equipment (PPE)
- Weigh boats or weighing papers
- Electronic balance or torsion balance with metric weights
- Spatulas
- Mortar card
- Ointment slab, parchment paper, or glass mortar and pestle
- Zinc oxide powder
- Cornstarch
- Glycerin
- White petrolatum
- 2-oz jar or tube for dispensing
- Label

- Auxiliary labels
- Zippered plastic storage bag (if desired)

Procedure
1. Gather all necessary supplies.
2. Ensure that equipment, supplies, and compounding area are clean and disinfected.
3. Organize materials on workbench.
4. Double-check recipe and calculations.
5. Wash hands and dry thoroughly.
6. Put on PPE.
7. Weigh zinc oxide, cornstarch, and white petrolatum on electronic balance or torsion balance.
8. Mix the zinc oxide and cornstarch together on an ointment slab or parchment paper.
9. Levigate zinc oxide and cornstarch mixture with a few drops of glycerin to form a paste.
10. Levigate equal amounts of white petrolatum with zinc oxide/cornstarch paste using an **S** pattern technique.
11. Levigate well.
12. Check product for uniformity and appearance.
13. Using a zippered plastic storage bag, package the paste into an ointment jar or ointment tube ensuring pharmaceutical elegance and weigh final packaged product.
14. Label product with all necessary information—including beyond-use date and auxiliary labels.
15. Document procedure and all necessary information on compounding log.
16. Clean equipment and put away.
17. Clean work area.

Packaging: Ointment jar or tube

Labeling: For external use only. Use only as directed.

BUD: Use USP <795> guidelines to determine BUD

Storage: Room temperature

Time needed to complete this activity: 45 minutes

Pharmacy Compounding Log					
Drug Name	Manufacturer	Mfg. Lot Number	Mfg. Expiration Date	Quantity Weighed/Measured	Technician Initials

BUD assigned: _____

392

28 Therapeutic Agents for the Hematologic System

Standard 1.4: Communicate clearly and effectively, both verbally and in writing.
Standard 2.5: Demonstrate basic knowledge of anatomy, physiology and pharmacology, and medical terminology relevant to the pharmacy technician's role.

REINFORCE KEY CONCEPTS

Terms and Definitions

Select the correct term from the following list and write the corresponding letter in the blank next to the statement.

A. Erythrocyte
B. Hemoglobin
C. Leukocyte
D. Phlebotomy
E. Plasma
F. Plasma protein
G. Serum
H. Thrombocyte
I. Whole blood

_____ 1. The oxygen-carrying component of red blood cells

_____ 2. Any of the dissolved proteins of blood plasma

_____ 3. Blood drawn from the body from which no constituent, such as plasma or platelets, has been removed

_____ 4. White blood cell

_____ 5. The transparent, yellowish fluid portion of the blood

_____ 6. A cell that contains hemoglobin and can carry oxygen to the body; also known as a *red blood cell*

_____ 7. A platelet

_____ 8. The clear, yellowish fluid obtained by separating whole blood into its solid and liquid components after it has been allowed to clot; plasma minus clotting factors

_____ 9. The act or practice of opening a vein by incision or puncture to remove blood

Select the correct term from the following list and write the corresponding letter in the blank next to the statement.

A. Absolute neutrophil count (ANC)
B. Albumin
C. Bone marrow
D. Colony-stimulating factor (CSF)
E. Cryoprecipitate
F. Erythropoiesis
G. Erythropoietin
H. Lymphoid organ
I. Splenectomy

_____ 10. The number of white blood cells that are neutrophils

_____ 11. A hormone that stimulates the bone marrow to synthesize hematopoietic cells

_____ 12. A hormone secreted by the kidney that stimulates the production of red blood cells by stem cells in bone marrow

_____ 13. The major protein found in plasma

_____ 14. Any precipitate that results from cooling; sometimes explicitly used to describe a precipitate rich in coagulation factor VIII obtained from the cooling of blood plasma

_____ 15. A component of the system of interconnected tissues and organs by which lymph circulates throughout the body

_____ 16. The tissue that fills the cavities in long bones, the source of red blood cells and many white blood cells

_____ 17. The formation of erythrocytes

_____ 18. Surgical removal of the spleen

393

Select the correct term from the following list and write the corresponding letter in the blank next to the statement.

A. Hydrostatic pressure
B. Idiopathic
C. Osmosis
D. Osmotic pressure
E. Pallor
F. Solute

_____ 19. The pressure exerted by water flowing through a semipermeable membrane separating two solutions with different concentrations of solutes

_____ 20. A term meaning "of unknown cause."

_____ 21. A substance dissolved in another substance; usually the component of a solution present in less amount

_____ 22. The pressure exerted by a fluid due to the force of gravity

_____ 23. A deficiency in color, particularly of the face

_____ 24. Diffusion of fluid through a semipermeable membrane from a solution with a low solute concentration to a solution with a higher solute concentration to achieve equilibrium

Select the correct term from the following list and write the corresponding letter in the blank next to the statement.

A. Anemia
B. Granulocytopenia
C. Hemophilia
D. Hypoxia
E. Leukemia
F. Leukopenia
G. Lymphoma
H. Neutropenia
I. Polycythemia
J. Thrombocytopenia
K. von Willebrand disease

_____ 25. A progressive, malignant disease of the blood-forming organs, marked by distorted proliferation and development of leukocytes and their precursors in blood and bone marrow

_____ 26. The most common inherited bleeding disorder, associated with a deficiency in the clotting protein von Willebrand factor

_____ 27. An oxygen supply reduction to a tissue despite adequate tissue perfusion

_____ 28. Abnormally low level of neutrophils in the blood

_____ 29. A decrease in the number of platelets in the blood

_____ 30. A hereditary coagulation disorder that leads to a decreased ability to clot normally

_____ 31. Cancer of the lymphatic system

_____ 32. An increase in the total cell mass of the blood

_____ 33. A reduction in granulocyte number, which encompasses specific types of white blood cells that contain "granules"

_____ 34. A reduction in the number of leukocytes (white blood cells) in the blood

_____ 35. A decrease in the number of red blood cells or hemoglobin, which impairs the blood's ability to carry oxygen to the tissues

True or False

Write T or F next to each statement.

_____ 1. Albumin is the major blood protein that maintains hydrostatic pressure in the vascular system.

_____ 2. The life span of a platelet is approximately 14 days.

_____ 3. Leukocytes, erythrocytes, and platelets form through hematopoiesis.

_____ 4. WBCs are cells of the immune system that help defend the body against infection.

_____ 5. The main function of the RBC is to carry oxygen to the tissues and organs.

_____ 6. Anemia is caused by a reduction in the total number of WBCs in the body or by a problem with the quality or quantity of hemoglobin present.

_____ 7. Pernicious anemia is the most common form of anemia worldwide.

_____ 8. Gastrointestinal bleeding can lead to iron deficiency anemia.

_____ 9. Hypoxia is a form of polycythemia that occurs in people who have a difficult time oxygenating their blood.

_____ 10. The principal treatment goal for thrombocytopenia is to prevent bleeding.

System Identifier

Components of Whole Blood

Identify each component in this system and enter the term next to the corresponding number.

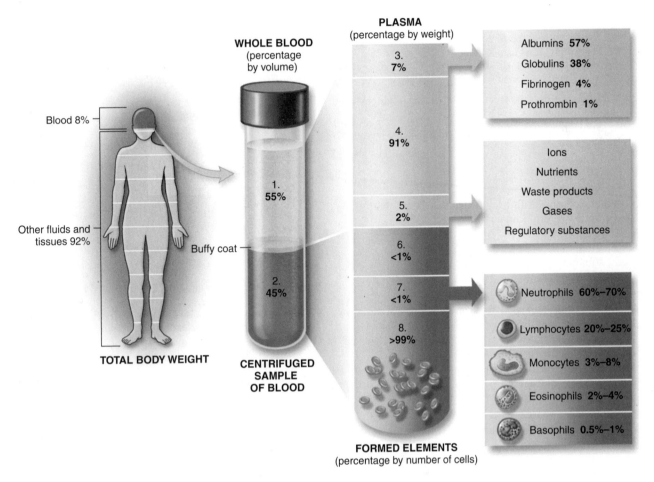

From Patton KT, Thibodeau GA: Anatomy and physiology, ed 8, St Louis, 2013, Mosby.

1. _____

2. _____

3. _____

4. _____

5. _____

6. _____

7. _____

8. _____

Multiple Choice

Complete each question by circling the best answer.

1. Which of following medications can cause iron deficiency anemia because of GI bleeding?
   A. Droxia (hydroxyurea)
   B. Naprosyn (naproxen sodium)
   C. FerrouSul (ferrous sulfate)
   D. Infed (iron dextran)

2. Mild anemia may be treated with dietary changes including an increase in:
   A. Spinach
   B. Broccoli
   C. Liver
   D. All of the above

3. Which of the following vitamins helps with the absorption of oral iron supplements?
   A. Vitamin A
   B. Vitamin B
   C. Vitamin C
   D. Vitamin D

4. _____ is indicated for iron deficiency anemia in people undergoing chronic dialysis and receiving epoetin alfa therapy.
   A. Ferrlecit (ferric gluconate)
   B. Slow Fe (ferrous sulfate)
   C. Neupogen (filgrastim)
   D. Droxia (hydroxyurea)

5. Drug therapy for polycythemia vera involves treatments aimed at minimizing the risk of thrombosis with a myelosuppressive agent such as:
   A. Vincasar (vincristine)
   B. bleomycin
   C. Hydrea (hydroxyurea)
   D. Efudex (fluorouracil)

6. Patients not responding to steroids, immunoglobulins, or splenectomy for thrombocytopenia treatment can take _____
   A. Rituxan (rituximab)
   B. Gleevec (imatinib)
   C. fludarabine
   D. Promacta (eltrombopag)

7. The primary drugs used in the treatment of neutropenia are recombinant growth factors known as _____
   A. antimetabolites
   B. antibiotics
   C. colony-stimulating factors
   D. miotic inhibitors

8. _____ can be used to treat idiopathic thrombocytopenic purpura (ITP).
   A. Neupogen (filgrastim)
   B. Promacta (eltrombopag)
   C. Leukine (sargramostim)
   D. Rheumatrex (methotrexate)

9. _____ are often used to treat leukemia.
   A. Antimetabolites
   B. Glucocorticoids
   C. Immunoglobulins
   D. Colony-stimulating factors

10. Treatment for von Willebrand's disease includes:
    A. Factor VIII concentrates
    B. DDAVP (desmopressin)
    C. Estrogen therapy
    D. All of the above

Fill in the Blanks

Answer each question by completing the statement in the space provided.

1. Phenytoin is an example of a drug that is highly bound to _____ and its use with other drugs that bind to albumin can lead to phenytoin toxicity.

2. Health professionals can use _____ for people with low RBC counts because of kidney disease or other medical conditions.

3. The first step in managing iron deficiency anemia should be identifying and/or ruling out _____ _____

4. Iron replacement therapy is the _____ treatment for iron deficiency anemia.

5. Severe _____ may necessitate activity restrictions such as limiting contact sports.

6. In immune-mediated thrombocytopenia, glucocorticoid medications can _____ the immune response.

7. The primary concern in a neutropenia patient is increased _____ risk.

8. A critical component of care for patients with chronic neutropenia includes regular dental care to prevent _____ and associated infection.

9. Because treatment results in bone marrow suppression, _____ is the leading cause of death in leukemia patients.

10. Hemophilia treatment involves _____ blood infusions or the use of recombinant Factor VIII or Factor IX products.

396

Matching

Match the following trade and generic drug names.

_____ 1. Slow Fe

_____ 2. Hydrea

_____ 3. Nipent

_____ 4. Ferrlecit

_____ 5. Promacta

_____ 6. Neupogen

_____ 7. Leukine

_____ 8. DDAVP

_____ 9. Epogen

_____ 10. Leukeran

A. pentostatin
B. filgrastim
C. epoetin alfa
D. hydroxyurea
E. eltrombopag
F. ferrous sulfate
G. sargramostim
H. chlorambucil
I. ferric gluconate
J. desmopressin

Match the following drugs with their classification.

_____ 11. Ferrex (iron polysaccharide)

_____ 12. Neulasta (pegfilgrastim)

_____ 13. Vesanoid (tretinoin)

_____ 14. Aranesp (darbepoetin alfa)

_____ 15. Gleevec (imatinib)

_____ 16. Cytarabine

_____ 17. Carboplatin

_____ 18. Purixan (mercaptopurine)

_____ 19. Rituxan (rituximab)

_____ 20. Trexall (methotrexate)

_____ 21. Daunorubicin

_____ 22. Toposar (etoposide)

_____ 23. Eldisine (vindesine)

A. Tyrosine kinase inhibitor
B. Antimetabolite
C. Purine nucleoside analogue
D. Oral iron salt
E. RBC stimulating agent
F. Alkylating agent
G. Vinca alkaloid
H. WBC stimulating agent
I. Monoclonal antibody
J. Anthracycline
K. Pyrimidine analogue
L. Topoisomerase II inhibitor
M. Retinoic acid derivative

Short Answer

Reply to each question based on what you have learned in the chapter.

1. List the classes of drugs used to treat leukemia.

   _____

   _____

2. List two agents, and side their effects, that cross the blood–brain barrier surrounding the central nervous system, which gives them the ability to treat cancers within the brain.

   _____

   _____

3. List five factors for the development of lymphoma.

   _____

   _____

   _____

4. List three combination therapies for Hodgkin's disease.

   _____

   _____

   _____

5. List three classes of drugs that have a common risk of drug-induced bleeding.

   _____

   _____

Research Activities

Follow the instructions given in each exercise and provide a response.

1. Access the website *http://www.hematology.org/Patients/ Blood-Disorders.aspx.*

   A. What are six common blood disorders that affect people?

B. To what type of physician would you be referred for the diagnosis of a blood disorder?

C. What are the benefits of participating in a clinical trial? Why is it important for females and minority patients to participate in a clinical trial? What clinical trials are currently available for blood disorders?

2. Access the website *https://www.cancer.gov/types.*

   A. List the many different types of blood cancers that are known.

   B. What types of treatment are available for blood cancers?

REFLECT CRITICALLY

Critical Thinking

Reply to each question based on what you have learned in the chapter.

1. Why is dental care important for those with neutropenia?

2. Many scientists claim that the cure for cancer lies in the plants of the world's greatest forests. These forests are disappearing because of the growth in the world's population and the use of land for mining or agriculture. Should governments get involved in plant-targeted cancer research? Why or why not? What can be done to foster research in this area? Present your case to your classmates.

Lab Scenarios

Therapeutic Agents for the Hematologic System

Objective: To review with the pharmacy technician terms associated with the components of the hematologic system and review the brand and generic names, indications, dosage forms, routes of administration, recommended daily dosage, and storage of medications used to treat disorders of the hematologic system

---

DID YOU KNOW?

- 3.4% of new cancer cases will be caused by leukemia.
- Approximately 100,000 Americans have sickle cell disease.
- 778,000 emergency room visits were made with anemia as the primary diagnosis.
- In 2017, 5,382 deaths occurred from anemias.

References:

National Center for Health Statistics. (2020, February 21). *Anemia or iron deficiency.* National Center for Health Statistics, Centers for Disease Control and Prevention. Retrieved September 12, 2020, from https://www.cdc.gov/nchs/fastats/anemia.htm

National Cancer Institute. (n. d.). *Cancer stat facts: Leukemia.* Surveillance Research Program, Division of Cancer Control and Population Sciences. Retrieved September 12, 2020, from https://seer.cancer.gov/statfacts/html/leuks.html

National Heart, Lung, and Blood Institute. (2020, September 1). *Sickle cell disease.* National Institute of Health, U.S. Department of Health & Human Services. Retrieved September 12, 2020, from https://www.nhlbi.nih.gov/health-topics/sickle-cell-disease

Lab Activity #28.1: Define the following terms associated with the hematologic system.

Equipment needed:
- Medical dictionary
- Pencil/pen

Time needed to complete this activity: 30 minutes

1. Acute lymphoblastic leukemia (ALL) _____

2. Acute myeloblastic leukemia (AML) _____

3. Aplastic anemia _____

4. Chronic lymphocytic leukemia (CLL) _____

5. Chronic myeloid leukemia (CML) _____

6. Folate deficiency anemia _____

7. Hemochromatosis _____

8. Hemolytic anemia _____

9. Iron deficiency anemia _____

10. Myelodysplastic syndrome _____

11. Myeloma _____

12. Pernicious anemia _____

13. Sickle cell anemia _____

14. Sideroblastic anemia _____

15. Thalassemia _____

Lab Activity #28.2: Using a drug reference book, identify the generic name, drug classification, indications, dosage forms, routes of administration, and recommended daily dosage of the most common medications used to treat conditions affecting the hematologic system.

Equipment needed:
- *Drug Facts & Comparisons* or *Physicians' Desk Reference*
- Pencil/pen

Time needed to complete this activity: 60 minutes

Generic Name	Brand Name	Classification	Indication(s)	Dosage Form(s)	Route(s)	Daily Recommended Dosage	Auxiliary Label(s)
Chlorambucil							
Cyanocobalamin							

Continued

Generic Name	Brand Name	Classification	Indication(s)	Dosage Form(s)	Route(s)	Daily Recommended Dosage	Auxiliary Label(s)
Dasatinib							
Ferrous fumarate							
Ferrous gluconate							
Ferrous sulfate							
Hydroxyurea							
Imatinib							
Iron polysaccharide							
Mercaptopurine							
Methotrexate							
Nilotinib							
Tretinoin							

Lab Activity #28.3: Using a drug reference book, identify the storage requirements and expiration date (at room temperature) for hematologic agents.

Equipment needed:
- *Handbook on Injectable Drugs*
- Pencil/pen

Time needed to complete this activity: 30 minutes

400

Brand Name (Generic Name)	Drug Classification	Indication	Dose Form	Route	Storage Requirements	Expiration Date
Aranesp (darbepoetin alfa)						
Campath (alemtuzumab)						
Cerubidine (daunorubicin)						
Cytosar (cytarabine)						
Cytoxan (cyclophosphamide)						
Infed (iron dextran)						
Eldisine (vindesine sulfate)						
Epogen (epoetin alfa)						
Ferrlecit (sodium ferric gluconate complex)						
Fludara (fludarabine)						
Idamycin PFS (idarubicin)						

Continued

401

Brand Name (Generic Name)	Drug Classification	Indication	Dose Form	Route	Storage Requirements	Expiration Date
Leukine (sargramostim)						
Leustatin (cladribine)						
Neulasta (pegfilgrastim)						
Neupogen (filgrastim)						
Nipent (pentostatin)						
Paraplatin (carboplatin)						
Rituxan (rituximab)						
Toposar (etoposide)						
Venofer (iron sucrose)						
Vincasar PFS (vincristine)						

29 Over-the-Counter (OTC) Medication

ASHP ACCREDITATION STANDARDS FOR PHARMACY TECHNICIAN EDUCATION AND TRAINING PROGRAMS

Standard 1.3: Demonstrate active and engaged listening skills.
Standard 1.4: Communicate clearly and effectively, both verbally and in writing.
Standard 1.10: Apply critical thinking skills, creativity, and innovation.
Standard 2.5: Demonstrate basic knowledge of anatomy, physiology and pharmacology, and medical terminology relevant to pharmacy technician's role.

REINFORCE KEY CONCEPTS

Terms and Definitions

Select the correct term from the following list and write the corresponding letter in the blank next to the statement.

A. Analgesic
B. Antiinflammatory
C. Antipyretic
D. Antitussive
E. Behind-the-counter drug
F. Circadian rhythms
G. Expectorants
H. Legend drugs
I. Nutraceutical
J. Over-the-counter (OTC) drugs
K. Pruritus

_____ 1. An itch.

_____ 2. Chemicals that loosen and thin sputum and bronchial secretions.

_____ 3. A drug that relieves pain.

_____ 4. A food or supplement with added health benefits.

_____ 5. Nonprescription medicines generally found outside the secure part of the pharmacy.

_____ 6. A drug that reduces fever.

_____ 7. A nonprescription medication kept behind the prescription counter that patients must buy at a pharmacy.

_____ 8. Medications that need a prescription.

_____ 9. A drug that reduces swelling.

_____ 10. 24-hour cycles of regular biological changes; often involves medications affecting sleep/wake cycles.

_____ 11. A drug that can decrease the coughing reflex.

True or False

Write T or F next to each statement.

_____ 1. Pharmacy technicians who familiarize themselves with the different ways pharmacies group or refer to over-the-counter medications can better help patients.

_____ 2. It is not important to include OTC drugs in the patient profile.

_____ 3. It is not necessary for parents to consult with their child's pediatrician before giving OTC medications, especially to children younger than 4 years.

_____ 4. Pregnant or breast-feeding women should always seek professional advice before taking an OTC product.

_____ 5. Patients widely use pain relievers for arthritis, headaches, and other aches and pains.

_____ 6. A potential and common side effect of NSAIDs is an increase in blood sugar.

_____ 7. The recommended duration for nonprescription sleep aids is 2 weeks maximum.

_____ 8. Diphenhydramine regularly causes next-day drowsiness in older adults.

_____ 9. Elderly patients may have multiple conditions that make self-treatment with OTC medication harmless.

_____ 10. The FDA recommends using measuring spoons or cups not included with OTC products when dosing infants and young children.

403

Multiple Choice

Complete each question by circling the best answer.

1. The number of OTC drugs available to consumers has increased since the:
   A. 1970s
   B. 1980s
   C. 1990s
   D. 2000s

2. The _____ houses published OTC drug monographs and outlines acceptable ingredients, dosages, formulas, and labeling.
   A. FDA
   B. GRASE
   C. *Federal Register*
   D. DEA

3. The same standards of safety and effectiveness that are placed on _____ also are similarly used to approve OTC drugs.
   A. legend drugs
   B. dietary supplements
   C. behind-the-counter drugs
   D. nutraceutical products

4. Considerations the FDA must take before approving an OTC product include all the following *except*:
   A. Labeling can be read, understood, and followed without the guidance of a health care provider
   B. OTC product is proved to be half as effective as the corresponding legend drug
   C. OTC product is safe and effective
   D. OTC product can be safely taken without a prescription

5. An OTC monograph includes:
   A. Acceptable ingredients
   B. Formulations
   C. Labeling
   D. All the above

6. Which condition cannot be treated with OTC drugs?
   A. High blood pressure
   B. Fever
   C. Cough
   D. Diarrhea

7. Children and teenagers should not take aspirin for chickenpox or flu because it has been associated with:
   A. Toxic shock syndrome
   B. Reye's syndrome
   C. Sudden infant death syndrome
   D. Acquired immunodeficiency syndrome

8. Taking too much _____ on a regular daily basis can lead to liver toxicity.
   A. Benadryl (diphenhydramine)
   B. Mucinex (guaifenesin)
   C. Motrin (ibuprofen)
   D. Tylenol (acetaminophen)

9. NSAID stands for:
   A. Nonsafety caps for AIDS patients
   B. Not safe as an IUD service
   C. Nonsteroidal antiinflammatory drug
   D. Nonsteroidal antiinflammatory disease

10. A common side effect of first-generation antihistamines is:
    A. Drowsiness
    B. Diarrhea
    C. Agitation
    D. Constipation

Fill in the Blanks

Answer each question by completing the statement in the space provided.

1. Only pharmacists can provide _____ advice about OTC medications.

2. Pharmacy technicians can _____ patients to the correct section.

3. Customers can buy over-the-counter products _____ a prescription.

4. Unless the prescriber writes a script for an OTC item, the pharmacist is not required to _____ patients on those products.

5. Patients on special diets, with allergies, diabetes, or interacting medications should use _____ in selecting an OTC medication.

6. When trying a new OTC medication, individuals should watch carefully for any _____ reactions that may occur.

7. To handle OTC products that were available before the NDA, the FDA set up the OTC _____ system.

8. Some medications have an OTC and _____ drug approval.

9. Taking extra time to listen to _____ patients and make them comfortable provides an avenue to a full medication history.

10. Most _____ products carry age- and/or weight-based dosage calculations.

Short Answer

Write a short response to each question in the space provided.

1. List four reasons why consumers use OTC products.

   A. _____

   B. _____

   C. _____

   D. _____

2. List three considerations consumers should address before buying and using OTC medications.

   A. _____

   B. _____

   C. _____

3. Give three examples of antiinflammatory products.

   A. _____

   B. _____

   C. _____

4. Give three examples of antihistamine uses.

   A. _____

   B. _____

   C. _____

5. List two examples of sleep aid products.

   A. _____

   B. _____

6. List two classes of drugs used to reduce or relieve gastric acid secretions.

   A. _____

   B. _____

7. List two antibiotics that should be taken with calcium-, magnesium-, and aluminum-containing antacids.

   A. _____

   B. _____

8. What is a common OTC product for gas?

   _____

9. What is a common OTC product for acne?

   _____

10. List two examples of special population groups that are at particular risk for receiving an inappropriate medication, the wrong dose, or the wrong drug product.

    A. _____

    B. _____

11. Give an example of an OTC product that is kept behind the pharmacy counter.

    _____

12. What OTC product is available to women for overactive bladder?

    _____

Matching

Match the OTC drugs with their medication class.

A. Stimulant laxative
B. Local anesthetic
C. Non-narcotic analgesic
D. Bulk laxative
E. NSAID
F. Antacid
G. H₂-blocker
H. Proton pump inhibitor
I. Antidiarrheal
J. Antifungal

_____ 1. Tinactin (tolfanate)

_____ 2. Zantac 150 (ranitidine)

_____ 3. Imodium A-D (loperamide)

_____ 4. Nexium (esomeprazole)

_____ 5. Lotrimin-AF (clotrimazole)

_____ 6. Lamisil (terbinafine)

_____ 7. Tylenol (acetaminophen)

_____ 8. Tagamet (cimetidine)

_____ 9. Prevacid (lansoprazole)

_____ 10. Milk of Magnesia (magnesium hydroxide)

_____ 11. Cepacol (benzocaine, glycerin)

_____ 12. Pepto-Bismol (bismuth subsalicylate)

_____ 13. Aleve (naproxen sodium)

_____ 14. Senokot (senna)

_____ 15. Tums (calcium carbonate)

_____ 16. Metamucil (psyllium)

_____ 17. Chloraseptic (benzocaine, menthol)

_____ 18. Motrin (ibuprofen)

_____ 19. Dulcolax (biscodyl)

_____ 20. Advil (ibuprofen)

Match the OTC drugs with their medication class.

A. Antihistamine (sedating)
B. Antihistamine (non-sedating)
C. Oral decongestant
D. Nasal decongestant
E. Ophthalmic decongestant
F. Nasal steroid
G. Expectorant
H. Antitussive
I. Topical antibiotic
J. Topical steroid

_____ 21. Neo-Synephrine (phenylephrine)

_____ 22. Sudafed (pseudoephedrine)

_____ 23. Delsym (dextromethorphan)

_____ 24. Neosporin (polymyxin B sulfate, neomycin, bacitracin)

_____ 25. Benadryl (diphenhydramine)

_____ 26. Opti-Clear (tetrahydrozoline)

_____ 27. Zyrtec (cetirizine HCl)

_____ 28. Mucinex (guaifenesin)

_____ 29. Allegra (fexofenadine)

_____ 30. Afrin (oxymetazoline)

_____ 31. Bacitracin (bacitracin)

_____ 32. Nasacort (triamcinolone)

_____ 33. Claritin (loratadine)

_____ 34. Flonase (fluticasone)

_____ 35. Cortisone-10 (hydrocortisone)

_____ 36. Clear Eyes (naphazoline)

_____ 37. Chlor-Trimeton (chlorpheniramine)

_____ 38. Rhinocort (budesonide)

Match the trade and generic drug names.

A. docusate sodium
B. terbinafine
C. famotidine
D. naproxen sodium
E. guaifenesin
F. pseudoephedrine
G. diphenhydramine
H. omeprazole
I. calcium carbonate
J. acetaminophen
K. ibuprofen
L. fluticasone
M. loratadine
N. dextromethorphan
O. ranitidine

_____ 39. Tums

_____ 40. Tylenol

_____ 41. Colace

_____ 42. Prilosec OTC

_____ 43. Lamisil

_____ 44. Flonase

_____ 45. Zantac 150

_____ 46. Aleve

_____ 47. Sudafed

_____ 48. Delsym

_____ 49. Mucinex

_____ 50. Advil

_____ 51. Claritin

_____ 52. Pepcid AC

_____ 53. Benadryl

Research Activities

Follow the instructions given in each exercise and provide a response.

1. Access the website *https://www.chpa.org/Switch.aspx*. Click on the link Switch List.

   A. What legend drugs have been converted to OTC status in the past 2 years? List the active ingredient, strength, product category, date of OTC approval, and product examples.

   B. What is the very first drug listed as making the switch from legend drug to OTC drug?

   C. How many OTC drugs are on the Rx-to-OTC switch list?

   D. Do you recognize any of the drugs listed? How many on the list have you taken yourself?

2. Access the website *http://www.fda.gov/Safety/MedWatch/default.htm*. What OTC products, if any, are listed in the MedWatch Safety Alerts in the last month? What is the safety concern with those products?

3. Access the website *https://www.fda.gov/drugs/drug-safety-and-availability/information-drug-class*. Click on the link Legal Requirements for the Sale and Purchase of Drug Products Containing Pseudoephedrine, Ephedrine, and Phenylephrine. What must buyers present to purchase pseudoephedrine? What must the seller verify when selling pseudoephedrine?

REFLECT CRITICALLY

Critical Thinking

Reply to each question based on what you have learned in the chapter.

1. In a chain store or mass merchandiser outlet, where is the pharmacy located? Why?

2. You have a sore throat, and none of the OTC lozenges are helping. You have been told to gargle with saltwater. How will this help your sore throat?

3. Sometimes people buy an OTC medication because someone they know tried it and it worked for that person. Why should you not base your decision to buy OTC medications on that reasoning?

4. The FDA recently allowed Patonal (olopatadine hydrochloride), a prescription eye antihistamine, to become an OTC product Pataday. What other drugs do you think should become OTC medications, provided they are safe and effective for patients? Present your possible OTC medication with reasons why you believe it should be an OTC product to your classmates.

5. What special considerations should be made for those suffering from high blood pressure? Which OTC products would not be recommended for those with this medical condition?

Lab Scenarios

Over-the-Counter (OTC) Medications

Objective: To introduce the pharmacy technician to various over-the-counter medications and their indication(s), warning(s), dosage form(s), and route(s) of administration

---

DID YOU KNOW?

- 81% of adults use OTC products as their first response to minor ailments.
- 70% of parents have given their child an OTC product in the middle of the night to help treat a sudden medical symptom.
- 75% of primary care physicians will recommend an OTC medication before prescribing a prescription.
- OTC product availability has created $142 billion in annual health care savings.

Reference:

Consumer Healthcare Products Association. (n. d.). *Statistics on OTC use.* Retrieved August 17, 2020, from https://www.chpa.org/MarketStats.aspx

Lab Activity #29.1: Visit a local pharmacy and familiarize yourself with the OTC section of the store. Complete the following table of OTC products.

Equipment needed:
- Retail pharmacy and/or Computer with Internet
- *Drug Facts and Comparison* or *Physician's Desk Reference*
- Pencil/pen

Time needed to complete the exercise: 60 minutes

1. What local pharmacy did you visit?

   Name: _____

   Address: _____

2. What signage or markers does the pharmacy use to differentiate each OTC section (e.g., Antacids, Analgesics, Allergy, etc.)?

3. Using the table below, list the active ingredients, strength of the active ingredient, indication, dose forms available, and section you found the OTC product.

Brand (Trade) Name	Active Ingredient(s)	Medication Strength and Indication	Dosage Form(s) Available	Section and/or Grouping
Abreva				
Advil				
Afrin				
Aleve				
Allegra				
Bayer Aspirin				
Benadryl				
Claritin				
Clearasil				
Delsym				
Dimetapp-DM				
Dulcolax				

Brand (Trade) Name	Active Ingredient(s)	Medication Strength and Indication	Dosage Form(s) Available	Section and/or Grouping
Ecotrin				
Flonase				
Gyne-Lotrimin				
Imodium A-D				
Lamisil				
Metamucil				
Mylanta				
Mylicon				
Nasacort				
Neosporin				
Nytol				
Pataday				
Pepcid A-C				
Pepto-Bismol				
Polysporin				
Preparation H				
Prevacid				
Prilosec				
Robitussin				
Sudafed PE				
Tagamet HB				
TheraFlu				
Tinactin				

Continued

Brand (Trade) Name	Active Ingredient(s)	Medication Strength and Indication	Dosage Form(s) Available	Section and/or Grouping
Triaminic				
Tums				
Tylenol				
Vicks Dayquil				
Vicks Nyquil				

Lab Activity #29.2: Using information learned and resources available, determine OTC therapeutic options the pharmacist may choose for each case. (Remember, only the pharmacist is legally allowed to counsel a customer.)

Equipment needed:
- Computer and Internet access
- *Drug Facts and Comparisons* or *Pocket Guide for Nonprescription Product Therapeutics*
- Pencil/pen

Time needed to complete the exercise: 30 minutes

1. A parent approaches the pharmacy counter stating they would like OTC product recommendations for their 8-year-old child's runny nose. Upon further questioning, they state the nasal discharge is clear and their child's nose itches. They also state their child sneezes often, is tired often, and does not have a fever.

    A. What may be wrong with this 8-year-old child? Why?

    _____

    _____

    B. What OTC products would help for this 8-year-old child? List the brand name(s) and generic name(s).

    _____

    _____

    _____

    C. Choose one of the products listed. What is the appropriate dose for this 8-year-old child?

    _____

    _____

D. What potential side effects may occur from taking this OTC product?

_____

_____

_____

E. Are there any other warnings or precautions that should be considered when taking this OTC product?

_____

_____

_____

2. A patient approaches the pharmacy counter stating their eyes feel irritated. Upon further questioning, they state that they often feel the need to rub their eyes and that it sometimes feels like there is sandpaper in them. They state that they do not have a history of allergies. You also notice that their eyes do look a little red. They would like to know if an OTC product would help their eyes feel better.

    A. What may be wrong with this patient? Why?

    _____

    _____

    B. What OTC products would help this patient? List the brand name(s) and generic name(s).

    _____

    _____

    _____

C. Choose one of the products listed. What is the appropriate dose for this patient?

_____

_____

D. What potential side effects may occur from taking this OTC product?

_____

_____

_____

E. Are there any other warnings or precautions that should be considered when taking this OTC product?

_____

_____

_____

3. A patient approaches the pharmacy counter stating they would like an OTC product recommendation for their feet. Upon further questioning, they state that their feet are itchy and sometimes burn. They also state that the symptoms began after they started attending the gym daily.

A. What may be wrong with this patient? Why?

_____

B. What OTC products would help for this patient? List the brand name(s) and generic name(s).

_____

_____

_____

C. Choose one of the products listed. What is the appropriate dose for this patient?

_____

_____

D. What potential side effects may occur from taking this OTC product?

_____

_____

_____

E. Are there any other warnings or precautions that should be considered when taking this OTC product?

_____

_____

_____

4. A patient approaches the pharmacy counter stating their stomach often feels upset after they eat, especially after eating tomatoes and acidic foods. Upon further questioning, they also state that it is sometimes worse if they lie down after eating. They also inform the pharmacy that they do not have a history of a heart condition.

A. What may be wrong with this patient? Why?

_____

B. What OTC products would help for this patient? List the brand name(s) and generic name(s).

_____

_____

_____

C. Choose one of the products listed. What is the appropriate dose for this patient?

_____

_____

D. What potential side effects may occur from taking this OTC product?

_____

_____

_____

E. Are there any other warnings or precautions that should be considered when taking this OTC product?

_____

_____

_____

Lab Activity #29.3: The FDA requires specific information to be on an OTC medication drug label. Using the OTC drug label given, answer the questions below.

Equipment needed:
■ Pencil/pen

Time needed to complete the exercise: 30 minutes

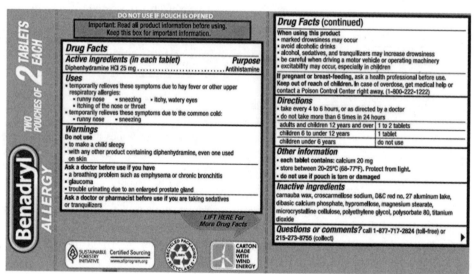

From NIH: US National Library of Medicine, *Daily Med,* https://dailymed.nlm.nih.gov/dailymed/index.cfm

1. What is the name of the product?

2. What is the generic name of the product (active ingredients) and strength?

3. What is the classification (purpose)?

4. What are the inactive ingredients?

5. What warnings are listed?

6. Who, if anyone, should not take this product?

7. What is the dosing schedule?

8. How should this product be stored?

30 Complementary and Alternative Medicine (CAM)

ASHP ACCREDITATION STANDARDS FOR PHARMACY TECHNICIAN EDUCATION AND TRAINING PROGRAMS

Standard 1.3: Demonstrate active and engaged listening skills.

Standard 1.4: Communicate clearly and effectively, both verbally and in writing.

Standard 1.5: Demonstrate a respectful and professional attitude when interacting with diverse patient populations, colleagues, and professionals.

Standard 1.6: Apply self-management skills, including time management, stress, and change management.

Standard 1.10: Apply critical thinking skills, creativity, and innovation.

Standard 2.4: Describe wellness promotion and disease prevention concepts.

Standard 2.5: Demonstrate basic knowledge of anatomy, physiology and pharmacology, and medical terminology relevant to pharmacy technician's role.

Standard 2.9: Describe investigational drug process, medications being used in off-label indications, and emerging drug therapies.

Standard 2.11: Support wellness promotion and disease prevention programs.

REINFORCE KEY CONCEPTS

Terms and Definitions

Select the correct term from the following list and write the corresponding letter in the blank next to the statement.

A. Alternative medicine
B. Ayurveda
C. Biofeedback
D. Chiropractic medicine
E. Complimentary medicine
F. Diagnosis
G. Herb
H. Homeopathy
I. Prophylaxis
J. Synthetic medicine
K. Traditional Chinese medicine

_____ 1. A physician's recognition of a condition or disease based on its outward signs and symptoms and/or confirming tests or procedures.

_____ 2. Any range of medical therapies not regarded as orthodox by Western medicine.

_____ 3. Complementary and alternative medicine whole medical system including a range of traditional medicine practices originating in China.

_____ 4. The use of electronic monitoring of an automatic bodily function to train someone to acquire voluntary control of that function.

_____ 5. A range of medical therapies that fall beyond the scope of Western medicine.

_____ 6. A therapeutic belief that dilutions of medicinal substances that cause a specific symptom can treat an illness that yields the same symptoms.

_____ 7. A holistic traditional medical system originating in India that emphasizes disease prevention.

_____ 8. A medication made in a laboratory from chemical processes.

_____ 9. Treatment or measure to prevent disease.

_____ 10. Manual manipulation of the joints and muscles.

_____ 11. Any plant that is valued for its aromatic, medicinal, flavorful, or other properties.

True or False

Write T or F next to each statement.

_____ 1. Traditional medicine has been in existence for thousands of years, whereas alternative approaches have been practiced for only a few hundred years.

_____ 2. Traditional medicine is the standard for the Western world.

_____ 3. Probiotics are used as complementary alternative medicine.

_____ 4. The use of daily multivitamins and other such supplementation is generally not considered CAM.

_____ 5. Herbs are considered a form of traditional medication.

_____ 6. Herbal medicines account for some of the first attempts to improve human health.

_____ 7. Many people do not report herbal use to health care providers.

_____ 8. Herbs that are brewed for teas usually are less potent than those prepared in capsule form.

_____ 9. The pharmacy technician does not need to know the most common interactions between herbal remedies and legend drugs.

_____ 10. Thousands of homeopathic remedies can be used for each illness.

Multiple Choice

Complete each question by circling the best answer.

1. Traditional medicine includes all the following *except*:
   A. Physician visits
   B. Prescription drugs
   C. Laboratory tests
   D. Visits to a chiropractor

2. Complementary alternative medicine includes all the following *except*:
   A. Herbs
   B. X-rays
   C. Acupuncture
   D. Yoga

3. Eastern medicine includes treatments originating from all the following *except*:
   A. Eastern Asia
   B. India
   C. Eastern United States
   D. Far East countries

4. A reason people may turn to alternative medicines is:
   A. Rising cost of health care
   B. Increasing age of the population
   C. Rising cost of traditional medications
   D. All the above

5. Which of the following is *not* considered a nondrug treatment?
   A. Massage
   B. Herbs
   C. Meditation
   D. Biofeedback

6. Herbs used in Chinese medicine can:
   A. Cure the body of illness
   B. Prevent future problems
   C. A and B
   D. None of the above

7. Biofeedback has proved effective for all the following *except*:
   A. Love life
   B. Heart rate
   C. Hypertension
   D. Gastrointestinal activity

8. Chiropractic treatment can include all the following *except*:
   A. Adjustments of the joints
   B. Heat therapy
   C. Massage
   D. Chemotherapy

9. The _____ oversees the manufacture of homeopathic drugs:
   A. NIH
   B. FDA
   C. *Homeopathic Pharmacopeia*
   D. NCCAM

10. Homeopathy is also sometimes referred to as:
    A. The placebo effect
    B. Law of opposites
    C. Law of similars
    D. Manipulation therapy

Fill in the Blanks

Answer each question by completing the statement in the space provided.

1. Many people use CAM to pursue _____ health.

2. Acupressure or acupuncture with prescription pain medication is a _____ strategy for pain.

3. Some patients believe because herbal products are "natural" they are not _____.

4. Herbs and herbal supplements are not regulated in the same way as drugs because they are considered _____ _____.

5. If someone is allergic to an herbal, then an herbal from the same family may cause an _____ response.

6. How companies prepare herbs determines the _____ _____ strength.

7. Mind and body CAM practices are based on the _____ between the brain, mind, body, and behavior.

8. Manipulative and body-based CAM practices focus on _____ and proper functioning of various structures and body systems.

9. A homeopathic drug must meet standards for strength, quality, purity, and other parameters established in the _____ _____.

10. All homeopathic agents must be _____ using good manufacturing practices (GMP).

Matching

Match the following herbs with their common uses.

A. Black cohosh
B. Chamomile
C. Cranberry
D. Echinacea
E. Garlic
F. Ginkgo biloba
G. Ginseng
H. Milk thistle
I. Saw Palmetto
J. Soy
K. St. John's wort

_____ 1. Urinary tract infections

_____ 2. Dementia, peripheral vascular disease, intermittent claudication

_____ 3. Hyperlipidemia, menopausal symptoms, osteoporosis prevention, cardiovascular disease prevention

_____ 4. Menopausal symptoms, premenstrual syndrome

_____ 5. Stimulant, diabetes, digestive aid

_____ 6. Immunostimulant, treatment of common cold and other respiratory infections

_____ 7. Depression, anxiety

_____ 8. Benign prostatic hyperplasia (BPH)

_____ 9. Hypertension, hypercholesterolemia, antimicrobial

_____ 10. Gastrointestinal upset, skin conditions

_____ 11. Antioxidant, toxin-induced liver damage, dyspepsia

Match the following CAM treatments with their correct description.

A. Acupressure
B. Acupuncture
C. Aromatherapy
D. Ayurveda
E. Biofeedback
F. Chiropractic medicine
G. Herbal remedies
H. Homeopathy
I. Traditional Chinese medicine

_____ 12. A learned technique that enables the self-control of various physiological responses of the body.

_____ 13. Through the sense of smell, various blends of fragrances result in relief of certain ailments.

_____ 14. Diagnosis is based on the person's dreams, tastes, sensations, smell, and other senses.

_____ 15. Treatment is based on the belief that the realignment of the body, specifically the spine, can remedy certain conditions.

_____ 16. Uses pressure to specific points on the body to unblock pathways carrying energy.

_____ 17. Uses a minute amount of "toxin" from which the patient is suffering to allow for the patient's body to fight the illness.

_____ 18. Uses needles to specific points on the body to unblock pathways carrying energy.

_____ 19. Available for the treatment of a variety of ailments and are frequently sold in pharmacies and health food stores.

_____ 20. Includes various postures, meditation, and massage; changing habits is a large part of this treatment.

SHORT ANSWER

Write a short response to each question in the space provided.

1. What are the three main goals of NCCAM?

   A. _____

   B. _____

   C. _____

2. List three prescription medications that can be affected by taking black cohosh and explain the potential interactions.

   A. _____

   B. _____

   C. _____

3. List three prescription medications that can be affected by taking echinacea and explain the potential interactions.

   A. _____

   B. _____

   C. _____

4. List three prescription medications that can be affected by taking garlic and explain the potential interactions.

   A. _____

   B. _____

   C. _____

5. List three prescription medications that can be affected by taking gingko biloba and explain the potential interactions.

   A. _____

   B. _____

   C. _____

6. List three prescription medications that can be affected by taking ginseng and explain the potential interactions.

   A. _____

   B. _____

   C. _____

7. List three prescription medications that can be affected by taking St. John's wort and explain the potential interactions.

   A. _____

   B. _____

   C. _____

Research Activities

Follow the instructions given in each exercise and provide a response.

1. Access the website _http://www.rxlist.com/_. Under the supplements tab, list the featured supplement.

   Featured supplement: _____

   A. Was this supplement discussed in the chapter?

B. By what other names is this supplement known?

2. Access the website *http://nccam.nih.gov/health* and access the Health Info.

  A. What resources are available for health care professionals?

C. What is the generic name and drug class?

  B. What resources are available for consumers?

D. How does the supplement work?

REFLECT CRITICALLY

Critical Thinking

Reply to each question based on what you have learned in the chapter.

E. What is the suggested dosing for each dosage form listed?

1. Alternative medicine has been on the rise the past few years. Many people are not aware that the FDA does not regulate many of the "natural" products being marketed. As a consumer, how can you be sure that these "natural" products really contain the ingredients reported on the labels? As a pharmacy technician, how can you help make consumers aware of "natural" products?

F. What are the dosing considerations for this supplement?

G. What are the side effect associated with this supplement?

2. In addition to the various therapies and herbal products discussed in the chapter, what other forms of alternative medicine are available?

H. What other drugs interact with this supplement?

3. Spiritual healing brings another dimension to alternative medicine. Why is it so different from the other forms discussed in the chapter?

I. What are the warnings and precautions for this supplement?

4. You are trying to convince your classmates that trying alternative medicine is better than seeing a physician every time you feel ill. How would you make your case for this form of therapy? What would be a case against it? What information is available to patients to help them make this decision? Present your case to your classmates and discuss how your communication of this information would be effective.

RELATE TO PRACTICE

Lab Scenarios

Complementary Alternative Medicine

Objective: To allow the pharmacy technician to promote wellness of mind and body for oneself, the pharmacy team, the community. To introduce the pharmacy technician to complementary alternative medicine and its usage in the prevention and treatment of illness

---

DID YOU KNOW?

Complementary and alternative medicine (CAM) is defined as "medical products and practices that are not part of standard care." Conventional medicine is medicine practiced by holders of M.D. and O.D. degrees and by all allied health professionals. Complementary and alternative medicine is gaining in popularity in the United States. As a member of the allied health team, pharmacy technicians need to be familiar with complementary and alternative medicine because of the changing demographics of our society.

Lab Activity #30.1: Using information learned from the chapter, answer the following questions about mind and body medicine.

Equipment needed:
- Computer with Internet access
- Pencil/pen

Time needed to complete this activity: 30 minutes

1. What, if any, mind and body practices have you tried before or currently practice? How did this practice affect your physical function and health? Would you recommend it others, why or why not? If you have not participated in a mind and body practice, would you consider participating in one on a regular basis, why or why not?
2. Explain potential benefits of participating in mind and body medicine on a regular basis?
3. How could you use the power of the mind and body practices to affect physical function and health positively?
4. Demonstrate to your classmates a mind and body practice that could be easily performed in the pharmacy to help relieve stress, when needed.
5. Explain the pharmacy technician's role in promoting wellness and disease prevention in the pharmacy and how it relates to CAM.

Lab Activity #30.2: Using the National Center for Complementary and Alternative Medicine website (*http://www. nccam.nih.gov*) or resources available, complete the following table of herbal products.

Equipment *needed*:
- Computer with Internet access
- Paper
- *PDR for Herbal Medicines*
- Pencil/pen

Time needed to complete this activity: 60 minutes

Herbal Product	Common Name(s)	Indication	Therapeutic Category	Approved Use	Unapproved Use	Dosage Forms Available	List Two Side Effects	Drug Interactions
Aloe vera								
Basil								
Belladonna								
Bilberry								

Herbal Product	Common Name(s)	Indication	Therapeutic Category	Approved Use	Unapproved Use	Dosage Forms Available	List Two Side Effects	Drug Interactions
Black cohosh								
Chamomile								
Cinnamon								
Cranberry								
Echinacea								
Elderberry								
Ephedra								
Eucalyptus								
Evening primrose								
Feverfew								
Flaxseed								
Garlic								
Ginger								
Ginkgo								

Continued

Chapter **30** **Complementary and Alternative Medicine (CAM)**

Herbal Product	Common Name(s)	Indication	Therapeutic Category	Approved Use	Unapproved Use	Dosage Forms Available	List Two Side Effects	Drug Interactions
Ginseng								
Green tea								
Ipecac								
Kava								
Lavender								
Licorice root								
Melatonin								
Milk thistle								
Oats								
Peppermint oil								
Psyllium								
Quinine								
Rosemary								
Sage								

Herbal Product	Common Name(s)	Indication	Therapeutic Category	Approved Use	Unapproved Use	Dosage Forms Available	List Two Side Effects	Drug Interactions
Saw palmetto								
Senna								
Soybean								
St. John's wort								
Turmeric								
Valerian								